Praise for *The Food Revolution*

"In what promises to be the publishing event of the decade, John Robbins provides both the information and the encouragement we need in order to reclaim the health of our bodies and our planet. Packed with political dynamite, this book will change your life. Forthright and fearless, thoroughly researched and engagingly presented, this is must reading for everyone who eats."

Joanna Macy, author of *Coming Back to Life*

"In *The Food Revolution*, John Robbins continues his groundbreaking research into the ill effects, both personal and collective, of the modern diet. Our food habits are the hardest addictions we face. Save your life. Save the world. Follow this book."

James Redfield, author of *The Celestine Prophecy*

"A person who leads me to eat in a way that cultivates spiritual awareness is my kind of prophet. John Robbins gives me a light at the end of the tunnel as well as providing a moral compass. The truth has few allies these days. I have deep respect for John Robbins and join him in the belief that the way we eat has profound environmental impact on our planet. I think it's high time we had a food revolution."

Woody Harrelson, movie and TV star

"With his brilliant and sharp pen/sword, John Robbins punctures the myths and lie balloons that lay millions of Americans in their graves every year. *The Food Revolution* will tell you how to save and extend your own life, show you how we can all easily work to reduce suffering on Earth, and give you a vibrant and vital sensation of life and health. This is one of those rare and truly transformational books: Buy it, read it, and share it with everybody you know!"

Thom Hartmann, author of *The Last Hours of Ancient Sunlight*

"Provocative and compelling, *The Food Revolution* delivers one of the most important messages of our time. Presented with clarity and conviction, Robbins leaves the reader sobered but inspired. He underscores the power that individuals can have when they vote with their knives and forks to save themselves and the planet. Nothing short of a call to action, this is a book to give to family, friends, and colleagues. I highly recommend it."

Suzanne Havala, author of the semin   1993 A
Dietetic Association position papers on v
Being Vegetarian for Dumr

D0032451

"This important book reminds us of the joys of aligning our personal choices with a concern for the environment. In my path of being vegan, my body, mind, heart, and spirit have all healed and grown stronger. And the incredible joy I receive from knowing that I am lessening my impact on this beautiful planet fulfills me in ways that a meat and dairy diet never could and never will."

Julia Butterfly Hill, environmental activist, author of *The Legacy of Luna*

"John Robbins has done it again. *The Food Revolution* is a riveting sequel to *Diet for a New America*. I started reading it and I couldn't put it down. I was especially impressed with the chapters on genetic engineering. Robbins explains the situation better than anyone I've ever heard. For the hundreds of thousands of people like me, whose lives have been forever changed by Robbins' work, *The Food Revolution* is a MUST READ. The word revolution is normally reserved in our society for guerrillas and telemarketers. THIS revolution is ours. It's a simple choice in the foods we eat that will have a radical effect on the world around us."

Adam Werbach, Former President, Sierra Club

"Beautifully written, *The Food Revolution* is a remarkable book by a remarkable man. It opened both my eyes and my heart. This is indeed a book that can save our lives."

Riane Eisler, author of *The Chalice and the Blade* and *Tomorrow's Children*

"The environmental health movement has become one of the most powerful grassroots movements of our time. With this book John Robbins continues his role as one of the movement's most outspoken and eloquent leaders."

Fritjof Capra, author of *The Web of Life*

"A vital and wonderful book, and easy to digest, this is a perfect read for anyone with a body, a mind, and a heart. *The Food Revolution* is the most positive book of the decade."

Ingrid Newkirk, President, People for the Ethical Treatment of Animals (PETA)

"*The Food Revolution* provides a cornucopia of arresting and revealing information. Robbins shows, in ways that both shock and fascinate, how the food we produce functions as a fateful link between our health as individuals and the health of the planet that gives us life. Particularly powerful is his well-documented account of the havoc wreaked by the "big cattle" industry on everything from our arteries to our aquifers."

Ed Ayres, Editorial Director, WorldWatch, author of *God's Last Offer*

"Once again, John Robbins enables us to find our way through the maze of information about food choices and the food industry. His impeccable research and visionary outlook are a gift to those of us who wish to make wise food choices. Personally, I found his reflections on many of the popular diets of our time to be extremely helpful."

Ann Mortifee, vocal artist and composer

"*The Food Revolution* will finish what *Diet for a New America* started. It is magnificent. Give a copy to everyone you care about!"

Howard Lyman, President, EarthSave, author of *Mad Cowboy*

"Revealing a host of astounding facts that the food industry would like to keep hidden, John Robbins shows how healthy eating is not only good for ourselves but also for the environment. Excellent and essential reading for all who want to live healthy lives and help make the world a better place."

Peter Russell, author of *Waking Up in Time* and *From Science to God*

"*The Food Revolution* has arrived in the nick of time to lead us toward healthy diets and healthy farms. Readable, poignant, brilliant, and amazing, this is the book to consult for the health of your family."

Brent Blackwelder, President, Friends of the Earth

"In *The Food Revolution*, John Robbins points out that the typical 'American diet' is not only associated with adverse effects on human health, but with the reprehensible treatment of animals and irreparable harm to our land and water. Packed with startling facts and provocative insights, *The Food Revolution* is compelling reading for anyone interested in nutritional health, the treatment of animals, or even, simply, the fate of the planet!"

David L. Katz, M.D., M.P.H., Yale University School of Medicine

"John Robbins' *The Food Revolution* is undoubtedly the most comprehensive and sophisticated study on the political, ethical, and sane choices for a healthy diet. His candor and compassion guide the reader through advertising misconceptions to propaganda perpetuated by our food industry. If you wish to learn how to give your body optimal health, you had better tune in to the messages in *The Food Revolution*."

Dave Scott, six-time Ironman Triathlon World Champion,
first inductee into the Ironman Hall of Fame, and
author of *Dave Scott's Triathlon Training*

"John Robbins does it again! *The Food Revolution* is a powerful and provocative expose of the political, economic, and social realities of our current food system. It challenges and inspires individuals to accept responsibility for our choices and to take action for positive change."

> Vesanto Melina and Brenda Davis, registered dietitians, co-authors of *Becoming Vegetarian* and *Becoming Vegan*

"*The Food Revolution* is the most comprehensive and persuasive argument ever assembled for a plant-based diet being proper human nutrition. Your life and the future of humankind may depend upon the spread of John Robbins' vital message."

> John McDougall, M.D., Medical Director of the McDougall Program at St. Helena Hospital, author of ten national bestselling books, and host of the nationally syndicated TV Show *McDougall, MD*

"In *The Food Revolution*, John Robbins once again opens our eyes and awakens our hearts. His vision of health-enhancing, Earth-friendly food choices offers hope and direction for a nourishing and sustainable tomorrow."

> Michael A. Klaper, M.D., Director, Institute of Nutrition Education and Research

"John Robbins is a wise man. In his engaging new book, *The Food Revolution*, John shares his wisdom in a way that touches our heart and mind. He makes us feel good about eating in a compassionate way that nurtures our body and soul. And his research into the dangers of genetically engineered foods is must reading for anyone concerned about health and the environment."

> Craig Winters, Executive Director, the Campaign to Label Genetically Engineered Foods

"Indispensable reading for the concerned consumer, John Robbins' book tells you how to vote, with your knife and fork, for a sustainable, healthy, and humane world."

> Ronnie Cummins, National Director Organic Consumers Association, and co-author of *Genetically Engineered Food*

"John Robbins has scored again. His writing style is engaging and sufficiently personal to make it MUST reading. And most importantly, he connects the dots that need connecting—environment, personal health, societal economics, and personal meaning. Scientific researchers also would do well to read what Robbins says."

> Colin Campbell, Senior Science Advisor, American Institute for Cancer Research, Professor of Nutritional Biochemistry, Cornell University

"*The Food Revolution* is John Robbins' opening salvo of the twenty-first century to save our health and our planet. It is a review packed with facts confirming how our health is held captive by the greed of industry. It is a must read and an excellent review source."

Caldwell Esselstyn, M.D.,
Preventative Cardiology Consultant, the Cleveland Clinic

"John Robbins shows the seamless integration between our food and our world. Diet and farming practices that are causing human disease are hurting animals and the planet. Now, genetic engineering, based on these damaging misunderstandings, is creating new dangers. Robbins clearly shows that the sensible path to restoring personal health is one with the path to restoring planetary health and with restoring moral relations with other living creatures."

Martha Herbert, M.D., Ph.D., Pediatric Neurology, Massachusetts
General Hospital, Vice-chair, Council for Responsible Genetics,
Instructor in Neurology, Harvard Medical School

THE
FOOD
REVOLUTION

THE FOOD

REVOLUTION

HOW **YOUR DIET** CAN HELP SAVE
YOUR LIFE AND OUR WORLD

JOHN ROBBINS

Foreword by **Dean Ornish, M.D.**

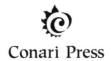

Conari Press

First published in 2001 by
Conari Press
an imprint of Red Wheel/Weiser, LLC
With offices at:
665 Third Street, Suite 400
San Francisco, CA 94107
www.redwheelweiser.com

Photo credits: 169: Earl R. Baker, U. S. Department of Agriculture, 170, 172, 184, 191, 193, 197, 201 (top), 215, 216: Courtesy of People for the Ethical Treatment of Animals (PETA), 175, 184, 187, 201 (bottom): Courtesy of Humane Farming Association (HFA), 215 (top), 216 (top): Courtesy of Jeff Nelson

Cover Illustration/Photography: © Viktor Balabanov/iStock.com
Cover Design: Stewart Williams
Book Design: Claudia Smelser
Author Photo: Mike de Boer

ISBN: 978-1-57324-487-9

Library of Congress Cataloging-in-Publication Data available upon request.

Printed in the United States of America on 100% recycled
(30% post-consumer) chlorine-free paper

MAL

10 9 8 7 6 5 4 3

The Food Revolution

Foreword

by Dean Ornish, M.D.

We tend to think of advances in medicine as a new drug, a new surgical technique, a laser, something high-tech and expensive. We often have a hard time believing that the simple choices we make each day—what we eat, how we respond to stress, whether we smoke, how much we exercise, and how well our social relationships support us—can make powerful differences in our health and well-being, even in our survival. But often they do.

I have spent most of my professional life using the latest high-tech medical technology to assess the power of low-tech and low-cost interventions. For the past twenty-five years, my colleagues and I at the non-profit Preventive Medicine Research Institute have, in collaboration with other institutions, conducted a series of scientific studies and randomized clinical trials demonstrating that the progression of even severe coronary heart disease can be stopped or reversed simply by making comprehensive changes in one's diet and lifestyle. These lifestyle changes include adopting a low-fat, plant-based, whole foods diet; stress management techniques (including yoga and meditation); moderate exercise; smoking cessation; and psychosocial group support.

When diet and lifestyle—often the underlying causes of poor health—are adjusted, the body has a remarkable capacity to begin healing itself, much more quickly than we had once thought possible. On the other hand, if we literally bypass the problem with surgery or figuratively with medications without also addressing its underlying causes, the same problem may recur, new problems may emerge, or we may be faced with painful choices—sort of like mopping up the floor around an overflowing sink without turning off the faucet first.

While our work at the Institute has focused primarily on the individual health benefits and cost effectiveness of choices in diet and lifestyle, there is a larger, more global context for lifestyle changes as well. John Robbins has for years been an eloquent spokesperson for these larger consequences of our personal choices. And, as he clearly describes in *The Food Revolution,* the personal and the global are deeply related. Your own body and the body politic affect each other—for better and for worse.

Sometimes the world's problems seem so overwhelming that all we can do is focus on our own lives and those of our families and friends. Maybe you aren't interested in running for political office, or writing a book, or conducting research, or endowing a foundation. But the choices you make each day in something as fundamental as what you eat have consequences that are far-reaching, not only for yourself but also for a much wider society. Some choices may lead to healing, whereas others may lead to suffering, both individually and globally.

Awareness is the first step in healing, whether personal or social. Understanding the connection between *when* we suffer and *why* is a fundamental step in having the freedom to make different choices. Awareness can help transform suffering into meaning and action and may even be a catalyst for healing. In this context, pain becomes information and motivation, not punishment.

Good science also can help increase our awareness. Scientific research linking smoking with serious health consequences such as heart disease, lung cancer, emphysema, and birth defects has caused many people to choose not to smoke. These social changes have occurred slowly—over a period of several decades—but look how far we've come! Fifty years ago, every office building, meeting room, and airplane was filled with cigarette smoke. What used to be acceptable and even cool or hip is now stigmatized.

Many people are confused by the conflicting information they hear. For example, first they are told, "Margarine is better than butter." Then, "Uh-oh—margarine isn't so good either; too many trans fatty acids." "High-protein diets are good." "Low-protein diets are good." People often get exasperated: "These damn doctors, they can't make up their minds, just bring out the bacon and eggs and quit worrying about it!"

News media report on what's new, and they like controversy. There can be a hundred studies showing, for example, that a diet high in fat and animal protein is unhealthful, but if a new study comes out purporting that a high-fat diet is good for you, often it makes headlines, however poorly designed the study might be.

After reviewing the scientific literature, however, it becomes clear that the evidence is mostly consistent, not controversial. There is more scientific evidence than ever that switching from a high-fat diet rich in animal protein and simple carbohydrates such as sugar to a whole foods, plant-based diet high in complex carbohydrates provides a double benefit: You significantly reduce your intake of disease-promoting substances such as cholesterol, saturated fat, and oxidants, and increase your intake of protective food substances.

There are in foods at least a thousand substances—phytochemicals, bioflavonoids, carotenoids, retinols, isoflavones, lycopene, genistein, and so on—that have anti-cancer, anti-heart disease, and anti-aging properties. Where are these important substances found? With few exceptions, they are in fruits, vegetables, grains, and beans, including soy products.

New studies provide additional mechanisms and insights to help understand why a plant-based diet is more healthful than one high in animal protein. For example, elevated blood levels of a substance called homocysteine may increase your risk of developing coronary heart disease. Animal protein in your diet increases your homocysteine levels, whereas folate and vitamins B-6, which are found in whole grains and green leafy vegetables, help reduce homocysteine levels.

Unfortunately, a globalization of illness is occurring. Many countries have copied the Western way of eating and living, and they are now copying the Western way of dying. Illnesses like coronary heart disease, which used to be very rare in countries such as Japan and other Asian countries, are becoming epidemics, causing huge drains on economies as well as personal suffering—much of which could be avoided. Japanese boys now have cholesterol levels as high as those of American boys. We need a globalization of health to counter these trends.

Sometimes, people tell me, "I don't care if I die sooner, I want to *enjoy* my life." They believe that eating a healthful diet is *borrrrr-ing.*

To me, there is no point in giving up something that I enjoy unless I get something back that's even better—and not thirty years from now, but after only a few weeks. When you change your diet, practice stress management techniques such as yoga and meditation, exercise, and quit smoking, the blood flow to your brain may improve. You may think more clearly, feel better, have more energy. (Remember a time when you had a rich Thanksgiving feast, and how tired and sluggish you felt afterward.) Also, when you make these changes in diet and lifestyle, the blood flow to your heart may improve. In our studies, we found an average reduction of 91 percent in the frequency of angina (chest pain) within just a few weeks. Even the blood flow to your sexual organs may increase when you make these changes in diet and lifestyle. As a result, sexual potency may improve. In addition, low-fat, plant-based foods can be both delicious and nutritious.

In the final analysis, of course, all of us are destined to die. The mortality rate is still 100 percent, one per person. So the most important question, to me, is not just how *long* we live but also how *well* we live. When we look back over our lives, how much distress did we cause? How much suffering did we help alleviate? How much love did we give, and how much did we receive? How many people did we help? These are profoundly spiritual questions; as such, they are often the most meaningful.

To the degree we can change our diets, we may be able to enhance our health, enjoy our lives even more fully, and reduce the suffering in our wake. We face a spectrum of choices every day; it's not all or nothing. You may not want to give up eating animal protein or fatty foods completely, but you may be able to consume them less frequently if you understand the benefits of cutting back, how quickly they may occur, and how far-reaching they may be.

John Robbins has dedicated his life to the journey of trying to make the world a better place for the next generation. Sometimes, he is intentionally provocative in order to get our attention and to make a point. Whether or not we agree with everything in this book (for example, McDonald's may deserve more credit for moving in the right direction) is less important than drawing our own conclusions based on the data and evidence that he and others provide. I greatly respect his intelligence and commitment; even more, I appreciate and remain inspired by his extraordinary compassion.

Dean Ornish, M.D.
Founder and President, Preventive Medicine Research Institute
Clinical Professor of Medicine, University of California, San Francisco
www.ornish.com
Sausalito, California, April 17, 2001

Acknowledgments

Many books are written and published, but how many are worth the dead trees they are printed on? If this book is worthwhile, it is because of the many wonderful people who have given their love and dedication to me, to this book project, and to the work for which they and I stand. I wish I could name them all.

I am infinitely grateful and appreciative to Deo Robbins, my partner, love, and friend for 34 years, who took care of 10,000 things so that I would have the time and space to write. Her brilliance and insight helped to shape *The Food Revolution,* and her ever-present faith in me has long been nectar for my heart.

Great thanks to Ocean and Michele Robbins, who read every word many times and provided whatever support I needed at every phase of the book's development. I cannot give enough acknowledgment to these two wonderful people—my son and daughter-in-love—whose hearts joined with Deo's in creating the external womb in which my writing, and my life, have taken shape.

I give thanks to Jeff Nelson, who played an indispensable role as a constant source of encouragement and information. He and his wife Sabrina are true warriors for the cause of life. Without them and their dedication, this book would never have been written.

I was tremendously fortunate to have Leslie Berriman as an editor. Her amazing support and clarity were constant sources of inspiration and renewal to me. Thanks, also, to Jenny Collins, Teresa Coronado, Sharon Donovan, Will Glennon, Brenda Knight, Rosie Levy, Heather McArthur, Leah Russell, Claudia Smelser, Pam Suwinsky, and the whole team at Conari Press. You could not find a more incredible bunch to work with.

A deep bow to Ed Ayres, Neal Barnard, Brenda Davis, Bruce Friedrich, Sue Havala, Brad Miller, and Craig Winters. They each read the manuscript at various stages, and it is a better book thanks to their generosity and expertise.

I am what I am and this book is what it is because of the allies, colleagues, confidantes, and friends who have given me so much support, love, and help. A special thank you to Richard Glantz, Earle Harris, Francis and Carol Janes, Shams Kairys, Michael Klaper, Howard Lyman, and Ian and Terry Thiermann, who have blessed me with their friendship and by their many kinds of contributions over the years to the nonprofit organization EarthSave.

I honor and thank the many others, too, who have poured their hearts, souls, and resources into EarthSave and given their efforts to shift our society in the direction of compassion, healing, and sustainability. Thanks from the bottom of my heart to Glenn and Amy Bacheller, Chris and Grace Balthazar, David Bernstein, John Borders, Patti Breitman, Susan Campbell, Patricia Carney, Deepak Chopra, Sue (Shanti) Cliff, Jerry Cook, Cynthia Cowen, Bob DiBenedetto, Gary and Emily Dunn, Mark Epstein, Larry Fried, Tom Gegax, Andrew Glick, Prem Glidden, Gail Goodwin, Jay Harris, Caryn Hartglass, Medeana Hobar, Sheila Hoffman, Stephanie Hoffman, Al Jacobson, Navin Jain, Alese Jones, Matt Kelly, Gabriele Kushi, Mary La Mar, Willy Laurie, Jim Littlefield-Dalmares, Steve Lustgarden, David Lustig, Pat Lynch, Cornell McClellan, Terrie and Paul Mershon, Kevin and Michelle Miller, Sandy Mintz, Marr Nealon, Audrey Nickel, Jules Oaklander, Kit Paraventi, Heart Phoenix, Mary Quillan, Tom Scholz, Michael Schwager, Mel Skolnick, Stewart Stone, Bert Troughton, Michael Tucker, Stacey Vicari, Eleanor Wasson, Marianne Williamson, Todd Winant, and the many, many others whom space doesn't permit me to mention. These are a few of the major contributors—the volunteers, directors, staff, and funders—who have played vital roles in EarthSave's work to discover, live, and communicate a world of compassion and healing. I thank them on behalf of our planet and all the life it holds, and I thank them on behalf of future generations that will have a more livable and peaceful home thanks to their devoted efforts.

I am forever grateful to Hal and Linda Kramer, friends for many years, publishers of many of my books, and great supporters of my work. Their caring and gifts have strengthened my spirit.

My gratitude to all those who have been responsible for the tremendous accomplishments of the nonprofit organization Youth for Environmental Sanity (YES!), including—in addition to Ocean and Michele Robbins—Johl Chato, Malaika Edwards, Ryan Eliason, Julia Butterfly Hill, Asha Goldstein, David Guizar, Tad Hargrave, Ivy Mayer, Maryam Roberts, Josh Sage, Malika Sanders, Levana Saxon, Aqeela Sherrills, Jessica Simkovic, Sol Solomon, Alli Starr, Karen Thompson, Sev Williams, and many other wonderful young people. And thanks also to all of the elders whose involvement as directors and funders has helped to make this remarkable phenomenon possible, including Richard Baskin, Masankho Banda, Brian Biro, Tom Burt, Tom Callanan, Lenedra Carroll, Aeeshah and Kokomon Clottey, Morty Cohen, Steve and Stephanie Farrell, Richard Glantz, Earle Harris, Wendy Grace and Michael Honach, Marion and Alan Hunt Badiner, Navin Jain, Darryl Kollman, Marta Kollman, Helaine Lerner, Joanna and Fran Macy, Josh Mailman, Sam Mills, Ani Moss, the folks at New Road Map, the Phoenix family, Horst Rechelbacher, Ann Roberts, Sunshine Smith, Ian and Terry Thiermann, Susie Tompkins, Michael Tucker, Lynne and Bill Twist, Paul Wenner, and many others.

My thanks and appreciation to the small group of remarkable people with whom I've been meeting regularly for the past year. Each of these people—Tom Burt, Catherine Gray, Tracy Howard, Joe Kresse, Catherine Parrish, Richard Rathbun, Ocean Robbins, Vicki Robin, Neal Rogin, Lynne Twist, and Mathis Wackernagel—has been tremendously successful in generating positive social change in their lives. Coming together with them to take the next step toward a thriving and sustainable world for all has been gratifying and inspiring.

I thank all those people I am grateful to call friends, including Karl and Jeanne Anthony, John and Kat Astin, Cris Bissonnette, Salima Cobb, Katchie Egger, Gypsy, Nadja Halilbegovich, Phil Kline, Ann Mortifee, Kali Rae, Craig and Heidi Schindler, Bobbi Spurr, Adrian Van Beveren, and the many others deserving of recognition. You know who you are. Your support means the world to me.

My thanks also to Sharon Gannon, Sandy Laurie, David Life, Jim Mason, Stan Sapon, Joanne Stepaniak, and the many others who have worked so hard and for so long to bring compassion and healing into our world.

A deep, slow bow to the memory of Cleveland Amory, David Brower, Cesar Chavez, John Denver, Raul Julia, Linda McCartney, Helen Nearing, River Phoenix, and Claire Townsend—dearly beloved soul companions and EarthSave and YES! board members—who have passed on in these last few brief years. I treasure their memories and the love they shared with me, and I stand on this Earth for the fulfillment of their dreams.

I have enormous gratitude and honor for the many men and women who work, often without recognition, for the greater healing for which we all pray. I thank all those on this Earth who have helped me or supported what I do. Again, you know who you are. With you, I offer myself in infinite gratitude to all things past, infinite service to all things present, and infinite responsibility to all things future.

Introduction to the
10th Anniversary Edition

For some years now, the U. S. Congress and the entire country have been engaged in an intense debate over health care reform. Although the debate has been at times vitriolic, most people agree that *something* has to be done. For one thing, the U.S. is the only industrialized country in the world that doesn't guarantee basic health care to all its citizens. Forty-seven million people in the country are without health insurance. And for another, the U.S. spends far more on health care than any other nation—nearly double that spent per capita in those countries that come closest to us in spending, such as Germany, Canada, Denmark, and France.

The annual health insurance premium paid by the average American family now exceeds the gross yearly income of a full-time minimum wage worker.[i] Every 30 seconds, someone in the U.S. files for bankruptcy due to the costs of treating a health problem.[ii]

Health care spending is so far out of control that not only individuals and families, but the entire economy is buckling under the strain. In 2007, General Motors was spending so much money for its employees' health care that Warren Buffet called the corporation "a health and benefits company with an auto company attached." That year, General Motors, like Ford and other U.S. automakers, paid more than $1,500 in health care costs for every car it made, while Japan's Honda paid only $150. Meanwhile, the chairman of Starbucks, Howard Schultz, was saying that his company was spending more money on insurance for its employees than it was spending on coffee.[iii]

It hasn't always been like this. In 2010, we spent more than $2.5 trillion on medical care. But as recently as 1950, Americans spent only about $8.4 billion ($70 billion in today's dollars).[iv] The increase has been mind-boggling. Now, adjusting for inflation, we spend as much on health care every ten days as we did in the entire year of 1950.

Perhaps such skyrocketing spending could be justified if the result was greatly improved health for the nation's citizens. But such, alas, has hardly been the case. It is not widely known, but our health has actually been declining in recent decades. According to a 2005 Johns Hopkins University analysis, "On most health indicators, the U.S. relative performance declined since 1960; on none did it improve."[v]

Despite spending far more per capita on health care than any other nation, the U.S. now ranks a dismally low 37th among nations in infant mortality rates, and 38th in life expectancy. In 2010, the World Health Organization assessed the overall health outcomes of different nations. It placed 36 other nations ahead of the United States.

It's striking to me that in all the heated debate about health care reform, one basic fact is rarely discussed, and that is the one thing that could dramatically bring down the costs of health care while improving the health of our people. Studies have shown that 50 to 70 percent of the nation's health care costs are preventable, and the single most effective step most people can take to improve their health is to eat a healthier diet. If Americans were to stop overeating, to stop eating unhealthy foods and to instead eat foods with higher nutrient densities and cancer protective properties, we could have a more affordable, sustainable, and effective health care system. And more importantly, we'd be less dependent on insurance companies and doctors, and more dependent on our own health-giving choices.

Today, we have an epidemic of largely preventable diseases. To these illnesses, Americans are losing not only their health but also their life savings.

Meanwhile, the evidence keeps growing that the path to improved health lies in eating more vegetables, fruits, whole grains, and legumes, and eating far less animal products.

At this point, the number of studies documenting the importance of eating more plant foods and fewer animal foods is enormous, and the data continues to pour in. The Physicians Committee for Responsible Medicine (PCRM) tracks such studies. Just in the six months before this edition of *The Food Revolution* went to press, PCRM noted, the following 13 studies were published in major medical journals:

Eating more fruits and vegetables increases survival rates in women with ovarian cancer. Women with the highest fruit and vegetable intakes have better ovarian cancer survival rates than whose who eat fewer of those foods, according to a study published in the March 2010 *Journal of the American Dietetic Association.* Researchers found that yellow and cruciferous vegetables (cabbage, broccoli, kale, collards, cauliflower, etc.) in particular contributed to longer survival, while consumption of dairy products and red and processed meats shortened lifespan. The authors concluded that low-fat, plant-based diets are not only beneficial for cancer prevention, they can also increase survival time in people diagnosed with cancer.[vi]

Eating more fruits, vegetables, and soy reduces the risk of breast cancer. Consumption of soy, fruits, and vegetables helps reduce the risk of breast cancer, according to a study published in the March 2010 issue of the *American Journal of Clinical Nutrition.* The research, based on more than 34,000 women in the Singapore Chinese Health Study, found that the longer the women had consumed these healthy foods, the less chance they had of developing breast cancer.[vii]

Animal protein is associated with decreased bone health. Animal protein is associated with decreased bone mineral density, according to a study published in the *British Journal of Nutrition* in March 2010. In a five-year study undertaken in Beijing, China, involving more than 750 girls, animal protein, particularly from meat and eggs, was found to weaken bones.[viii]

Soy protects against lung cancer. A report based on a major Japanese study involving more than 76,000 participants was published in the February 2010 issue of the *American Journal of Clinical Nutrition*. It found a significantly lower risk of lung cancer in non-smoking men and women who consumed the most soy, compared to those who consumed the least.[ix] Soy foods in the study included miso soup, soymilk, tofu, and fermented soybean products.[x]

A low-fat vegetarian diet and healthy lifestyle rejuvenates coronary arteries. Researchers reporting in the February 2010 edition of the *American Journal of Cardiology* found that men and women who followed a low-fat vegetarian diet, along with a moderate exercise program and stress management, measurably improved the function of their endothelium (the inner lining of arteries that is key to preventing heart attacks).[xi]

Chicken implicated in urinary tract infections. Bacteria from chicken products are a major cause of urinary tract infections, according to a study published by the Centers for Disease Control and Prevention in January 2010. Researchers examined urine samples from women who had urinary tract infections and traced the E. coli pathogens in the samples to contaminated foods. They found that most of the E. coli was ingested through meat products, 61 percent of which were chicken products. The authors concluded that chicken was the main source of urinary tract infection-causing E. coli. They also warned that E. coli from animal products are increasingly drug-resistant, due to the widespread misuse of antibiotics in modern livestock production.[xii]

Animal protein increases diabetes risk. Researchers analyzed the diets of more than 38,000 Dutch participants in the European Prospective Investigation into Cancer and Nutrition study. Their report, published in the January 2010 issue of the medical journal *Diabetes Care*, found a strong correlation between the amount of animal protein consumed and the risk of developing diabetes. Increased animal protein intake also coincided with increased body mass index, waist circumference, and blood pressure. Increased vegetable protein intake, on the other hand, was not associated with diabetes risk.[xiii]

Soy increases breast cancer survival. In a report published in the December 2009 issue of the *Journal of the American Medical Association*, researchers found that women diagnosed with breast cancer who consumed soy products such as soymilk, tofu, or edamame have a 32 percent lower risk of recurrence and a 29 percent decreased risk of death, compared with similar women who consume little or no soy. The report was based on the largest population-based study of breast cancer survival, the Shanghai Breast Cancer Survival Study, which followed more than 5,000 women for four years.[xiv]

Going vegetarian improves mood. Omnivores who cut meat out of their diets experience mood improvements, according to a report presented in December 2009 at the annual conference of the American Public Health Association. Researchers at Arizona State University divided omnivorous participants into three dietary groups: control (made no changes in diet); fish (consumed three to four servings of fish per week and no other meat); and vegetarian (consumed no meat or eggs). The vegetarian group experienced improvements in both tension and confusion categories, while the meat-eating and fish eating groups showed no significant changes in mood.[xv]

Pregnant women's diet affects their babies' risk of diabetes. In a study published in *Pediatric Diabetes* in October 2009, researchers found that women who consumed the least amount of vegetables during pregnancy were more likely to have babies who developed type 1 diabetes. Compared with women who ate vegetables daily, those consuming vegetables only three to five times per week had a 71 percent increased risk of having a child with diabetes.[xvi]

Meat consumption increases the risk of diabetes. According to a systematic review published in the October 2009 issue of the medical journal *Diabetologia*, intakes of red meat and processed meat were associated with 21 and 41 percent increased risk of diabetes, respectively.[xvii]

Soy intake decreases risk of hip fractures. In a study published in the October 2009 issue of the *American Journal of Epidemiology*, intake of soy products reduced the risk of hip fracture as much as 36 percent among women who consumed the greatest amount of soy. The study was part of the Singapore Chinese Health Study, involving more than 63,000 adults.[xviii]

Red meat increases risk of prostate cancer. In a study of more than 175,000 men published in the *American Journal of Epidemiology* in October 2009, the men who consumed the most red meat had a 30 percent increased risk of prostate cancer, compared to those who consumed the least.

Healthy People, Healthy Planet

The financial and health implications of our diets are nearly impossible to overstate. And there are other compelling reasons that we need a food revolution. President Herbert Hoover famously promised "a chicken in every pot and a car in every garage." But as bestselling author and health advocate Kathy Freston points out: "With warnings about global warming reaching feverish levels, many are having second thoughts about all those cars. It seems they should instead be worrying about the chickens."

Kathy Freston's comments appeared in her provocatively titled article, "Vegetarian is the New Prius."[xix] She wrote it in the wake of a seminal report published in 2007 by the Food and Agriculture Organization (FAO) of the United Nations.[xx] Titled *Livestock's Long Shadow*, the report states that meat production is the second or third largest contributor to environmental problems at *every* level and at *every* scale, from global to local. It is a primary culprit in land degradation, air pollution, water shortage, water pollution, species extinction, loss of biodiversity, and climate change. Henning Steinfeld, a senior author of the report, stated, "Livestock are one of the most significant contributors to today's most serious environmental problems. Urgent action is needed to remedy the situation."

Comparing eating little or no animal products with driving a Prius, and likewise comparing eating meat with driving a Hummer, may seem farfetched. But this comparison, as striking as it is, actually understates the amount of greenhouse gases that stem from meat production. In 2006, a University of Chicago study found that a vegan diet is far more effective than driving a hybrid car in reducing our carbon footprint.[xxi]

The scientists who did the calculations said that a Prius driver who consumes a meat-based diet actually contributes more to global warming than a Hummer driver who eats low on the food chain.

As Ezra Klein wrote in the *Washington Post* in 2009, "The evidence is strong. It's not simply that meat is a contributor to global warming; it's that it is a huge contributor. Larger, by a significant margin, than the global transportation sector."[xxii]

One of the reasons is methane. Some people find it difficult to take cow burps and flatulence seriously, but livestock emissions are no joke. Methane comes from both ends of the cow, and in such enormous quantities that scientists increasingly view it as one of the greatest threats to our earth's climate.

And there's more. The United Nations' FAO report states that livestock production generates fully 65 percent of the nitrous oxide (another extremely potent greenhouse gas) produced by human activities. The FAO concludes that overall, livestock production is responsible for 18 percent of greenhouse gas emissions, a bigger share than all the SUVs, cars, trucks, buses, trains, ships, and planes in the world combined.

Similarly, a 2009 report published in *Scientific American* remarked that "producing beef for the table has a surprising environmental cost: it releases prodigious amounts of heat-trapping greenhouse gases."[xxiii] The greenhouse gas emissions from producing a pound of beef, the study found, are 58 times greater than those from producing a pound of potatoes.

Some people thought the Live Earth concert handbook was exaggerating when it stated that, "Refusing meat is the single most effective thing you can do to reduce your carbon footprint," but it wasn't. This is literally true. Even Environmental Defense, a group hardly known for taking radical stands, calculates that if every meat eater in the U.S. swapped just one meal of chicken per week for a vegetarian meal, the carbon savings would be equivalent to taking half a million cars off the road.

Not surprisingly, the U.S. meat industry has claimed that livestock production isn't to blame for global warming, and has tried to persuade the public, opinion leaders, and government officials that the FAO indictment of meat is overstated. But in 2009, the prestigious Worldwatch Institute published a landmark report that made the FAO report seem ultra-conservative in comparison.[xxiv] This thoughtful and meticulously thorough study, written by World Bank agricultural scientists Robert Goodland, who spent 23 years as the Bank's lead environmental advisor, and Jeff Anhang, an environmental specialist for the Bank, came to the staggering conclusion that animals raised for food actually account for more than half of all human-caused greenhouse gases. Eating plants instead of animals, the authors conclude, would be by far the most effective strategy to reverse climate change, because it "would have far more rapid effects on greenhouse gas emissions and their atmospheric concentrations—and thus on the rate that the climate is warming—than actions to replace fossil fuels with renewable energy."

A Time for Action

A growing and overwhelming body of evidence tells us that there is a tremendous correlation between the food choices that are the healthiest, and those that are most socially and environmentally responsible. But this information does us little good if we keep right on doing the same thing.

While efforts to use government policy for social impact are controversial, there might be a place for it here. Why don't we tax the things that are bad for the world and that cost our society in the long run? What if we were to lower taxes on income, for example, while raising taxes on unhealthy and environmentally destructive activities? This could be a revenue-neutral way of encouraging steps towards a healthier population and a healthier world.

Could it be that the time has come for creating fiscal incentives that support people in making lifestyle choices that are healthier for the planet and that reduce the risk of the chronic diseases that are imposing an intolerable burden on us financially? What if we taxed agrochemicals, and used the revenue to subsidize organic and other safe forms of growing food? What if we taxed junk food and used the income to subsidize fresh fruits and vegetables? What if we taxed high fructose corn syrup, and used the income to subsidize and thus lower the price people pay for fresh vegetables? What if we taxed products that are responsible for a disproportionate share of greenhouse gases, like meat, and used the money to subsidize vegetable gardens and fruit orchards in every school and neighborhood in the country?

And government aside, what if the business community got on board? What if health insurance companies educated their members about the health benefits of a plant based diet, or lobbied for healthier food in such formative places as schools and hospitals? Might they realize payout savings, thus being able to reduce their member's premiums? What if large companies gave their employees bonuses and incentives to take steps towards a healthier lifestyle, and found that they reduced their health insurance costs in the process?

And without depending on government, business, or anyone else, what would happen if each of us took steps towards a healthier diet and a healthier life? What if we stopped eating the most saturated fat and junk food of any large population in the history of the world, and started on the path to a healthier diet, a healthier life, and a healthier world?

The results would be impressive: We'd have genuinely happy meals, because we'd be eating far better and at far less expense. We'd be so much healthier as people that the amount we'd save in medical bills would go a long way toward solving the crisis in the health care system and toward stabilizing our precarious economy. And we'd dramatically reduce our emissions of greenhouse gases and thus have a more stable climate.

What do you say? Food revolution, anyone?

John Robbins
Soquel, CA

chapter 1

Introduction

What Is the Food Revolution?

I was born into ice cream. Well, not literally, but just about. My father, Irv Robbins, founded, and for many years owned and ran what would become the world's largest ice cream company: Baskin-Robbins (31 Flavors). Along with my uncle, Burt Baskin, he built an empire, with thousands of stores worldwide and sales eventually measuring in the billions of dollars. We had an ice cream cone-shaped swimming pool, our cats were named after ice cream flavors, and I sometimes ate ice cream for breakfast. Not all that surprisingly, many people in the family struggled with weight problems, my uncle died of a heart attack in his early fifties, my father developed serious diabetes and high blood pressure, and I was sick more often than not.

None of that showed up on the balance sheets, however, and my father was grooming me to succeed him. I was his only son, and he expected me to follow in his footsteps. But things did not develop that way. I chose to leave behind the ice cream company and the money it represented, in order to take my own rocky road. I walked away from an opportunity to live a life of wealth to live a different kind of life, a life in which, I hoped, I might be able to be true to my values and learn to make a contribution to the well-being and happiness of others. It was a choice for integrity. Instead of the Great American Dream of financial success, I was pulled forward by a deeper dream.

Explaining that kind of thing to my father, a conservative Republican businessman who sometimes drove a Rolls Royce and never to my knowledge went a day without reading the *Wall Street Journal*, was not easy. At one point I told him, "Look, Dad, it's a different world than when you grew up. The environment is deteriorating rapidly under the impact of human activities. Every two seconds somewhere on Earth a child dies of starvation while elsewhere there are abundant food resources going to waste. Do you see that for me, under these circumstances, inventing a thirty-second flavor just would not be an adequate response for my life?"

My father was not pleased. He had worked hard his whole life and had achieved a level of financial success most people can only fantasize about, and he wanted to share his success and his company with his only son. From his point of view, I am sure, he got the only kid in the country who would turn down such a golden opportunity.

But turn it down I did, and, hungering for connection to the natural world and life's deeper rhythms, I moved with my wife, Deo, in 1969, to a little island off the coast of British Columbia. There we proceeded to build a one-room log cabin, where we lived for the next ten years, growing most of our own food. We were financially poor, some years spending less than $1,000 total, but we were rich in love. Four years into our time on the island, our son Ocean was born into my hands. Deo and I are still lovingly together all these years later, by the way—a rarity in our generation.

During this time we began to live by the values that would culminate, in 1987, with the publication of my book *Diet for a New America*. I was learning to perceive the immense toll exacted by the standard North American diet—and the benefits that might be gained by a shift in a healthier direction. I was learning that the same food choices that do so much to prevent disease—that give you the most vitality, the strongest immune system, and the greatest life expectancy—were also the ones that

took the least toll on the environment, conserved our precious natural resources, and were the most compassionate toward our fellow creatures.

In *Diet for a New America* I described what it was that pulled me
away from the path my father had envisioned and prepared for me, and
set me instead on the one I took:

> "It's a dream of a success in which all beings share because it's founded
> on reverence for life. A dream of a society at peace with its conscience
> because it respects and lives in harmony with all life forms. A dream of a
> people living in accord with the natural laws of Creation, cherishing and
> caring for the environment, conserving nature instead of destroying it. A
> dream of a society that is truly healthy, practicing a wise and compassion-
> ate stewardship of a balanced ecosystem.
>
> "This is not my dream alone. It is really the dream of all human beings
> who feel the plight of the Earth as their own, and sense our obligation to
> respect and protect the world in which we live. To some degree, all of us
> share in this dream. Yet few of us are satisfied that we are doing all that is
> needed to make it happen. Almost none of us are aware of just how pow-
> erfully our eating habits affect the possibility of this dream becoming a re-
> ality. We do not realize that one way or the other, how we eat has a
> tremendous impact."

In *Diet for a New America*, I attempted to show in full detail the nature of this impact on our health, and in addition on the vigor of our society, on the health of our world, and on the well-being of its creatures. I
had no idea, while writing that book, that it would become a bestseller. I
never suspected that I would receive 75,000 letters from people who
read the book or who heard me speak about its message. And even if I
had known how widely the book would be read, and how deeply it
would impact the course of many people's lives, I don't think I could
ever have imagined that it might help to impact choices on a larger
scale. In the five years immediately following the book's publication,
beef consumption in the United States dropped nearly 20 percent.

But in the last few years there's been a backlash. Fad diet books have
sold millions of copies telling people they can lose weight and obtain
optimum health while eating all the bacon and sausage they want. The
U.S. meat industry has managed to divert attention away from the fact

that the animals raised in modern factory farms are forced to endure conditions of almost unimaginable cruelty and deprivation. The USDA is proposing to irradiate increasing numbers of foods to combat the deadly food-borne diseases such as E. coli 0157:H7 that increasingly breed in today's factory farms and slaughterhouses.

Rather than clean up the conditions that produce these pathogens in the first place, the U.S. meat industry has strongly supported food disparagement laws that make it illegal to criticize perishable food products, and then has used such legislation to sue those who challenge their control over your wallet. They even sued Oprah Winfrey for saying that, based on what she'd learned about meat production in the United States, she was never going to eat another burger.

Meanwhile, the chemical industry has mounted an aggressive campaign to discredit organic food. And without the knowledge or consent of most Americans, two-thirds of the products on our supermarket shelves now contain genetically engineered ingredients.

The debate about animal products and genetically engineered foods, and about their impact on our health and our world, is not going to go away. It will be fought in courtrooms and the media, but it will also be fought in people's minds, hearts, and kitchens. In the process, those seeking a more humane and sustainable way of life—for themselves and for our society—will be criticized and attacked by the industries that profit from activities that are harming people and the planet.

As the discussion intensifies, so will the amount of information floating around. Some of it will be valid and rigorously accurate. And some of it will be the product of the public relations machinery of the industries that are selling unhealthy food and exploiting our world. I have written *The Food Revolution* because I believe that, given a chance, most people can tell the difference between the propaganda of industries whose entire intention is to promote and sell products, and data from researchers and scientists whose focus is the public interest.

I have written *The Food Revolution* to provide solid, reliable information for the struggle to achieve a world where the health of people and the Earth community is more important than the profit margins of any industry, where basic human needs take precedence over corporate greed. I have written this book so that you might have clear information on which to base your food choices. It will show you how to attain greater health and respond more deeply from your connection to all of life.

There is still strong in our society the belief that animals and the natural world have value only insofar as they can be converted into revenue. That nature is a commodity. And that the American dream is one of unlimited consumption.

There are many of us, on the other hand, who believe that animals and the natural world have value by virtue of being alive. That Nature is a community to which we belong and to which we owe our lives. And that the deeper American dream is one of unlimited compassion.

In 1962, Rachel Carson dedicated *Silent Spring* to the "host of people" who are "even now fighting the thousands of small battles that in the end will bring victory for sanity and common sense." I have written *The Food Revolution* because I believe that virtually every one of us, if given a chance, would choose to be one of those people and would make our lives, if we knew how, into statements of caring and compassion.

I believe there is within every human being a desire to make choices that help create a healthier future for ourselves, for our children, and for our beleaguered planet and all the life it holds. This desire may be buried, it may be twisted, bent, and broken, it may seem all but destroyed, but it still remains, driving each of us even if from afar, hungering for an opportunity to be seen and heard and felt.

Judging by what appears in the mass media, it would be easy to think that people are only interested in the most shallow and trivial of concerns, that all we want is to eat our burgers, that we couldn't care less about how our food is produced and what the consequences will be to our health and to the wider Earth community. But that's a grievous lie, and it dishonors who we are. The truth is, most people care about world hunger, they are deeply concerned about global warming, they abhor cruelty to animals, they know the planet is in crisis, they sense much of the food we eat in this society is unhealthy, they are alarmed about the uncertainties of genetic engineering, and they are looking for ways to express their caring and concern.

I don't care whether you call yourself a vegetarian, a vegan, or an asparagus. I care whether you live in accord with your values, whether your life has integrity and purpose, whether you act with compassion for yourself and for all of life.

I don't care whether your diet is politically correct. I care whether your food choices are consistent with your love. I care whether they bring you health, uphold your spirit, and help you to fulfill your true nature and reason for being alive.

The truth, as has been said countless times, will set you free. But what is said far less often is that sometimes it first will make you confront habits of behavior and thought that might be limiting you, so that you might attain the awareness to use your freedom for the benefit of your greater self and all of life.

Not that long ago, the average American mother would have been more concerned to learn that her son or daughter was becoming a vegetarian than to learn that he or she was taking up smoking. Not that long ago, organic food products could only be found in specialty stores. Blood cholesterol levels of 300 milligrams per deciliter were considered normal, and patients in hospital coronary care units were fed bacon and eggs, and white toast with margarine and jam for breakfast. Not that long ago, people who ate food that was healthy, environmentally friendly, and caused no animals to suffer were considered health nuts, while those who ate food that caused disease, took a staggering toll on the resource base, and depended on immense animal suffering were considered normal. But all this is changing.

The revolution sweeping our relationship to our food and our world, I believe, is part of an historical imperative. This is what happens when the human spirit is activated. One hundred and fifty years ago, slavery was legal in the United States. One hundred years ago, women could not vote in most states. Eighty years ago, there were no laws in the United States against any form of child abuse. Fifty years ago, we had no Civil Rights Act, no Clean Air or Clean Water legislation, no Endangered Species Act. Today, millions of people are refusing to buy clothes and shoes made in sweatshops and are seeking to live healthier and more Earth-friendly lifestyles. In the last fifteen years alone, as people in the United States have realized how cruelly veal calves are treated, veal consumption has dropped 62 percent.

I don't believe we are isolated consumers, alienated from what gives life, and condemned to make a terrible mess of things on this planet. I believe we are human beings, flawed but learning, stumbling but somehow making our way toward wisdom, sometimes ignorant but learning through it all to live with respect for ourselves, for each other, and for the whole Earth community.

I have written *The Food Revolution* in the belief that—wounded and human as we are—we can still create a thriving and sustainable way of life for all. The restorative powers of both the human body and the Earth are immense.

When I walked away from Baskin-Robbins and the money it represented, I did so because I knew there was a deeper dream. I did it because I knew that with all the reasons that each of us has to despair and become cynical, there still beats in our common heart our deepest prayers for a better life and a more loving world.

When I look out into the world, I see the forces that would bring us disaster. I see the deep night of unthinkable cruelty and blindness. But I also look within the human heart and find something of love there, something that cares and shines out into the dark universe like a bright beacon. And in the shining of that light, I feel the dreams and prayers of all beings. In the shining of that beacon I feel all of our hopes for a better future, and the strength to do what we are here to do.

May all be fed. May all be healed. May all be loved.

PART I

Food and Healing

chapter 2 **Healthy Heart, Healthy Life**

Has anyone in your life ever had a heart attack or suffered from serious heart disease? If you answered Yes to that question, you're not alone. In fact, most people in our society would be with you.

I would. I'm thinking at the moment about my uncle. Burton Baskin was my father's brother-in-law, and also his business partner. Together, they founded, owned, and ran the Baskin-Robbins Ice Cream Company. A talented man with a great sense of style, my Uncle Butch, as we called him, touched countless lives with his expansive spirit. His fatal heart attack struck while he was still in his early fifties, with a loving wife, two incredible kids, a wildly successful business, and everything in the world to look forward to.

Tact was never my strong suit, and maybe I should never have mentioned it, but a few years later I asked my father whether he thought there could be any connection between the amount of ice cream my uncle had eaten and his fatal heart attack. Given that my uncle had weighed something like 220 pounds and that he had certainly enjoyed the family product, the question seemed a reasonable one. But my father was not particularly interested in such reflections. "No," he said. "His ticker just got tired and stopped working."

I can now understand why my father would not have wanted to consider the question. He had by that time manufactured and sold more ice cream than any other human being who had ever lived on this planet, and he most definitely did not want to think that ice cream might be harming anyone, much less that it might have contributed to my uncle's death. Besides, not nearly as much was known, then, about the effects of saturated fat and cholesterol on the human cardiovascular system.

To this day there are a number of people in my family who are angry at me for mentioning any of this in public. They tell me that when I bring this up I am dishonoring my uncle's memory. But I disagree. Burton Baskin loved life, and I believe that he would want his story told, if in the telling it might help others to be more aware of the choices they are making, and more able to live in a way that brings greater health and happiness into their lives.

Similarly, it's poignant that Ben & Jerry's ice cream cofounder Ben Cohen needed to undergo quadruple bypass surgery in 2001, at age 49, due to serious coronary artery disease.

Am I saying that an ice cream cone is going to kill you? Of course not. What I am saying, though, is that ice cream is very high in saturated fat and sugar; and the more saturated fat and sugar you eat, the more likely you are to have a heart attack. This is not a value judgment, and it's not just my opinion. It is a statistical reality, arrived at by the most comprehensive and conscientious body of medical research in world history. What we eat does matter.

The irony is that my father, who like many men of his generation did not believe there was much connection between diet and health, ended up suffering from severely high blood pressure and diabetes, two conditions which also are directly linked with the kind of high-saturated fat, high-sugar diet he ate for most of his life. Thankfully, however, when he was in his late seventies, he changed his diet in the direction I've long been advocating, and he experienced major improvements in his overall health. I cannot tell you how grateful I was the day he told me, "Thank God some of us have lived long enough to learn a few new things."

Many of us, though, will go on eating bacon and eggs for breakfast, and hamburgers and milkshakes for lunch, until the day we wind up in a hospital, hurting badly. We won't change until we get hit over the head.

Some of us, it seems, only know how to learn from pain. I can remember more times than I like to admit when I resisted learning new things with stunning tenacity, and held on to my opinions and behavior patterns despite insurmountable evidence that I was harming myself by doing so. I have been able, under a wide variety of circumstances, to remain loyally committed, despite everything, to my familiar ways of behaving, even when they no longer served any conceivable good purpose. Having acquired a great deal of experience that way, however, I now want to understand the messages life sends me and embrace the changes that are called for, without necessarily having to go through ungodly amounts of pain first.

The philosopher Nietzsche said it well: "He who will, the fates lead; he who won't, they drag."

What keeps us stuck? What keeps us from recognizing the power that we have to make choices that honor our spirits and enrich our lives? What keeps us passive and distant from our greatness? What keeps us closed down when we could be vibrant and creative? The same thing that keeps the animal in his cage, even when the door is opened and he has the chance to walk free. Habit.

When it comes to food choices, habit is stupendously powerful. Our familiar foods give us comfort, reassurance, and a sense of identity. They are there for us when the world may not be. They can be our best friends, loyal and true. It does not take effort or creativity to do the same thing over and over again. There is ease and relaxation in doing what we have always done. And if our habits are continually reinforced by the society around us, they can become even more powerful and alluring.

On the other hand, it does take effort to question whether our conventional ways of thinking and acting truly serve us. It takes effort to ask whether our lives are in alignment with the prayers and deeper purposes of our hearts. It takes effort to consciously make choices that deviate from the cultural norms, yet bring us closer to our wholeness and true health.

We all know people who eat with great care and still get sick, and we all know others who eat any old thing and seem to thrive. But does this change the fact that we have far better odds for healthy lives and vibrant bodies that express our living spirit when we eat more consciously and make healthier choices?

If I told you that you could join either group A, in which one out of every two men and one out of every three women would die of heart disease, or group B, in which heart disease deaths would be practically unknown and people would be healthier in every other way as well, which group would you join? Group B, of course. You'd be nuts to choose otherwise. And yet, tragically, the vast majority of people in our society are in fact members in good standing of group A. Eating the standard American diet that's based on meat and dairy products, with plenty of white flour and white sugar, one-third of the women and one-half of the men in the U.S. population die of heart disease. Meanwhile, medical research is telling us that vegetarians and vegans (vegetarians who consume no dairy products or eggs) not only have far less heart disease, but also have lower rates of cancer, hypertension, diabetes, gallstones, kidney disease, obesity, and colon disease.[1] They live on average six to ten years longer than the rest of the population, and in fact seem to be healthier by every measurement we have of assessing health outcomes.

I know what some of you are thinking. Maybe vegetarians don't actually live longer; maybe their lives are so boring it only seems that way. You're thinking, Being a vegetarian is like being celibate; it might work for some people, but not for me. But I want to ask you a question: How much pleasure is there in illness? Who do you think enjoys life more, the person who is flourishing in vibrant health, eating a deliciously prepared yet simple meal of wholesome foods, or the person who is burdened by weight problems and high blood pressure, gorging on steak and ice cream?

I'll tell you this: If you want to know what health is worth, ask the person who has lost it.

Scientific Data or Industry Propaganda?

The meat and dairy industries, naturally, disagree with everything I'm saying. They tell us repeatedly that their products are the cornerstones of a balanced and complete diet. They say we need the foods they produce to have adequate protein, calcium, iron, B-12, riboflavin, and zinc. They say that without the consumption of animal products, human health would decline dramatically.

What I think any sane person would want to know is this: Opinions aside, what does the hard data indicate? Does it support the contention of vegetarians and vegans that they have lower rates and less risk of heart disease, and indeed for almost all of the "diseases of affluence" that plague our culture? Is there sound science behind the claims that vegetarians are leaner and more fit people who outlive the rest of the population by six to 10 years? Or is this simply the fuzzy rhetoric of radical extremists?

The National Cattlemen's Beef Association and the National Dairy Council tell us again and again that we jeopardize our health and well-being if we do not consume the products they provide. Impartial researchers and nonprofit public health organizations such as the World Health Organization, the American Institute for Cancer Research, the American Heart Association, the Physicians Committee for Responsible Medicine, the National Cancer Institute, and the Center for Science in the Public Interest, however, have a different perspective.

It can get contentious. . . .

Is that so?

"[It's a] myth [that] people who eat vegetarian diets are healthier than people who eat meat."

—National Cattlemen's Beef Association[2]

"Studies indicate that vegetarians often have lower morbidity and mortality rates. . . . Not only is mortality from coronary artery disease lower in vegetarians than in nonvegetarians, but vegetarian diets have also been successful in arresting coronary artery disease. Scientific data suggest positive relationships between a vegetarian diet and reduced risk for . . . obesity, coronary artery disease, hypertension, diabetes mellitus, and some types of cancer."

—American Dietetic Association Position Paper on Vegetarian Diets[3]

When we see industry statements juxtaposed nakedly against those from more objective sources, it is possible to see the contrast, get a sense of the differences, and appraise which is more likely to be true. But in everyday life, we are hardly ever given the opportunity to compare the messages we receive from industries promoting the sale of their food products with messages from more reliable sources.

The statements of the meat and dairy industries are important to evaluate because, even though they are no more true than any other form of advertising, they are broadcast so pervasively in our culture that they very likely have insinuated themselves into your mind. The meat and dairy industries in the United States spend literally billions of dollars annually, not only on advertising, but on thousands of other ways by which they influence what you think and how you spend your money. They provide free educational materials to schools. They issue a constant stream of public service announcements to radio and TV stations. They continually flood newspapers and magazines with press releases. They promote their products heavily to doctors, nurses, and dieticians. And they typically proceed with a veneer that implies they're doing all this for your own good.

The amount of money spent on food in our culture is phenomenal, and these dollars are, of course, highly coveted. There are whole industries with massive budgets whose entire goal is to sell their products. From their point of view, if their products are healthy, great, and if not, they'll find another marketing angle. They typically spend the most money promoting the very foods that are most harmful. They'll want you to be more concerned with what's cool or what other people are doing than what's healthy. And they'll tell you that their foods are healthy even when they're not.

This is not just misinformation. It is really affecting people's lives, and probably yours. There are industries profiting from keeping you ignorant, confused, and misinformed, buying and consuming products that lead to unnecessary suffering and death for you and your loved ones.

Today, heart disease is the number one killer of Americans.[4] More people die from heart and blood vessel diseases each year in the United States than from all other causes of death combined.

What is the single greatest risk factor for heart disease? A high blood cholesterol level.[5] And what is the single most important factor in raising blood cholesterol levels? The consumption of saturated fat. The correlations between cholesterol levels, saturated fat intake, and heart disease are among the strongest and most consistent in the history of world medical research. This is why every authoritative health body in the world, from the American Heart Association to the World Health Organization to the National Heart, Lung and Blood Institute, is calling for reductions in saturated fat consumption.

It is also, however, why the meat and dairy industries sometimes have not been happy with what has been learned. . . .

Is THAT SO?

"Who says meat is high in saturated fat? This politically correct nutrition campaign is just another example of the diet dictocrats trying to run our lives."
—Sam Abramson, CEO, Springfield Meats[6]

"Meat contributes an extraordinarily significant percentage of the saturated fat in the American diet."
—Marion Nestle, Chair of the Nutrition Department, New York University[7]

Take hamburgers, for example. . . .

What WE KNOW

Percentage of adult daily value for saturated fat in one Double Whopper with cheese: 130 percent

Percentage of eight-year-old child's daily value for saturated fat in one Double Whopper with cheese: More than 200 percent

Scientists at the Center for Science in the Public Interest have studied the American diet for years, and have sought to give people sound information on which they can base healthy food choices. Recognizing the saturated fat in hamburgers, they have been outspoken about the health consequences of such food. "If you had to pick a single food that inflicts the most damage in the American diet," they said in their newsletter in 1999, "ground beef would be a prime contender. Whether it's tacos, meatloaf, lasagna, or the ubiquitous hamburger, Americans stuff themselves with ground beef without a second thought about its consequences. 'Billions and billions served' means 'billions and billions spent'—on doctor's visits and hospital bills."[8]

How has the U.S. meat industry responded? Some of its representatives have called the Center for Science in the Public Interest "food fascists," "culinary dictators," and similar names.[9] This gives me pause. Name-calling has never impressed me as a valid form of argument. I suppose it shows the frustration of an industry with increasingly reduced scientific grounds on which to defend its products. Still, I would think these people could grasp that there is an enormous difference between dictating your food choices, which is a form of coercion, and providing education as to what science has learned about diet and health, so you can make informed choices about matters that affect your health.

Others, a little more thoughtfully, have pointed out that there are some kinds of saturated fat that don't raise cholesterol levels. Red meat, for example, contains a type of saturated fat—stearic acid—that has little effect on cholesterol levels. But these comparatively rare types of saturated fat are almost always accompanied by the kinds of saturated fat that do raise cholesterol levels. Red meat is very high in another kind of saturated fat—palmitic acid—that is notorious for raising cholesterol levels.

With what we've learned about diet and heart disease, it is not easy to defend animal fat consumption today. Even the American Meat Institute and National Dairy Council acknowledge that the primary suppliers of saturated fat in the American diet are animal products—beef, cheese, butter, chicken, milk, pork, eggs, and ice cream. They like to point out, however, that their products are not the only culprits. There are a few other foods that are also high in saturated fat, such as palm and palm kernel oil, hydrogenated oils, margarine, and chocolate.

They are correct. But the producers of chocolate aren't trying to convince you and me and the rest of the public that the foods they sell should be the mainstays of our diets. You won't see famous actors and celebrities in expensive ad campaigns telling you that palm kernel oil is "real food for real people." James Garner, speaking for the American beef industry, said that about beef. That was just before the actor, who was so fond of beef, was hospitalized for a quintuple bypass heart operation.

Wʜᴀᴛ ᴡᴇ ᴋɴᴏᴡ

Drop in heart disease risk for every 1 percent decrease in blood cholesterol: 3–4 percent[10]

Blood cholesterol levels of vegetarians compared to non-vegetarians: 14 percent lower[11]

Risk of death from heart disease for vegetarians compared to non-vegetarians: Half[12]

Blood cholesterol levels of vegans (vegetarians who eat no meat, eggs, or dairy products) compared to non-vegetarians: 35 percent lower[13]

Most of us grew up believing that animal protein is superior to plant protein, and that if we don't eat animal protein we are risking our health. This is ironic given that animal proteins, in particular, have been found to raise cholesterol levels.[14] Soy proteins, on the other hand, have consistently been found to lower cholesterol levels.[15]

Meanwhile, the meat, dairy, and egg industries in the United States continue to tell you that you should eat their products. And medical researchers continue to say something else.

Iꜱ ᴛʜᴀᴛ ꜱᴏ?

"[It's a] myth [that] the risk of death from heart disease can be greatly reduced if a person avoids eating a meat-centered diet."
—National Cattlemen's Beef Association[16]

"Vegetarians have the best diet; they have the lowest rates of coronary heart disease of any group in the country."
—William Castelli, M.D., Director, Framingham Health Study, the longest-running study of diet and heart disease in world medical history[17]

It reminds me of the three stages any new truth always goes through. First, it is ignored. Second, it is violently opposed. And third, it is accepted as self-evident.

When it comes to the benefits of a plant-based diet for heart disease, we seem today to be in the middle of the violent opposition stage.

IS THAT SO?

"The fallacy . . . is that animal foods are the critical elements in the diet that are causing coronary heart disease."
—National Cattlemen's Association[18]

"In regions where . . . meat is scarce, cardiovascular disease is unknown."
—Time magazine[19]

"[Advocates of plant-based diets] lack a firm scientific basis. . . . No study . . . has demonstrated that changing diet prevents coronary artery disease."
—Dairy Bureau of Canada[20]

"A large and convincing body of evidence from studies in humans . . . shows that diets low in saturated fatty acids and cholesterol are associated with low risks and rates of atherosclerotic cardiovascular disease."
—U.S. National Research Council, in "Diet and Health, Implications for Reducing Chronic Disease Risk"

The meat, dairy, and egg industries are having a hard time. They can't dispute that the primary dietary sources of cholesterol are eggs, shellfish, chicken, beef, fish, pork, cheese, butter, and milk. Nor can they dispute the fact that no plant food contains any cholesterol. Sometimes the chicken industry will imply that chicken is lower in cholesterol than beef. But that simply isn't true. Chicken has about as much cholesterol as beef. There is simply no escaping the correlation between meat consumption and cholesterol levels.

WHAT WE KNOW

Intake of cholesterol for non-vegetarians: 300–500 milligrams/day[21]

Intake of cholesterol for lacto-ovo vegetarians: 150–300 milligrams/day[22]

Intake of cholesterol for vegans: Zero[23]

Average cholesterol level in the United States: 210[24]

Average cholesterol level of U.S. vegetarians: 161[25]

Average cholesterol level of U.S. vegans: 133[26]

Blood cholesterol levels are of course not the only dietary factor affecting the risk of heart disease, but the advantages of having a lower level are enormous. William Castelli, M.D., Director of the Framingham Health Study, says that when people keep their cholesterol levels below 150, they are virtually assured of never suffering a heart attack. "We've never had a heart attack in Framingham in 35 years in anyone who had a cholesterol under 150."[27]

It can be stunning how quickly people with heart disease improve when they adopt a low-fat vegan diet. Patients enrolled in the Mc-Dougall Program at St. Helena Hospital in Santa Rosa, California, consistently show dramatic improvement after only two weeks on a very low-fat vegan diet.

Faced with evidence like this, the meat, dairy, and egg industries persist nonetheless in trying to defend their products. Sometimes they attempt to shift responsibility onto your genes. It's not what you eat that matters most, they say, it's your DNA, so you may as well go ahead and have a steak. . .

Is THAT SO?

"Your genetics are a prime determinant of whether you will get atherosclerosis and heart disease. If your parents and grandparents had it, then you are a candidate; if they didn't have it, your risk is much lower."
—The Beef-Eaters Guide to Modern Meat[28]

"It's true that a small percentage of patients have a hereditary form of arteriosclerosis in the sense that in their immediate family and their parents' and grandparents' families, there is a high incidence of atherosclerosis and coronary heart disease. . . . But that only constitutes about five percent of the cases. Most people (who develop heart disease) don't really have a hereditary disease."
—Michael Debakey, M.D., Director, Cardiovascular Research Center, pioneer in heart transplants, bypasses, and the artificial heart[29]

The meat, dairy and egg industries have had a difficult time in recent years, as study after study has confirmed the link between their products and heart disease. In the effort to exonerate their products, they have often tried to make much of what is, in fact, very little.

In 1999, a study appeared in the *Archives of Internal Medicine* that has since been widely touted by the U.S. meat industry. This study, they say, "proves" that red meat should be part of a healthy diet. The reason for the industry's enthusiasm is that participants in the study who ate lean red meat lowered their cholesterol levels by 1 percent.[30]

People who eat low-fat, near-vegan, plant-based diets, on the other hand, regularly lower their cholesterol levels by 10 to 35 percent.[31]

Another important risk factor in determining your risk of heart disease is the ratio of your total cholesterol to your HDL (high-density lipoprotein) level. The higher the ratio, the greater your danger of heart disease. The ideal ratio of total cholesterol to HDL is 3.0 to 1 or lower.[32]

The average American male's ratio is 5.1 to 1.[33] The average vegetarian's ratio, on the other hand, is 2.9 to 1.[34]

When it comes to heart disease, the evidence against animal products has today become so convincing and so thorough that even many in the livestock industry can see the handwriting on the wall. Dr. Peter R. Cheeke is a professor of animal science at Oregon State University and serves on the editorial boards of the *Journal of Animal Science* and *Animal Feed Science and Technology*. In his widely used animal science textbook, he says,

> "Many studies, involving hundreds of thousands of people, have shown . . . a positive relationship between coronary heart disease and serum (blood) cholesterol. The higher the serum cholesterol, the higher the risk for coronary heart disease. Populations in which the average serum cholesterol level is (low) . . . are those on the lower end of the per capita meat consumption scale, while those (with high cholesterol levels) are populations with high intakes of animal products. . . . It's more useful to the livestock industries and animal scientists to come to grips with the demonstrated relationships among saturated fat and cholesterol intakes and coronary heart disease, than to claim that there is no relationship or that there's some sort of conspiracy against animal products by the medical community."[35]

Treating Heart Disease

For many heart attack victims, the first sign that anything is wrong is a searing pain, followed by a fatal heart attack. The more fortunate victims of heart disease have advance notice. They develop chest pain, called angina, and/or other symptoms that tell them something is seriously wrong. They are alerted by these signals to the reality that their arteries have become dangerously clogged, and that the flow of oxygen and nutrition carried by the blood throughout their cardiovascular system has become seriously impeded.

This year, more than 1 million Americans will undergo coronary bypass surgery or angioplasty to relieve pain by enlarging the opening in clogged arteries. The national cost for these two operations will be $15.6 billion.[36] This, of course, is only the dollar cost, which takes no account of the agony and anxiety that will be experienced by these patients and their families. Nor does it say anything of the unwanted side effects and trauma they will endure.

WHAT WE KNOW

Risk of dying during bypass surgery: 4.6–11.9 percent[37]

Risk of permanent brain damage from bypass surgery: 15–44 percent[38]

Recipients of bypass surgery for whom it prolongs life: 2 percent[39]

Risk of death during angioplasty: 0.4–2.8 percent[40]

Risk of major complications developing during angioplasty: 10 percent[41]

Studies that have found that angioplasty prolongs life or prevents heart attacks: Zero[42]

Patients undergo bypass and angioplasty operations primarily to relieve angina and improve blood flow to the heart. Yet there is a 25 to 50 percent likelihood that within six months their blood vessels will again become blocked, and their chest pain will recur—assuming they continue to eat a meat-based diet.[43]

On the other hand, three-quarters of the patients who follow the renowned program for reversing heart disease developed by Dean Ornish, M.D., clinical professor of medicine and attending physician at the School of Medicine, University of California, San Francisco, experience marked and long-lasting reduction in angina—without surgery.[44]

The Ornish program is made up of five basic components:

1. A very low-fat, whole foods, vegetarian (near-vegan) diet

2. Half an hour a day of walking or other exercise

3. Half an hour a day of stretching, meditation, relaxation, stress reduction, etc.

4. Psychological and emotional support groups

5. No smoking

Of course, there are people with heart disease who won't follow these kinds of guidelines. They want it to be easier. They don't want to change their lifestyles that much. Accordingly, the American Heart Association has come up with a program that includes some low-fat animal products and utilizes high doses of cholesterol-lowering drugs. I find it fascinating to compare the results patients obtain from these two programs.

> How many patients on the American Heart Association program achieve discernible reversal of atherosclerosis? One out of every six.[45]
>
> How many patients on Dr. Dean Ornish's program achieve discernible reversal of atherosclerosis? Three out of every four.[46]
>
> What kind of change do patients on average see in arterial blockage in five years on the American Heart Association program? A 28 percent increase.[47]
>
> What kind of change do patients on average see in arterial blockage in five years on the Ornish program? An 8 percent *reduction*.[48]

There is a reason why more than forty insurance companies now cover all or part of the Ornish program. Nearly 80 percent of patients with severely clogged arteries who follow the Ornish program for a year or more are able to avoid bypass or angioplasty.[49]

Despite (or maybe because of) such outstanding results, the Ornish program has been the subject of massive controversy. Some say his approach is too drastic, and we should stick to more medically conservative methods. Ornish's reply is simple and difficult to argue with: "I don't understand why asking people to eat a well-balanced vegetarian diet is considered drastic, while it's medically conservative to cut people open or put them on powerful cholesterol-lowering drugs for the rest of their lives."

Some people in the meat and dairy industries, as you might imagine, have not been overly fond of Dr. Dean Ornish's approach. They might have cringed when *Newsweek,* heralding his breakthrough approach, put his photo on the cover of an issue. They were not pleased when there were rumors he might be appointed Surgeon General. They have criticized his program from any angle they could find. Among other things, they have said that diet and lifestyle changes might be okay for younger people who aren't all that sick, but they won't work for older people and those who have severe heart disease.

The reality, however, is that people who follow the Ornish program consistently show dramatic improvements, regardless of how old or ill they are.[50]

Critics of Ornish's program have countered that it is not clear whether the improvements patients experience are due to the diet or to the other health-supporting components in the program. This is true. Ornish's approach is essentially holistic, which means that all of the various pieces of the program work together to produce the intended effect. He has never had an intention to isolate the various components.

Interestingly, however, Cleveland Clinic general surgeon and researcher Caldwell B. Esselstyn, M.D., has demonstrated comparable results using a low-fat near-vegan diet, without employing the other factors in the Ornish program. Reporting in the *American Journal of Cardiology,* Esselstyn wrote, "In this study, patients become virtually heart-attack proof. We achieved these excellent results without structured exercise, meditation, stress management, and other added lifestyle changes."[51]

Not ones to give up easily, meat and dairy industry advocates tried to refute Esselstyn's work by saying that it's not clear whether these kinds of results will continue over the long term, and besides, maybe his patients weren't that sick to begin with.

Hardly. All of the patients in Esselstyn's study had severe heart disease at the outset, yet after twelve years on his program, 95 percent of them were alive and well. How sick were they to begin with? The patients in Esselstyn's study had experienced 48 serious cardiac events in the eight years before they joined the study. But in the 12 years after they joined the study, those patients who were compliant with the program experienced a grand total of zero cardiac events.[52]

Yes, said those holding court for the meat industry, but the diet is too restrictive for most people to comply with for any length of time. You just can't ask people to be that restrictive in their diets and expect very many of them to comply.

This sounds reasonable. But what percentage of the patients in Esselstyn's 12-year study do you think were compliant?

Ninety-five.[53]

Does his program ask too much of people? Is an exclusively plant-based diet too radical? Esselstyn doesn't think so. "Some criticize this exclusively plant-based diet as extreme or draconian," he writes. "Webster's dictionary defines draconian as 'inhumanly cruel.' A closer look reveals that 'extreme' or 'inhumanly cruel' describes not plant-based nutrition, but the consequences of our present Western diet. Having a sternum divided for bypass surgery or a stroke that renders one an aphasic invalid can be construed as extreme; and having a breast, prostate, colon, or rectum removed to treat cancer may seem inhumanly cruel. These diseases are rarely seen in populations consuming a plant-based diet."[54]

From every direction, the evidence keeps piling up. Twenty-five years ago, the region of the world with the worst heart disease problem was North Karelia, in Eastern Finland. Today, the region of the world with the fastest dropping rates of heart disease is the very same North Karelia. What happened? The area adopted a "get fit" program, based on reducing cholesterol and smoking through government-sponsored media campaigns, labeling meats and other foods as to their saturated fat and cholesterol levels, and converting farms that had been producing animal products to growing vitamin-rich fruits and vegetables. How much difference did it make? In the past twenty-five years, heart disease deaths in North Karelia have been reduced by an astonishing 65 percent.[55]

How to Lower Blood Pressure

In Western societies, many of us would like to eat our bacon and eggs for breakfast, and then, if need be, take a cholesterol-lowering pill to lessen our risk of heart disease. We don't want to change our lifestyles. We don't want to question what we eat.

Even the most conscious of us may not realize what we are doing to ourselves, and may not see when we are harming ourselves.

I'm thinking, at the moment, of one of the great spiritual mentors of our time, *Be Here Now* author Ram Dass. After he read *Diet for a New America,* Ram Dass told me, "You've really made it hard for me to eat chicken now. I've always liked chicken. But you've left me no excuse. You've made it clear what I need to do." He wrote an endorsement, stating, "John Robbins' extraordinary book points out in an uncompromising fashion that our cultural dietary habits are killing us in spirit and body, and leaves little doubt as to the inevitable course of our actions." Ram Dass was kind enough to serve for nearly ten years on the board of advisors for EarthSave, the nonprofit organization I founded to channel the public response to *Diet for a New America* into sustained, positive, and effective action.

But like many of us, Ram Dass has had food habits that might not be in keeping with his own best interest. He returned, in time, to eating chicken and ice cream and other such foods—and probably too much of them for his own good. He continued, even though his blood pressure was too high and his weight a challenge.

It does not dishonor this man, who has given so much of such value to so many, to acknowledge that he is human, and that he too has had struggles learning to care for himself and eat in accord with his optimal health and well-being. One of the things that has endeared Ram Dass to millions and made his message so meaningful over the years has been that he doesn't pretend to be perfect or act as if he has it all together. I've always appreciated this about him, because it's helped me, too, to be more fully human, and more fully honest with my own struggles.

Eventually, and tragically, he suffered a stroke. I love Ram Dass dearly, and am sad that he has had to suffer as a result of his stroke. I have only admiration for the courage with which he has sought to find meaning in his pain and to transform his suffering into growth. He is one of the people referred to in the saying, "Things tend to turn out the best for those people who make the best of things, however they turn out."

After his stroke, Ram Dass finished writing his book *Still Here,* a moving guide to the final phases of life. In it, he talks about his stroke, which left him in a wheelchair and with limited speech. "One of the reasons for the stroke was that I had been ignoring my body. I had spent most of my life keeping my Awareness 'free of my body,' as I thought of it then; but I can see now that I was also ignoring my body, pushing it away. By forgetting to take my blood pressure medicine, I showed how I was disregarding my body."[56]

We may never know why Ram Dass' blood pressure was too high, nor what role his diet might have played in the stroke. We cannot know whether or not this dear man's stroke would have happened if he had eaten more healthfully. But people with high blood pressure are seven times more likely to suffer a stroke, four times more likely to have a heart attack, and five times more likely to die of congestive heart failure than people with normal blood pressure.

It is certainly sad that so many people suffer from the consequences of high blood pressure without knowing how much of this is preventable through different food choices. Today, a greater portion of people are taking medication for high blood pressure than have ever taken medicine for any illness ever encountered in human history.

WHAT WE KNOW

Most common problem for which people go to doctors in the United States: High blood pressure

Ideal blood pressure: 110/70 or less (without medication)[57]

Average blood pressure of vegetarians: 112/69[58]

Average blood pressure of non-vegetarians: 121/77[59]

Definition of high blood pressure: The top number (systolic) is consistently over 140, or the bottom number (diastolic) is consistently over 90, while the person is at rest

Incidence of high blood pressure in meat eaters compared to vegetarians: Nearly triple[60]

Incidence of very high blood pressure in meat eaters compared to vegetarians: 13 times higher[61]

Patients with high blood pressure who achieve substantial improvement by switching to a vegetarian diet: 30–75 percent[62]

What patients are typically told when prescribed medications for high blood pressure: "You'll probably need to take these for the rest of your life."

Patients with high blood pressure who are able to completely discontinue use of medications after adopting a low-sodium, low-fat, high-fiber vegetarian diet: 58 percent[63]

Incidence of high blood pressure among senior citizens in United States: More than 50 percent[64]

Incidence of high blood pressure among senior citizens in countries eating traditional low-fat plant based diets: Virtually none[65]

Breaking Free

We know today that the same diets that help to prevent most heart attacks also help to prevent most cases of high blood pressure. And we know that these same diets also do wonders for those who, unfortunately, have already developed these problems. This is marvelous news, for it places in our hands the means to prevent massive amounts of unnecessary suffering.

Not everyone, however, is pleased that this knowledge has been attained. There are those who, perhaps a little biased by their own self-interest, say and do some remarkable things. . . .

Is THAT SO?

"We must be eternally vigilant to guard against those who would undermine confidence in the health benefits of eating meat. If meat-eaters have higher blood pressure, it's from the stress of having to defend the perfectly reasonable desire to chow down on a thick sirloin against the misguided and intrusive efforts of the food police."

—Sam Abramson, CEO, Springfield Meats[66]

"Blood pressure fell within hours of starting the (very low-fat vegan diet) McDougall Program. Twenty percent of the people were on blood pressure medications the day they began the program. In almost every case the medications were stopped that day. Yet the blood pressure dropped (significantly) by the second day. This data is from over 1,000 participants at the McDougall Program at St. Helena Hospital in the Napa Valley of California."

—John McDougall, M.D.

The irony is that many of us still think we must eat animal products in order to have balanced diets and be healthy. We still think heart attacks and high blood pressure are regrettable but more or less inevitable byproducts that come with living well and growing old. We think that the best we can do for heart attacks is to take cholesterol-lowering drugs, and that the best we can do for high blood pressure is take medication to bring it under control. These illnesses have become so much a part of the American scene as to virtually be institutions. We don't realize to what extent our destinies lie in our own hands, and on our own plates. We don't realize how powerfully and inexorably our food choices lead us toward or away from these afflictions.

Many of us feel confused. There is so much information about diet and health all around us. How do we sort it out? Our task is not made easier when those who sell the foods that contribute to heart disease, high blood pressure, and many other diseases are doing everything they can, and spending billions of dollars in the effort, to influence how we think and what we eat.

Confused and disempowered, we too often end up *not* making the food choices that could dramatically improve the health of our cardiovascular systems, greatly reduce our risk of heart disease and high blood pressure, and vastly improve the quality of our lives. We complain, we feel bad, we get sick, but we don't do the one thing that could in fact go far to restore our inner vitality and the unimpeded circulation of our bloodstreams.

It's a shame that we allow people and industries to keep us bewildered and alienated from our personal power. It's a shame that we allow them to keep us ignorant of the enormous health advantages that would be ours with a shift toward a more healthy plant-based diet.

Fortunately, more and more of us are every day realizing we can choose a way of life, and a way of eating, that free us to our highest health potential and lead us to a far more fulfilling experience of our bodies and our lives. We can experience the joy of healthy cardiovascular systems and healthy hearts, and naturally healthy blood pressure levels. We don't need any longer to clog our arteries with saturated fat and cholesterol, but can feed our bodies with wholesome natural food so we can truly live to the heights of our potential. We can break out of the habits that tell us to conform and stay put, and say No to the lies of industries that profit from our pain.

We can do what gives us power, energy, and aliveness. We can say Yes to our vitality and passion. Leaving behind the standard American meat-based diet in favor of a healthy plant-based diet can be like breaking free from chains, to become, perhaps for the first time, truly free.

Dick Gregory, the human rights activist and devoted vegetarian, has said that when you eat consciously and cleanse your body of toxins and fears, something truly wonderful happens. "You are really at home with Mother Nature and happily at peace with life in Mother Nature's World. You can shout the words of the familiar freedom phrase and they will have a meaning only you will truly realize: 'Free at last!'"[67]

chapter 3 # Preventing Cancer

I am, it is certainly true, a proponent of each of us taking as much responsibility for our own health as we can. I am, without a doubt, in favor of each of us making food choices that are in alignment with our highest good, and developing relationships to food that serve the natural unfolding of our well-being. I do not believe that, in this society, we can become fully compassionate, conscious beings without deeply questioning the food we eat.

But that does not mean any of us are to blame for the illnesses we might experience. I'm talking about greater self-responsibility here, not greater guilt. None of us should ever be made to feel a failure for becoming sick, or for failing to cure ourselves. None of us should ever be made to feel that we are letting ourselves or anyone else down if we become ill. Eating healthfully raises your odds of being well. It greatly reduces your risk of many diseases, and it opens the door to experiencing new levels of joy and passion and purpose in your body. But it can not guarantee that you won't become ill.

If I have learned anything about our true power, it is this: It does not come from our opinions. Our true power comes from responding to and nurturing life.

Our beauty does not come from dominating and conquering and winning. It comes from blessing and appreciating and loving. Our glory does not come from being right or being in charge. Our glory comes from being who we really are.

This life we lead may be hard, may be downright agonizing at times, but it's not about finding fault. It's about finding a way of life that honors your living spirit. It's not about blame. It's about coming to a deeper understanding of who you are, and of the love and power that lie within you. It's not about pointing fingers. It's about pointing the way, whenever possible, to a thriving, healthy, and compassionate life.

We live in a Judeo-Christian cultural context that has historically shown a stupendous ability to produce feelings of guilt. Many of us have been taught to see God as a punishing parent. It's easy for us to see illness as a punishment for wrongdoing, or wrong thinking. It's easy for us to see the ill as responsible for their own suffering. It's easy to blame ourselves for our woes, to see our suffering as proof that we have sinned.

To me this is, to speak frankly, cruel. As if being sick weren't enough of a travail, we add to it the further burden of responsibility for having gotten sick in the first place. If you have cancer, it must be because you repressed your anger, or because you don't really want to get well, or because you have eaten the wrong foods.

We don't need this.

Treya Wilber cofounded the Cancer Support Community, a non-profit organization that provided support groups, educational programs, and special events, all free of charge, for people with cancer and their families. She wrote movingly of her struggle with this very concept:

"Five years ago I was sitting at my kitchen table, having tea with a friend, when he told me that, some months earlier, he had learned he had thyroid cancer. I told him about my mother who had surgery for colon cancer fifteen years ago and has been fine ever since. I then described the various theories my sisters and I had come up with to explain why she had gotten cancer.

"We had a number of explanations, our favorite being that she had been too much my father's wife and not enough of her own person. (For example, had she not married a cattleman, we speculated, she might have become a vegetarian and avoided the dietary fats linked to colon cancer.) We also theorized that her family's difficulty expressing emotions had played a role. . . .

"My friend, who obviously had thought deeply about the implications of his illness, then said something that shook me deeply. 'Don't you see what you're doing?' he asked. 'You're treating your mother like an object, spinning theories about her. Other people's theories about you can feel like a violation. I know, because in my case the reasons my friends have come up with about why I have cancer have felt like an imposition and a burden. I don't feel they're offered solely out of concern for me. Rather, the thought of my having cancer must have frightened them so much they needed to find a reason, an explanation, a meaning for it. The theories were to help them, not to help me, and they cause me a lot of pain.'

"I was shocked. I had never looked at what was behind my theorizing, never speculated about how my theories affected my mother. Even though none of us in the family ever told her about our ideas, I'm quite certain she sensed how we felt. That kind of climate, I realized, wouldn't encourage trust or openness. I suddenly saw that my attitude had kept me distant from my mother during the greatest crisis of her life.

"That incident with my friend opened a door. It was the beginning of a shift toward my becoming more compassionate toward people who are sick, more respectful of their integrity, more kindly in my approach—and more humble about my own ideas. I began to see the judgment only partly hidden behind my theorizing and to recognize the unacknowledged fear that lay deeper still. The implicit message behind such theories began to emerge. Instead of saying, 'I care about you; what I can do to help?' I was actually saying, 'What did you do wrong? Where did you make your mistake? How did you fail?' And, not incidentally, 'How can I protect myself?'"[1]

Treya wrote these words as someone who herself had cancer and who wanted to know where her true responsibility lay. She continued,

"I'm certain that I played a role in my becoming ill, a role that was mostly unconscious and unintentional, and I know that I play a large role, this one very conscious and intentional, in getting well and staying well. I try to focus on what I can do now; unraveling the past too easily degenerates into a kind of self-blame which makes it harder, not easier, to make healthy, conscious choices in the present.

"As a correction to the belief that we are at the mercy of larger forces or that illness is due to external agents only, this idea that we create our own reality and therefore our own illnesses is important and necessary. But it goes too far. It is an overreaction, an oversimplification. It is more accurate to say we *affect* our own reality. This leaves room both for effective personal action and for the wondrous rich mysteriousness of life.

"I try to use my own setbacks and weaknesses and illnesses to develop compassion for others and for myself, while remembering not to take serious things too seriously. I try to stay aware of the opportunities for psychological and spiritual healing around me in the very real pain and suffering that ask for our compassion."[2]

Sadly, the author of these beautiful words, Treya Wilber, died of breast cancer. And meanwhile, the numbers of people with cancer keeps rising. . . .

The Search for a Cure

It was in 1971 that President Richard Nixon declared war on cancer, pledging to spend whatever it would take to find a cure for the disease. The United States had put a man on the moon, and the belief in technology was at an all-time high. The power of antibiotics seemed to suggest that any disease could be conquered if only the right drug were found. In the following years, hundreds of billions of dollars were poured into chemotherapy research and treatment.

Although patients who were given chemotherapy suffered tremendously, extended remissions were achieved for some forms of childhood cancer, most notably acute lymphocytic leukemia, as well as for some cancers, such as Hodgkin's disease, that struck primarily adolescents. It became possible to cure a number of childhood cancers that had previously been fatal. Further, chemotherapy contributed to the successful treatment of other rare kinds of cancer, such as Burkitt's lymphoma, choriocarcinoma, lymphosarcoma, Wilms' tumor, and Ewing's sarcoma.

There were breakthroughs in the use of chemotherapy for testicular cancer, and promising signs of an ability to prolong life in cases of ovarian cancer.

The belief was widespread that with enough money, researchers would eventually discover how to conquer the more common cancers, the solid tumors. Surely, these cancers would be the next to fall. One leading chemotherapy advocate called the effort to defeat cancer "the greatest mobilization of resources . . . ever undertaken to conquer a single disease."[3]

It was a time of grand hope.

Unfortunately, as the years passed, the successes remained isolated to a few relatively rare forms of cancer. Campaigns to raise money for cancer research kept saying we could "see the light at the end of the tunnel," but the light never reached the ever-increasing millions of people with cancer and their families. The hoped-for breakthrough in the war against cancer was always "just around the corner," and it never really materialized.

With it all, there was little real improvement in survival rates for the vast majority of cancers. The sober truth was that for most people with cancer chemotherapy continued to be a disappointment. The inescapable fact that researchers could never manage to circumvent was that the amount of chemotherapy necessary to kill every last cancer cell in a human body was almost invariably lethal for the body itself.

As time went along, the bad news began to be announced in scientific journals. In 1985, a professor at the Harvard University School of Public Health, John Cairns, M.D., published a seminal article on the war on cancer in *Scientific American,* in which he showed that chemotherapy was able to save the lives of only 2 to 3 percent of cancer patients. Despite the overwhelming investment the medical community had made in chemotherapy, he said, it was not capable of defeating any of the common cancers.[4]

The next year, the former editor of the *Journal of the National Cancer Institute,* John C. Bailar, M.D., published a landmark study in the *New England Journal of Medicine.* Simply looking long and hard at the data, Dr. Bailar said, had compelled him to lose faith in chemotherapy, and indeed in the entire war on cancer. "Some 35 years of intense and growing efforts to improve the treatment of cancer," he wrote, "has not had much overall effect. . . . Overall, the effort to control cancer has failed, so far, to attain its objectives."[5]

It was becoming increasingly difficult to ignore the painful contrast between the great hopes that had once been held for chemotherapy and the dismal reality that had thus far come to pass.

Meanwhile, the number of deaths due to cancer was continuing to grow. By the mid-1990s, more than half a million Americans were dying of cancer yearly. The numbers showed a continual and significant increase even after adjusting for the growth and aging of the population.

The breakthroughs that had occurred with chemotherapy were mostly in childhood cancers. And yet by 1997, cancer had become the leading cause of death due to disease among U.S. children.

With cancer rates rising, and attempts to find a cure problematic at best, the need to prevent cancer could not be more urgent.

Focus on Prevention

In 1997, the American Institute for Cancer Research, in collaboration with its international affiliate, the World Cancer Research Fund, issued a major international report, *Food, Nutrition and the Prevention of Cancer: A Global Perspective.*[6] This report analyzed more than 4,500 research studies, and its production involved the participation of more than 120 contributors and peer reviewers, including participants from the World Health Organization, the Food and Agriculture Organization of the United Nations, the International Agency on Research in Cancer, and the U.S. National Cancer Institute. Since its publication, the report has been hailed by scientists around the world and has helped establish a new foundation for research and education efforts related to cancer prevention.

The report finds that 60 to 70 percent of all cancers can be prevented by staying physically active, not smoking, and most important, by following the report's number one dietary recommendation: "Choose predominantly plant-based diets rich in a variety of vegetables and fruits, legumes, and minimally processed starchy staple foods."[7]

The study included a panel of 15 of the world's leading researchers in diet and cancer who reviewed more than 200 case-controlled studies on the link between fruits and vegetables and cancer. An astounding 78 percent of these studies were found to show a statistically protective effect in regard to one or more kinds of cancer. Only 22 percent showed no significant link. None showed an increase of cancer with consumption of these foods.

The report by the World Cancer Research Fund and the American Institute for Cancer Research concludes its analysis of vegetarian diets and cancer by stating simply, "Vegetarian diets decrease the risk of cancer."[8]

T. Colin Campbell, the former Senior Science Advisor to the American Institute for Cancer Research, is outspoken on the diet/disease connection. He says, "The vast majority of all cancers, cardiovascular diseases, and other forms of degenerative illness can be prevented simply by adopting a plant-based diet."

The cattlemen, however, have their own point of view. . .

Is THAT SO?

"The basic reason why heart disease and cancer have become the number one and number two causes of death in the U.S. and other affluent countries is that people are living longer. What has allowed us to live long enough to run these risks? Meat, among other things."

—National Cattlemen's Association[9]

"Now some people scoff at vegetarians, but they have only 40 percent of our cancer rate. They outlive us. On average they outlive other men by about six years now."

—William Castelli, M.D., Director, Framingham Heart Study; National Heart, Lung, and Blood Institute[10]

Researchers have found that the likelihood of a vegetarian reaching the age of 80 is 1.8 times greater than that of the general population—even after adjusting for smoking.[11] And cancer rates for vegetarians are 25 to 50 percent less than those of the general population—even after controlling for smoking, body mass index, and socioeconomic status.[12]

It was in recognition of this that the American Cancer Society, in 1996, released guidelines calling for a reduction in meat intake to lower the risk of cancer. The American Meat Institute responded by saying: "Guidelines go too far when they begin to dictate food choices."[13]

But no one had been proposing dictating food choices. The American Cancer Society was simply telling people what they could do to lower their risk of cancer. The facts are simply the facts. Indeed, a few years later the *British Medical Journal* reiterated, "What is remarkable about the diet-cancer story is the consistency with which certain foods emerge as important in reducing risks across the range of cancers. Millions of cancer cases could be prevented each year if more individuals adopted diets low in meat and high in fruits and vegetables."[14]

When Prevention And Profits Don't Mix

In 1998, the National Cancer Institute announced with much fanfare that a breakthrough in prevention had occurred. A drug that had been used for chemotherapy for two decades, called Tamoxifen, had cut the occurrence of new breast cancer by 45 percent in a group of 13,388 women who were believed to have a high risk for the disease.[15] An excited spokesperson for the FDA said "potentially tens of millions of women" could be candidates for Tamoxifen treatment.[16]

Unfortunately, Tamoxifen may not deserve such acclaim. According to recent data, for every 1,000 women who take the drug for five years, 17 breast cancers are avoided. However, in the same 1,000 women, it causes an additional 12 endometrial (uterine) cancers, and at least 10 potentially fatal blood clots. There are reductions in bone fractures, but there are also increases in strokes and eye cataracts.[17]

Tamoxifen is now being touted as a cancer preventative drug, but critics have pointed out that it's an odd kind of prevention that calls for treating people with toxic drugs year after year.

Zeneca Pharmaceuticals, the company that sells Tamoxifen under the brand name Nolvadex, has mounted an aggressive sales effort on behalf of the drug, widely promoting it as a means of preventing breast cancer. Since Tamoxifen costs more than $1,000 a year, tens of millions of women taking it would mean tens of billions of dollars in annual sales to Zeneca.

You might think Zeneca Pharmaceuticals would know something about breast cancer prevention, for Zeneca is the very company that sponsors the highly publicized annual Breast Cancer Awareness Month. But a closer look reveals something different.

Breast Cancer Awareness Month was launched in 1987 by Zeneca's parent company, Imperial Chemical Industries (ICI). This highly publicized event takes place every October, and is "focused on educating women about early detection of breast cancer"—with a particular focus on mammograms. Its trademark slogan, "Early Detection Is Your Best Prevention," seems convincing at first, but it is actually absurd. By the time a cancer can be detected, it already exists, so it's too late to prevent it. Breast Cancer Awareness Month says it's about prevention, but by focusing so much on mammograms, many people believe it diverts attention away from real prevention.[18]

What are we to make of the almost total absence of concern for real prevention in Breast Cancer Awareness Month? ICI/Zeneca has been the sole financial sponsor of Breast Cancer Awareness Month since the event's beginnings. In return for its investment of many millions of dollars, the corporation has been allowed to approve—or veto—every poster, pamphlet, and advertisement Breast Cancer Awareness Month uses.[19]

The problem is that ICI is one of the world's largest manufacturers of pesticides and plastics, and one of the world's most notorious chemical polluters.[20] Zeneca Pharmaceuticals, the ICI spin-off that now exclusively funds and controls Breast Cancer Awareness Month, earns more than $300 million a year from the sale of a carcinogenic herbicide (acetochlor) while simultaneously marketing Tamoxifen, which has now become the world's bestselling cancer therapy drug.[21]

With so much concern and passion arising about the epidemics of cancer, with women marching to raise money for breast cancer research, with huge campaigns to get women to have mammograms, and with all kinds of people wearing pink ribbons to demonstrate solidarity with the effort, it's sad how little understanding most people actually have of the steps they can take to reduce their risk of cancer. Poignantly, there is not a word in the literature of Breast Cancer Awareness Month to suggest the role diet can play in cancer prevention, nor is there any mention of how to decrease other forms of exposure to carcinogens.

Yet people need to know that the primary route through which many environmental carcinogens enter the human body is through food, and specifically through animal products. If we eat high on the food chain today, we expose ourselves to levels of environmental toxicity that have never before existed on Earth.

There are many environmental factors that can contribute to cancer. The list includes exposure to radiation, pesticides, and xenoestrogens (synthetic chemicals which mimic or block estrogen in the human body), and many others. Much of the damage is caused by "persistent organic pollutants" (POPs), a group of highly toxic, long-lived, bio-accumulative chemicals. The harmful effects of these long-lasting compounds have only begun to be discovered in recent years, because they can emerge years (and sometimes generations) after exposure.

> "Scientists are only now discovering that many of these chemicals cause irreversible damage in people and animals at levels that were dismissed as inconsequential by the experts less than a decade ago. The catalog of the destructive effects of POPs is long and growing, from cancer and reproductive health effects to learning disorders and reduced immunity. People receive about 90 percent of their total intake of these compounds from foods of animal origin. Something as common as a McDonald's Big Mac carries 30 percent of the World Health Organization's recommendation for daily dioxin intake." (Worldwatch Institute, 2000)[22]

Dioxin is an extraordinarily carcinogenic and perilous threat to the health and biological integrity of human beings and the environment. A prestigious group of German scientists concluded in 1998 that dioxin may be responsible for 12 percent of human cancers in industrialized societies.[23] Dr. Diane Courtney, head of the Toxic Effects Branch of the EPA's National Environmental Research Center, told Congress that "dioxin is by far the most toxic chemical known to mankind."[24] Dioxin is obviously not a substance you'd want on your plate. Yet the EPA says that up to 95 percent of human dioxin exposure comes from red meat, fish, and dairy products.[25]

As if to prove the point, in June 1998, *Consumer Reports* published test results that found alarming levels of dioxin in the meat-based baby foods sold by all the major baby food brands.[26]

So great is the contamination of animal products today with dioxin that even those meat and dairy companies that are trying to offer healthier products find it nearly impossible today to provide pure foods. Ben & Jerry's, for example, seeks to be environmentally aware and to use milk from family farms. The company's promotional literature and Web site states that "dioxin is known to cause cancer, genetic and reproductive defects and learning disabilities. . . . The only safe level of dioxin exposure is no exposure at all."

Yet so pervasive is dioxin in dairy, meat, and fish products today that in November 1999, a level of dioxin 200 times greater than the "virtually safe (daily) dose" determined by the EPA was found in Ben & Jerry's Vanilla Ice Cream.[27] In fact, a study presented at the "Dioxins 2000" conference in August 2000, found "levels of dioxin in a sample serving of Ben & Jerry's brand ice cream are approximately 2,200 times greater than the level of dioxin allowed in a 'serving' of wastewater discharged into San Francisco Bay from the Tosco Refinery."[28]

In view of findings like this, there is one question the meat, dairy, and chemical companies do not want people to ask. It is a question, however, that I find important. How much less cancer and suffering would there be if people were spreading information about true prevention with the same passion and zeal with which they are telling women to get mammograms and raising money for chemotherapy research?

Breast Cancer

The incidence of breast cancer in the United States began climbing steadily in the early 1970s, and is now the highest ever seen in human history. Nearly 50,000 American women die of the disease every year. In the face of this tragedy, a great deal of attention has been given to genetics, but the presence of the breast cancer susceptibility gene, called BRCA-1, only accounts for at most 5 percent of breast cancers.

Exercise is very important to breast cancer risk. In fact, women who exercise (walk) for four hours per week lower their risk by 33 percent. And women who exercise more than that lower their risk even further.[29]

But diet, it turns out, is even more important. . .

What we know

Death rate from breast cancer in the United States: 22.4 (per 100,000)

Death rate from breast cancer in Japan: 6.3 (per 100,000)

Death rate from breast cancer in China: 4.6 (per 100,000)

Primary reasons for difference: People in China and Japan eat more fruits and vegetables and less animal products, weigh less, drink less alcohol, and get more exercise than people in the United States.

Breast cancer rate for women in Italy who eat a lot of animal products compared to women in Italy who don't: 3 times greater[30]

Breast cancer rate for women in Uruguay who eat meat often compared to women in Uruguay who rarely or never eat meat: 4.2 times greater[31]

Breast cancer rate for affluent Japanese women who eat meat daily compared to poorer Japanese women who rarely or never eat meat: 8.5 times greater[32]

Impact on breast cancer risk for adult women who are 45 pounds overweight: Double[33]

American women who are aware that there are any dietary steps they can take to lower their chances of developing breast cancer: 23 percent[34]

American women with less than high school educations who are aware that there are any dietary steps they can take to lower their risk of developing breast cancer: 3 percent[35]

American women who believe that mammograms prevent breast cancer: 37 percent[36]

Lung Cancer

I have a good friend, Patrick Reynolds, who is the grandson of R. J. Reynolds of tobacco and aluminum fortune and fame. Patrick's grandfather died of emphysema and his father died of lung cancer, no doubt from smoking the family product. Patrick upset many in his family when he decided not only to sell all his tobacco stocks, but to speak out in congressional hearings about the dangers of tobacco and to mount an anti-smoking campaign.

We've done many TV shows together. They call us "rebels with a cause."

Once, a TV anchor asked Patrick whether he felt guilty about the enormous amount of damage his family's tobacco products had caused to the health of millions. He was quick to respond: "No, I throw guilt out the window! I'm here to change things now!"

I'm glad Patrick "throws guilt out the window." Feeling guilty wouldn't do a thing to help matters. But taking action, such as he has done, makes a difference.

Taking your power is not about guilt. It's about the privilege of responsibility. It's about living what you've woken up to, making your life congruent with the visions you have had of how best to live. It's not about feeling bad about the past. It's about creating a positive future.

I have no desire to look down on people who still smoke. I don't want to make their lives any more difficult. That wouldn't help a thing. And I have no interest in judging or criticizing people who still eat meat with every meal. No one needs that, no one wants that, no one is helped by that.

And yet being respectful of another's path doesn't mean colluding with that person in patterns to which we are opposed. It means honoring the heart of those with whom we differ. We don't have to understand or agree with other people's decisions in order to respect and uphold the worthiness of their lives.

I don't always find it easy to love people when they make choices I disagree with, but I know it's incredibly important to do so. And it's also important to me to provide people with clear and accurate information from which to make their choices. My role is to support people in understanding and clarifying their choices using reliable information. I have far too much respect for the vastness and mystery of the human journey to attempt to make anyone's choices for them. My prayer, and that of many, is that we all have the courage to change the things we can, the serenity to accept the things we can't, and the wisdom to know the difference.

WHAT WE KNOW

Most common cause of cancer mortality worldwide: Lung cancer

Number of lives lost to lung cancer each year in the United States: 150,000

Impact of smoking on lung cancer incidence: So overwhelming that even people exposed to secondhand smoke are at heightened risk

Impact on risk of lung cancer for people who frequently eat green, orange, and yellow vegetables: 20–60 percent reduction[37]

The vegetable with the strongest protective effect: Carrot[38]

Impact on risk of lung cancer among people who consume a lot of apples, bananas, and grapes: 40 percent reduction[39]

Rate of lung cancer in British vegetarian men compared to the general British population: 27 percent[40]

Rate of lung cancer in British vegetarian women compared to the general British population: 37 percent[41]

Rate of lung cancer in German vegetarian men compared to the general German population: 8 percent[42]

As you might imagine, the meat and dairy industries are not entirely pleased with what is being learned about diet and cancer rates. They may not have science on their side, but that hasn't stopped them from spending millions of dollars a day to broadcast their opinions, influence what we think, feel, and do, and maintain their control over U.S. food policies.

These industries, of course, have a right to express their points of view. But the more I listen to them, the more I'm reminded of the old adage: "Never ask a barber whether you need a haircut."

Is THAT SO?

"Reported links between diet and cancer have been mostly hypothetical. . . . No single dietary factor, including fat or meat, could possibly account for more than a small fraction of cancer in the U.S."

—National Cattlemen's Association[43]

"A low-fat plant-based diet would not only lower the heart attack rate about 85 percent, but would lower the cancer rate 60 percent."

—William Castelli, M.D., Director, Framingham Health Study; National Heart, Lung, and Blood Institute

Prostate Cancer

The year 2000 was an eventful one for New York City Mayor Rudolph Giuliani. He began the year running for senator against Hillary Clinton, but withdrew when he learned that he had prostate cancer. His marital problems became front-page news. And satirical anti-dairy billboards appeared portraying him with a milk mustache, asking, "Got Prostate Cancer?"

The mayor denied there was any connection between his cancer and his consumption of dairy products, and even kept a glass of milk by his side during public events arising from the controversy.

No one likes to think they have brought their misfortunes upon themselves. And it's true; we don't know with certainty what the connection might be between Guiliani's eating habits and his illness. It's rarely possible to unravel the past and determine with certainty what caused a particular disease. In addition to diet, there are so many other influences, including upbringing, genetics, and exposure to toxic chemicals. The list is long. But just as the data indicate a strong connection between consumption of animal fat, high blood pressure, and stroke, so too does the evidence suggest stunning correlations between dairy consumption and prostate cancer.

WHAT WE KNOW

Most common cancer among American men: Prostate cancer

Risk of prostate cancer for men who consume high amounts of dairy products: 70 percent increase[44]

Risk of prostate cancer for men who consume soy milk daily: 70 percent reduction[45]

Risk of prostate cancer for men with low blood levels of beta-carotene: 45 percent increase[46]

Best sources of beta-carotene: Carrots, sweet potatoes, yams

Risk of prostate cancer for men whose diet is abundant with lycopene-rich foods: 45 percent reduction[47]

Best sources of lycopene: Tomatoes

Amount of beta-carotene and lycopene in meats, dairy products, and eggs: None

Risk of prostate cancer for men whose intake of cruciferous vegetables (broccoli, Brussels sprouts, cabbage, cauliflower, collards, kale, mustard greens, and turnips) is high: 41 percent reduction[48]

American men who are aware of a link between animal products and prostate cancer: 2 percent[49]

We may not be able to pin down the causes of a particular case of cancer. But there is one thing we can predict with near certainty. The meat and dairy industries will continue to resist the medical research that finds correlations between consumption of their products and cancer rates.

That's what they've done in the past, and that's what they will continue to do. No one wants to be accused of contributing to a disease that is causing such an enormous amount of suffering. And of course, they have their profits to protect. But if we are to learn from this suffering and take the steps necessary to lessen or prevent it, to whom should we listen, the meat industry or independent researchers?

Is THAT SO?

"[It's a] myth [that] beef contributes to cancer."
—National Cattlemen's Beef Association[50]

"If you step back and look at the data [on beef and cancer], the optimum amount of red meat you eat should be zero."
—Walter Willett, M.D., Chairman of the Nutrition Department, Harvard School of Public Health, and director of a study of 88,000 American nurses that analyzed the link between diet and colon cancer[51]

Colon Cancer

The colon is another name for the large intestine, the lower half of the digestive tract. Obviously, the food you eat has a great impact on the health of your colon. Of all forms of cancer, colon cancer may be the most strongly linked to diet.

WHAT WE KNOW

Number of lives lost to colon cancer each year in the United States: 55,000

Risk of colon cancer for women who eat red meat daily compared to those who eat it less than once a month: 250 percent greater[52]

Risk of colon cancer for people who eat red meat once a week compared to those who abstain: 38 percent greater[53]

Risk of colon cancer for people who eat poultry once a week compared to those who abstain: 55 percent greater[54]

Risk of colon cancer for people who eat poultry four times a week compared to those who abstain: 200–300 percent greater[55]

Risk of colon cancer for people who eat beans, peas, or lentils at least twice a week compared to people who avoid these foods: 50 percent lower[56]

Impact on risk for colon cancer when diets are rich in the B-vitamin folic acid: 75 percent lower

Primary food sources of folic acid: Dark green leafy vegetables, beans, and peas

---

Ratio of colon cancer rates for white South Africans compared to black South Africans: 17 to 1[57]

Explanation for this vast discrepancy (according to the *American Journal of Gastroenterology*): South African blacks are protected from colon cancer by the absence of animal fat and animal protein, and by the resulting differences in bacterial fermentation[58]

Americans who are aware that eating less meat reduces colon cancer risk: 2 percent[59]

What We Hear

Fortunately, there are some voices within the meat industry who face the facts. They speak with regret about the associations between meat consumption and cancer, but they acknowledge them. Peter R. Cheeke, professor of animal science at Oregon State University and the author of the textbook, *Contemporary Issues in Animal Agriculture*, writes,

> "Rates of colorectal cancer in various countries are strongly correlated with per capita consumption of red meat and animal fat, and inversely associated with fiber consumption. Even the most dedicated Animal Scientist or meat supporter must be somewhat dismayed by the preponderance of evidence suggesting a role of meat consumption in the etiology of colon cancer."[60]

But voices like Cheeke's are rarely the ones the American public hears. You and I and the rest of the country are still bombarded with the prevailing viewpoints of the meat and dairy industry. They speak to us in billboards, TV ads, magazine ads, newspaper ads. They flood our daily papers with op-ed pieces and "news" articles, and in a thousand other ways use their money and the sophistication of their public relations companies to keep us hooked on their products.

You have to give them credit. They have not always been able to avoid stumbling over the truth, but they always seem to manage to pick themselves up and carry on as if nothing had happened.

Is THAT SO?

"The associations between cancer and meat-eating are overblown. Genetics are more important than diet."

—*The Beef-Eaters Guide to Modern Meat*[61]

"Five to ten percent of all cancers are caused by inherited genetic mutations. By contrast, 70 to 80 percent have been linked to [diet and other] behavioral factors."

—Karen Emmons, M.D., Dana-Farber Cancer Institute, Boston[62]

_____

"If a person accepts the theory that a low-fat diet will help prevent cancer, beef should probably be in that person's diet, because modern beef is lower in fat and calories."

—National Cattlemen's Association[63]

"The beef industry has contributed to more deaths than all the wars of this century, all natural disasters, and all automobile accidents combined. If beef is your idea of 'real food for real people,' you'd better live real close to a real good hospital."

—Neal Barnard, M.D., President, Physicians Committee for Responsible Medicine

My Friend Mike

My commitment not to judge the food choices of others was sorely tested when a friend of mine came down with colon cancer. Not that my relationship with Mike had ever been particularly easy. He could be, to be perfectly frank, a bit of a pain. When we would go out to eat, he would always, knowing full well that I was a vegetarian and had written on the subject, ask me whether I felt more like a steak or a hamburger. He always made a point of telling me during the meal how fabulous his meat or ice cream tasted, and made a display of offering to share it with me, all the while acting as if his doing so was motivated entirely by affection and generous concern for my well-being.

It wasn't only at restaurants that this kind of thing went on. When he would outrace me in the long distance runs we sometimes took together, he would announce triumphantly that his prowess was entirely due to the bacon he had eaten that morning. He did this, I am sure, even on those days when his breakfast had been granola.

But I was not about to let him get my goat. I'd just smile, and inwardly vow that next time I would win. Not that I ever did. He had been a champion cross-country runner in high school, and was naturally gifted. I, on the other hand—well, let's just say I tried hard.

Still, I worried about him. Perhaps because things physical had always come easy to Mike, he seemed to take his health for granted. Aside from our runs, he didn't exercise much, and as time passed, and he gained quite a bit of weight, he became less and less interested in running and eventually stopped altogether. I told him it was obvious that he was terrified of losing to me and simply wanted to avoid the inevitable. His reply wasn't particularly subtle. "My ass, Mr. Bean-sprouts-for-breakfast. You couldn't beat me if I had to hop on one leg." Of course he was wrong. I've never once eaten bean sprouts for breakfast.

Once I spoke to him about *ahimsa*, the practice of nonviolence, the practice of living with compassion for all creatures. "That sounds great," he answered. "I'm into ahimsa, ahimsa for myself. I'm not going to do violence to myself by denying myself a nice thick slice of roast beef. Want to join me?"

"No, thanks," I answered, softly. I didn't say any more. I didn't feel like arguing with him. I didn't want to create any more separation. I thought he was creating quite enough all by himself.

"No problem," he responded. "But don't forget that plants have consciousness, too." He pointed to my salad. "You're murdering those poor lettuce leaves."

On another occasion I told him that I was concerned about his health. "I don't want to see you get sick." I mentioned that people who ate the way he did very often developed chronic diseases like cancer.

"Maybe," he answered. "But I've been to the health food store. The people there are all skinny and sickly. If it's in the cards, that's what's going to happen."

When Mike gained ever more weight and stopped exercising entirely, his wife Carol became concerned. "He isn't happy in his work," she told me, "and he's becoming increasingly irritable and short-tempered. What's worse, he doesn't talk to me anymore about what he's feeling, and spends all his free time on his computer."

We were seeing each other less and less, until one day Mike called, and said he needed to talk to me. Could I come over? My first thought was I had better things to do, but there was something in his voice that seemed somehow different. I said Yes, I'd be right over.

When I arrived, the atmosphere in their house was heavy and dark. Mike had been to the doctor, he and his wife told me, and had been diagnosed with a very serious form of colon cancer—Dukes' D, it's called, which means the cancer has already spread quite widely through the body. The prognosis with Dukes' D is terrible. The five-year survival rate is about 5 percent, at best maybe 20 percent if liver metastases can be surgically removed.

They were scared. I listened, and my heart felt sick. Oh Mike, I thought, Oh Mike! Why didn't you listen? Didn't I tell you? Outwardly, I tried to listen and be supportive, but inside I was angry and hurt. Angry at Mike for not taking better care of himself, angry at God for letting this happen, and angry at myself for not having been able to prevent it.

I listened as attentively as I could, and asked a few questions. They talked about his treatment options, and about the financial pressures they were dealing with. Not a word about diet. I stayed for dinner. Mike had a thick slab of beef. At least this time he didn't offer me any. The truth, though, is that night, for the first time ever, I was wishing he would. Not that I'd have taken it. I just wanted him to be his old, stupid, teasing self. He might have been a jerk, but we were buddies, pals, compadres, friends. Oh, Mike.

I was hurting and I was in denial. I didn't want to face what was happening. I wanted the old Mike back, even if he was a jerk.

In the weeks that followed, Mike underwent surgery and, then chemotherapy. He was having a terribly hard time with nausea, abdominal pain, vomiting, diarrhea, and a host of other kinds of distress, but he and Carol pinned their hopes for a cure on the drugs. They made it clear that they didn't want to discuss alternative treatments.

It was hard for me not to be judgmental. When Mike complained about how helpless he felt, I tried to be understanding and to help him make intelligent and grounded choices, but inside I was thinking, "Why didn't you think about that before? What do you expect when you eat the way you have?" He said he was at last cleaning up his diet, but I wasn't convinced. He was still going to McDonald's and Burger King.

Mike's last days weren't pleasant or comfortable. But there was one thing that happened that, now when I look back on that time, stands out for me. I don't want to make too much of this, but to me it feels important.

One of the last times I saw him, Mike said to me, "Thank you for not pushing your trip on me. I hate vegetables, that's all there is to it."

"You can say that, but honestly, Mike, I feel bad that I wasn't more assertive. Maybe it would have done some good."

"No, it wouldn't have. I was set in my ways. I've always been set in my ways. I wouldn't have listened." He paused, and reached for my hand. "I felt your love, John. I always felt your love. Do you know what that's meant?"

"No."

"More than you'll ever know, carrot brain."

I can't remember the rest of the conversation. I was weeping too hard.

chapter 4

The Great American Diet Roller Coaster

Not too long after my book *Diet for a New America* came out, in the days before Rush Limbaugh and Dr. Laura became famous, I got a call from a man representing a radio show. He told me he worked for the Tom Leykis show, out of Los Angeles, and they would like me to come on as his guest. That's very nice, I thought, but I don't want to go to Los Angeles. The air's bad, the traffic's terrible, and the city's obsessed with image and glitz.

Before I had a chance to speak, though, he proceeded to tell me that Tom had the largest listening audience of any talk show in the country. Suddenly I remembered that I'd wanted to go to Los Angeles for a long time. Such a fabulous city. So full of life and vitality. People there are great; they don't get hung up being serious and deep; they know how to have fun.

We proceeded to make the arrangements. I was told that Tom wanted me in the studio early, because he wanted to spend time with me personally before we went on air. I was also told that this never happened, that every author in the country wanted to be on his show but he almost never had guests.

I had never heard of the show. I didn't know that Tom Leykis was not only the most popular talk show host in the country at that time, but also the most controversial, known far and wide for being sexist, abrasive, and, whenever he felt like it, downright obnoxious. When he didn't like a statement made by the singer Cat Stevens, he made a large pile of Cat Stevens' recordings, rented a tractor, and, on air, drove over them.

He was, however, very nice to me. In fact, he treated me with great respect. The people on his staff just stared in disbelief. They told me they had never, ever, seen him treat anybody like that before.

It turns out that he had been talking to Casey Kasem, the famous Top 40 DJ, and Casey had told Tom that he just had to read my book and had given him a copy. Tom said this impressed him. Given who Tom was, and the fact that he had the ability to generate huge publicity for books, everyone was always telling him about *their* books, *their* schtick, trying to get him to promote *their* work. But here was Casey, not trying to use Tom to advance his own career, talking not about his own books, but about mine. Tom liked that.

Before reading *Diet for a New America*, Tom told me and his listening audience, he thought nothing of having a 24-ounce steak for lunch. After reading it, he decided he would no longer eat anything that came from something that had a face. It was that simple. He told his audience that following that decision and as a direct result of reading my book and heeding its advice, he had lost 70 pounds.

Within a few days after the show, I received more than a thousand letters from people who wanted copies of my book and who wanted to lose weight. And overall, I've since received more than 10,000 letters from people telling me about the excess weight they have lost after reading my books. A relative of mine who likes to play with numbers tells me that this leads him to certain conclusions. Taking into account that for each of those letters there are undoubtedly others who have had similar experiences but didn't write me, he says I must be responsible for the loss of several thousand tons of excess fat from the bodies of my readers.

The truth, however, is that my work has never been primarily oriented toward weight loss. It's about healthy, compassionate, and conscious eating. But it is certainly true that it also leads, for many people who have been carrying too much weight, to the weight loss they have been wanting, often, for years.

I objected when my publisher wanted to give my first book the title *Diet for a New America*, because I didn't particularly like the word *diet*.

It brought to my mind images of austerity, restriction, and deprivation, and then, like clockwork, the inevitable backlash, the bingeing and gorging, and the gaining back of every pound that had been lost, if not more. It made me think of the $30 billion weight loss industry, and how predictable it is that people who lose weight on these programs soon thereafter gain it back.

As well, the word *diet* reminds me how cruel our society can be to people, particularly females, whose bodies don't fit the cultural ideal.

We are deluged with messages on TV, in movies, magazines, and in all kinds of advertisements, telling us that in order to be attractive and be loved, a woman has to be thin. This is a great way to make women dissatisfied with themselves. If you wanted to produce negative body images and eating disorders, could you think of a better way than to create a show like *BayWatch*? How many girls and women can compare themselves to this cultural beauty standard and feel good about themselves and their bodies? How many are that thin? It enrages me that our media makes many girls and women feel like the most important thing in life is the size bathing suit they wear.

So I had a real aversion to the word *diet*. Not that it mattered to my publisher. They titled the book what they thought would sell. And diet books, they told me, sell. They made the title choice, and *Diet for a New America* it was.

Thus I became a "diet" book author. It wasn't so bad. I'm sure it was less than 17 million times that I had to answer interviewers who, knowing only the title of my book, asked me to explain the meaning of my patriotic weight loss program.

The reality, though, is that I don't teach a step-by-step, follow-the-rules program to lose weight. I'm not particularly interested in obsessive attempts to trim pounds. What I propose is the development of a healthy and wholesome relationship to your body and to food, so that unhealthy weight naturally drops off on its own.

That's important, and not just for cosmetic reasons. Let's put issues of appearance aside for a moment. There are very real health reasons not to be overweight. The number of Americans who die prematurely each year as a result of being overweight is nearing the number who die prematurely from cigarette smoking. But there is a difference. The number of cigarettes smoked per person in the United States is on the decline, while obesity is on the rise. It is apparently only a matter of time until deaths from obesity-related illnesses exceed those related to smoking.[1]

WHAT WE KNOW

Americans killed annually by diseases due to excess weight: 280,000[2]

Increased risk of heart disease for obese people: Double to triple[3]

Increased risk of gallstones for obese people: Double to triple[4]

Increased risk of colon cancer for obese people: Triple to quadruple[5]

Increased risk of diabetes for very obese people: 40 times greater[6]

Obesity rate among the general U.S. population: 18 percent[7]

Obesity rate among vegetarians: 6 percent[8]

Obesity rate among vegans: 2 percent[9]

Average weight of vegan adults compared to non-vegetarian adults: 10–20 pounds lighter[10]

U.S. children who are overweight or obese: 25 percent[11]

U.S. vegetarian children who are overweight or obese: 8 percent[12]

U.S. children who eat the recommended levels of fruits, vegetables, and grains: 1 percent[13]

U.S. vegan children who eat the recommended levels of fruits, vegetables, and grains: 50 percent[14]

Fat in a single foil-packaged restaurant serving of butter: 6 grams[15]

Fat in a Burger King Whopper: 40 grams[16]

Fat in a Double Whopper with cheese: 67 grams[17]

Fat in the average veggie burger found in U.S. supermarkets and natural food stores: 3 grams[18]

The relative slimness of vegetarians was brought home to me recently when I spoke to a prominent liposuction surgeon. Liposuction—the surgical removal of fat—is the leading form of cosmetic surgery in the United States today. In fact, more than 1,000 liposuction operations are performed per day in this country.[19] Scott Jones, M.D., has specialized in this type of surgery for many years. He told me, "I perform liposuction procedures on patients daily, and have done so for many years. In the process, I always discuss diet with my patients. In all this time, I don't know that I've ever operated on a vegetarian."

Weight Loss Programs

On any given day, a huge number of Americans are on diets, diligently trying to control what they eat in order to lose weight. Author Geneen Roth, who has helped many people deal consciously and compassionately with weight issues, describes her experience:

"When I was in college, I went on a diet a friend told me about: nothing but fried chicken for breakfast, lunch, and dinner. It seemed like an unusual way to lose weight, but it sounded reasonable as well as delicious, because I had heard of the 'mono-food' theory as a way of reducing. According to this approach, if you ate only one food, no matter what it was—ice cream, fudge, potato chips, bananas—you'd lose weight. My boyfriend Lee, who was not fat but loved me very much, accompanied me on my daily search for restaurants that served fried chicken for breakfast. Lunch and dinner were easier. When I was five days into the diet, three pounds heavier and nauseated by the sight of anything that could have come from a chicken, the same friend who had told me about the diet came back with some unhappy news: she had gotten the story wrong. On the diet she had read about, fried chicken was the only thing you couldn't eat. 'So sorry,' she said. 'I hope I didn't add to your problem.'

"Every week, from ten to twenty-five women call me with similar stories. Each session of the workshops I lead is filled to capacity with people who have tried every procedure ever advanced for losing weight and are still uncomfortable with their bodies. Food is the pivot around which their lives revolve. All of them describe themselves as fat, no matter what their body weight. All of them dislike their bodies.

"They are not unusual."[20]

People who don't feel good about their bodies are easy prey for those who hawk the latest diet fad. Sadly, there have been many self-described experts who have authored books that have sold millions, despite having little or no legitimate scientific basis.

My criticism is not of people who try these diets in hope of losing weight. My argument is not with people who try these diets desiring to become more attractive. Nor is it with people who try these diets in hope of feeling better, or wanting to become healthier. In fact, I have great appreciation for people who have the courage to try new things and eat in new ways in order to see how their bodies respond and how they feel.

My complaint is not even with those people who are the authors of fad diet books. I have met many of them, and I am sure that most of them genuinely believe in what they are doing. But the fact that they are sincere and well meaning doesn't mean their diets have merit. It is helpful now and again to remember that the damage done by sincere and well-meaning zealots throughout history is considerable.

My quarrel is with diet regimens that have only their authors' belief in and opinions about them, but no sound science to back them up. My criticism is with diet regimens that provide seeming short-term benefits but do so with profound negative long-term health consequences. My problem is with fad diets that make great promises, and end up causing great harm.

Fad diets typically promise a "quick fix," or to "melt fat in just two weeks." They ignore the reality that sustained health comes from making gradual, long-term, balanced adjustments to diet and overall lifestyle. Fad diets distract people from the discipline and joy of creating a genuinely healthy and empowering way of eating.

Many high-fat, high-protein, low-carbohydrate diets have come and gone from the American scene in the last few decades. Some have been very popular. Most of them have cost their adherents dearly in long-term health impacts. Their names include Dr. Atkins' New Diet Revolution, the Beverly Hills Diet, Protein Power, the Carbohydrate Addict's Diet, the Scarsdale Diet, Charles Hunt's Diet Evolution, and the Quick Weight-Loss Diet.

These diets have several things in common. None is advertised as a low-calorie diet, and yet that is what all of them turn out to be. They all prescribe a daily caloric intake that is well below average requirements.

As a result, they may seem to work in the short run, but they do not sustain long-term health. Most of these diets are deficient in major nutrients, such as dietary fiber and carbohydrates, as well as in specific vitamins, minerals, and protective phytochemicals. Further, they put the body on a low-calorie diet roller coaster. When the body is starved for calories, it loses weight, but it also goes into survival mode—slowing metabolism and burning fewer calories. When normal caloric intake is resumed, rapid weight gain almost always results.

Countless organizations are opposed to high-protein, high-fat, low-carbohydrate diets, including the World Health Organization, the American Heart Association, the American Cancer Society, the American Dietetic Association, the office of the Surgeon General of the United States, and the American Institute for Cancer Research.

Noting that these diets increase the risk of constipation and other gastrointestinal difficulties, heart disease, kidney diseases, osteoporosis, and some forms of cancer, the American Dietetic Association describes them as "a nightmare."[21]

Dr. Atkins' Diet—Good Advice or Carbo Phobia?

On the cover of *Dr. Robert Atkins' New Diet Revolution,* we are told that with this "amazing weight-loss plan" you can "enjoy a cheeseburger when you're hungry." We are told "eating rich foods can be your path to weight-loss." We are told you will "see amazing results in 14 days." And we are told there are more than 6 million copies in print.[22]

This is the classic profile of a fad diet scam. Promise people they can eat whatever they want, tell them this is a new and amazing revolution, promise them that it won't take any effort, tell them the results will be nearly instantaneous, and make sure they think that everybody else is doing it. Who could resist such hype?

If only it were true.

In actuality, the primary mechanisms by which the Atkins diet causes weight loss are caloric restriction and ketosis. *Ketosis* occurs when there is an imbalance in fat metabolism, such as occurs in diabetes or starvation. In ketosis, the body begins to metabolize muscle tissue instead of fat. Authors of these diets advocate "taking advantage" of ketosis to lose weight.

Dr. Atkins bases his entire program on ketosis. He says, "Ketosis is an indicator used at the Atkins Center as a marker for whether a person is staying on the diet. . . . The Atkins diet is a lifelong nutritional philosophy. . . . The important thing is you are in ketosis."[23]

He doesn't say, however, that the consequences of extended ketosis include muscle breakdown, nausea, dehydration, headaches, light-headedness, irritability, bad breath, kidney problems, and increased risk of heart disease.[24] Nor does he mention that a potential consequence of extended ketosis in pregnancy is fetal abnormality or death. Nor that a danger of extended ketosis for diabetics is death.

When the prestigious American Institute for Cancer Research evaluated Atkins' diet, they didn't mince words. "Atkins' diet," they wrote, "can lead to the kind of rapid weight fluctuations that adversely affect the heart. Moreover, the breakdown of fatty acids that occurs during ketosis may also increase the risk of heart disease. One of the basic tenets of Atkins' diet is that sugar causes cancer. Such misleading pronouncements are essentially scare tactics, meant to direct the dieter towards foods on the Atkins plan. Finally, nothing about this plan encourages the dieter to learn some very basic weight management strategies like portion control and serving sizes, let alone develop the skills necessary for a lifetime of balanced nutrition."[25]

What we know

Atkins and other advocates of high-protein, high-fat, low-carbohydrate diets claim: All high glycemic index carbohydrates (like bread and potatoes) produce heightened blood sugar levels and insulin response, and should not be eaten.

Scientific reality: Any harmful effect of high glycemic index carbohydrates is reduced by eating them together with low glycemic index foods[26]

Atkins and other advocates of high-protein, high-fat, low-carbohydrate diets claim: High insulin levels are to blame for hypertension, heart disease, and just about every other health problem people can experience, including weight gain and obesity

Scientific reality: Being obese causes high insulin levels, not the other way around[27]

Atkins and other advocates of high-protein, high-fat, low-carbohydrate diets claim: For people with insulin resistance, eating carbohydrates will raise insulin levels, causing weight gain and heart disease

Scientific reality (published in the *American Journal of Cardiology*): Among people with insulin resistance, three weeks on a high-complex carbohydrate diet, along with exercise, reduced insulin levels by 30 percent. Additional benefits included a 4 percent decrease in weight, and more than 20 percent reductions in cholesterol and triglycerides, indicating greatly reduced heart disease risk[28]

Atkins and other advocates of high-protein, high-fat, low-carbohydrate diets claim: High-protein diets improve all aspects of our lives

Scientific reality (published in the *International Journal of Obesity Related Metabolic Disorders*): High-protein diets impair mental functioning[29]

Atkins says, "My diet will correct most of the risk factors for heart disease."[30] But a study published in the *Journal of the American Dietetic Association* found quite the opposite. People who followed the Atkins diet for 12 weeks showed significant increases in LDL ("bad" cholesterol), and substantial reductions in HDL ("good" cholesterol), indicating markedly increased risk for heart attacks.[31]

For 30 years, Atkins has been claiming his diet reverses heart disease. During that entire time, not a single study has been published that substantiates his claim.

In fact, in all these years Atkins has never published a single study in any medical journal. He has, however, funded one study. Unfortunately, the study found that on the Atkins diet, 70 percent of people become constipated, and 65 percent develop bad breath.[32]

Two foods that appear regularly in Atkins' recipes and recommendations are pork rinds and sausage. Dean Ornish, M.D., is Professor of

Medicine at the University of California, San Francisco, and founder and president of the Preventive Medicine Research Institute. The physician who developed an astoundingly successful heart disease prevention and treatment program, he is appalled by Atkins' promises that such foods will help people's hearts. "Telling people that pork rinds and sausage are good for you is an appealing way to sell books," he says, "but it's irresponsible and it's dangerous for people who follow this advice."[33]

Other foods that are encouraged on the Atkins diet are bacon, pork, steak, seafood, eggs, butter, cream, and artificial sweeteners. As Atkins says, "The Atkins Diet is heavily weighted on eggs, meat, chicken and fish." A typical Atkins breakfast is a cheese/broccoli omelet, with bacon and/or sausage.

People who don't want to alter the eating habits that are endangering their health flock to regimens like this. But the scientific reality, published in thousands of peer-reviewed medical journal articles, is clear. The foods on which the Atkins diet is based are the very foods that contribute to our most common causes of disease, disability, and death.

People do often lose weight on the Atkins diet, at least for a while. But they do so at great cost to themselves and to their long-term health. James Anderson, M.D., is Professor of Medicine and Clinical Nutrition at the University of Kentucky School of Medicine. He has studied the Atkins Diet, and his evaluation is forthright:

"People lose weight, at least in the short term. But this is absolutely the worst diet you could imagine for long-term obesity, heart disease, and some forms of cancer. If you wanted to find one diet to ruin your health, you couldn't find one worse than Atkins. We have 18 million diabetics in this country, 50 million people with high blood pressure. They can have kidney problems, and high protein intake will bring them on faster. The diet is thrombogenic, meaning the fat will tend to form lipid particles in your blood after meals, which could lead to blood clots, meaning heart attack or stroke. We worry about this, because many of the people who love these diets are men aged 40 to 50, who like their meat. They may be 5 years from their first heart attack. This couldn't be worse for them. Did you know that for 50 percent of men who die from heart attacks, the fatal attack is their first symptom? They will never know what this diet is doing to them."[34]

In 2000, doctors at the Bassett Research Institute in Cooperstown, New York, published a study on the Atkins diet and weight loss. They found that when people lose weight on the Atkins diet, it is only because they are consuming fewer calories. In fact, in the Atkins ongoing weight-loss phase, dieters eat an average of only 1,500 calories a day, and even less during its more restrictive phases. The study's lead author, Dr. Bernard Miller, said patients felt tired and were nauseated on the plan. Allan Green, director of the Institute, noted, "Weight loss is still calories in and calories out. . . . We're not recommending this diet to anyone."[35]

Dean Ornish's opinion of the weight-loss results of Atkins' diet is equally direct: "You can lose weight in lots of ways that aren't healthy. You can take chemotherapy or get cancer or AIDS or be an alcoholic and lose weight. . . . The problem with high animal protein diets is that even if you can lose weight, you're mortgaging your health in the process."[36]

There's a strange irony to the Atkins story. Atkins said in 2000 that he had been on his own diet for 36 years.[37]

Yet Dr. Atkins himself is so overweight that he exceeds the upper limits of weight recommended by federal guidelines.[38]

Entering the Zone—An Honest Look

Barry Sears' *Enter the Zone* is another bestselling book that advocates a high-protein and relatively high-fat diet.[39] It is not nearly as extreme as Atkins' regimen, and seems comparatively sane. But like Atkins' diet, it is seriously flawed.

Sears claims that our epidemic of obesity stems from the advice of health experts to eat less fat. He writes,

> "The message, from top scientists, nutritionists and the government, was simple. Americans were told to eat less fat and more carbohydrates. . . . We're now 15 years into the experiment, and one doesn't have to be a rocket scientist to see it isn't working. . . . The country has experienced an epidemic rise in obesity. . . . People are eating less fat and getting fatter."[40]

The reality, however, is a little different. Yes, there has been a dramatic rise in obesity. And yes, nutrition authorities have been telling people to eat less fat. But despite the urgings of health experts, the percentage of calories eaten as fat by the average American has barely changed in the past 15 years. The reason there has been a huge rise in obesity and overweight problems is that we are eating (on average) several hundred more calories per day and exercising less than we were in the mid-1980s.[41]

Sears repeatedly says that Americans are eating far less fat than ever. But according to the USDA, since 1989 American's daily fat intake has actually risen from 89 grams to 101 grams for men, and from 62 grams to 65 grams for women.[42]

Like Atkins, Sears promises that if you follow his diet, you will achieve permanent weight loss, increased energy, and improved health—all without restricting calories.[43] The reality, however, is that the Zone diet's weight-loss phase typically supplies only 1,200–1,600 daily calories, far less than even a 100-pound woman needs for daily maintenance.

Is that so?

"This is not a calorie deprivation program."

—Barry Sears[44]

"It's painfully clear, in spite of Sears statements to the contrary, that the foundation of the Zone is extreme calorie restriction. In the short term, such a very low calorie diet will indeed lead to weight loss, but most of it is water loss. In the long term, it will cause nutritional deficiencies and a decreased metabolic rate, making it even harder to maintain a healthy weight."

—Jennifer Raymond,
noted author and nutrition specialist[45]

What we know

Daily calories recommended by the National Academy of Sciences for a 128-pound woman: 2,000

Daily calories consumed by some females following the Zone diet (according to Sears): 1,100[46]

Daily calories recommended by the National Academy of Sciences for a 175-pound man: 2,900

Daily calories consumed by some males following the Zone diet (according to Sears): 1,400[47]

Food that Sears says to avoid eating because it could put you into what he calls "carbohydrate hell": Carrot[48]

Foods Sears says are acceptable in the Zone diet, as long as you add low-fat cottage cheese: Haägen-Dazs ice cream, Snickers bars, 12-ounce bottles of beer, Boston cream pie[49]

Studies published by Barry Sears in any medical journal ever: None

---

Sears often sounds scientific. But his books have no footnotes, so there is no way to track the sources he says substantiate his remarks. And he has never published any supporting research of his own.

The expert Sears cites to support his theory that eating more carbohydrates raises blood insulin, which causes weight gain—and so the way to lose weight is to eat more protein and fat and less carbohydrates—is Stanford University's Gerald Reaven, M.D.[50] But Dr. Reaven does not agree with Sears' theories. He says,

> "I disagree strongly with the notion that having high blood insulin, by itself, makes you gain more weight. There are so many studies showing that if you decrease calories, people lose weight, and it doesn't matter if you do it by cutting fat, protein or carbohydrate."[51]

Very often, Sears' remarks seem to be without any scientific basis whatsoever. For example, Sears says, "Humankind has been genetically unable to cope with . . . grains."[52] It is hard to imagine how he can manage to overlook the indisputable reality that the vast majority of the human race has for thousands of years relied on grains for most of its food energy.

Many of Sears other basic tenets are equally fanciful. He says repeatedly, "For cardiovascular patients, a high-carbohydrate diet may be hazardous to their health."[53] It remains a mystery how he can ignore the spectacular results in reversing heart disease reliably obtained by cardiovascular patients on the high-carbohydrate near-vegan diet programs developed by Dean Ornish, M.D., Caldwell Esselstyn, M.D., John McDougall, M.D., and many others.

Alice Lichtenstein, of the U.S. Department of Agriculture Human Nutrition Research Center on Aging at Tufts University, was asked about the scientific validity of Sears work. Her opinion is succinct: "Although Sears hides it, the book advocates a low-calorie diet. . . . Sears relies on studies that have never been published, peer-reviewed, or adequately controlled. It's science-fiction. . . . He's preying on vulnerable people."[54]

In some cases, Sears' dietary advice strikes me as truly off the wall. "You must treat food as if it were a drug," he says. "You must eat . . . as if it were an intravenous drip. . . . The best time to eat is when you're not hungry." And on the back cover of his book he actually announces, nakedly and without shame, "You can burn more fat watching TV than by exercising."[55]

Sears also seems to have an odd obsession with precise protein consumption. "My daily protein requirement," he says, "calculates to be 100 grams. If I eat any less than that amount, I'll be protein malnourished. If I eat more than 100 grams of protein, that will be too much."[56]

WHAT WE KNOW

Barry Sears' height: 6 feet 5 inches

Sears' daily protein intake (according to his own statements): 100 grams

Calories from 100 grams of protein: 400

Total daily caloric intake for someone who is consuming 400 calories a day from protein, and following Sears' recommendations for 30 percent of calories from protein, 30 percent of calories from fat, and 40 percent of calories from carbohydrates: 1,330 calories

Reality of 1,330 calories a day for a 6-foot 5-inch man: A starvation diet

IS THAT SO?

"Within 2 weeks you will notice that your clothes are fitting much better. . . . Judge your success by the fit of your clothes."

—Barry Sears[57]

"Barry Sears' The Zone . . . is another diet craze. . . . Sears' advice will probably help you lose weight, but only because you'll be eating fewer calories, not because his untested theories about protein, carbohydrates and insulin will put you into what he calls 'The Zone.' And to experts who have seen miracle diets come and go like hemlines, hair-dos, and celebrity romances, that's nothing new. . . . The Zone and other 'carbo-phobia' diets are based on an eensy-weensy kernel of truth—blown way out of proportion by theory, not evidence."

—Center for Science in the Public Interest[58]

To its credit, the Zone diet has helped sedentary, overweight people to lose weight. Its emphasis on small meals eaten frequently makes sense, as does its suggestion to reduce sugar consumption. It is probably an improvement over the standard American diet. But in one area, particularly, this diet has in my judgment done considerable harm.

Since more than 70 percent of a typical Zone diet's protein comes from animal sources, Sears' books and his theories about protein have reinforced the widespread misconceptions that only animal proteins can provide sufficient levels of essential and nonessential amino acids, and that vegetarians must carefully combine their proteins. He states, "About one-third of Americans are . . . suffering from protein malnutrition."[59]

The American Dietetic Association, in a formal position paper on the subject, makes it clear that these beliefs, while commonly held, have no scientific backing whatsoever: "Plant sources of protein alone can provide adequate amounts of the essential and nonessential amino acids. Conscious combining of these foods within a given meal as the complementary protein dictum suggests is unnecessary."[60]

Although Sears has tried in a later book (*The Soy Zone*) to assist vegetarians to fit into his diet regimen, his calling for such high protein loads has in fact turned many seeking to follow his advice toward animal products. Regrettably, there is the likelihood that these people will suffer harmful effects. Sears, remember, calls for 30 percent of your calories to be from protein. The World Health Organization doesn't think this is a good idea, telling us that "there are no known health advantages from increasing the proportion of energy derived from protein, and high intakes may have harmful effects.[61]

Perhaps the best summation of the damage done by the kind of protein consumption Sears advocates comes from the prestigious Worldwatch Institute.

> "The adverse health impacts of excessive meat-eating stem in part from what nutritionists call the "great protein fiasco"—a mistaken belief of many Westerners that they need to consume large quantities of protein. This myth has resulted in Americans and other members of industrial societies ingesting twice as much protein as they need. Among the affluent, the protein myth is dangerous because of the saturated fats that accompany protein in meat and dairy products. Those fats are associated with most of the diseases of affluence that are among the leading causes of death in industrial countries: heart disease, stroke, and breast and colon cancer." (Worldwatch Institute)[62]

WHAT WE KNOW

Protein in human mother's breast milk (as percentage of total calories): 5 percent[63]

Human minimum protein requirement (according to the World Health Organization): 5 percent of total calories[64]

U.S. Recommended Dietary Allowance for adult protein intake: 10 percent of total calories[65]

World Health Organization international guidelines for optimum protein intake: 10–15 percent of calories[66]

Barry Sears' recommended protein intake: 30 percent of total calories

---

Primary disease linked to inadequate protein consumption: Kwashiorkor

Number of cases of kwashiorkor in the United States: Virtually none

Primary diseases linked to excess protein consumption: Osteoporosis and kidney disease[67]

Number of cases of osteoporosis and kidney disease in the United States: Tens of millions

---

Barry Sears cites the athletic achievements of the legendary triathlete Dave Scott as testimony to the value of his diet. "My Zone-favorable diet," he brags, "helped Dave Scott—known as the godfather of triathletes—finish second in the 1994 Gatorade Ironman Triathlon—at the age of forty, and after a layoff of five years."[68]

As it happens, Dave Scott is a friend of mine, and I asked him whether this was true. He minced no words: "That's the biggest false statement ever. I've never read Sears' book. I've never tried Sears' diet. It's been awful having to refute this lie for the past five years. I called and left a message for Sears and sent him an e-mail, and he never replied."

Sears has a problem with credibility, and not just because he has never published any research to support his theories. The front cover of his bestseller *Enter the Zone* tells us the book is a "dietary road map to lose weight permanently," and the back cover promises that you will "achieve permanent fat loss." Ironically, in his own book, Sears admits he is overweight.[69]

Eat Right for Your Type?

The book *Eat Right for Your Type* by Peter J. D'Adamo proposes that there are four different ideal diets, one for each blood type: A, B, AB, and O. Follow the diet that is "right for your type," he says, and you can lose weight, cure ear infections, fight off cancer, heal yourself from Chronic Fatigue Syndrome, and much, much more. By "eating right for your type," D'Adamo asserts, you will be eating like your prehistoric ancestors did.[70]

This may sound very appealing. In a time when we have strayed so far from a natural way of eating, a guide to eating like your prehistoric ancestors could be quite helpful. And, indeed, many have been attracted by D'Adamo's promises.

But according to the *Tufts University Health and Nutrition Letter*, D'Adamo has his blood typing all wrong. "It's a fallacy even to speak of 'original' type O's or 'original' type A's because blood types did not originate with humans," explains Dr. Stephan Bailey, a nutritional anthropologist at Tufts University. "They came on the biologic scene long before humans did. Furthermore, there is no anthropologic evidence whatsoever that all prehistoric people with a particular blood type ate the same diet."[71]

D'Adamo has come up with 16 different food groups, further divided into "Highly beneficial," "Neutral," and "Avoid" foods, depending entirely on what blood type you are. Type A's, for example, are told they do well on vegetarian diets, but they should avoid cabbage, potatoes, eggplant, olives, peppers, and tomatoes, among many other foods. They are, however, advised to eat snails.[72]

Type O's, on the other hand, are told to base their diets heavily around red meat. They are told to avoid oranges, apples, wheat, peanut butter, avocados, cabbage, and potatoes, but encouraged to eat veal, ground beef, and beef heart.

D'Adamo tells Type B's to eat a lot of dairy products, including frozen yogurt. He tells them to avoid sunflower seeds, garbanzo beans, pinto beans, whole wheat bread, corn, pumpkin, tofu, tempeh, and tomatoes, but encourages them to eat rabbit, lamb, and mutton.

Type AB's are told to avoid corn, peppers, olives, sunflower seeds, sesame seeds, and lima beans, but encouraged to eat jam, jellies, rabbit, and turkey.

Many people who have tried D'Adamo's diet have lost weight. There is a reason, but it isn't the one he gives. In actuality, the diets recommended for all four blood types are each extremely low in calories. Some day's plans have only 1,000 calories, half the caloric needs of an adult woman.

Nevertheless, for D'Adamo, virtually everything in life comes down to whether you are an A, B, AB, or O blood type. According to him,

"(ABO) blood type can determine so many things: how much and how often we should eat; what our optimal daily schedule should be; what our best sleep/rest patterns are; how stress affects us and how to combat it; how to maximize our health; how to overcome disease; how we deal with aging; and even our degree of emotional well-being."[73]

D'Adamo believes that people who are type O and type B must eat meat daily to be healthy. When confronted with the fact that vegetarian diets have been consistently shown to produce lower rates of cancer, heart disease, hypertension, diabetes, gallstones, kidney disease, obesity, and colon disease, and to enable people to live longer and more healthfully, he explains that type A's do well on vegetarian diets. It is, however, mathematically impossible that the health advantages seen in vegetarians could be accounted for only by type A's benefiting from the absence of meat. According to the Red Cross blood bank, the population of the United States is approximately 39 percent type A, 46 percent type O, 11 percent type B, and 4 percent type AB.[74] There is no possible way that the consistent superiority of vegetarian diets that has been demonstrated repeatedly by world medical research could be due to vegetarian diets having health advantages only for type A's, who are, after all, a minority of the population.

Similarly, D'Adamo's explanation for the success of Dr. Dean Ornish's program of reversing heart disease, which includes putting people on a near-vegan diet with no meat, is that it has only worked for type A's. It does not, he says, help type O's, type B's, or type AB's.[75]

I asked Lee Lipsenthal, M.D., the vice president and medical director of Dr. Dean Ornish's Preventive Medicine Research Institute, whether this might be possible. He replied,

"There is no evidence in the scientific literature associating blood typology with nutrient needs. Although heart disease almost invariably gets worse, even when patients follow the American Heart Association recommendations, most of our patients have shown actual reversal of their disease, and the vast majority have shown measurable improvement in many areas—improved physical function on exercise tests, improved blood flow to the heart muscle, improved mood and sense of vitality, improved cholesterol levels, improved blood pressure, improved sleep patterns, and improved social function. We've had many hundreds of patients show dramatic improvements, and all this has been measured by objective tests. I don't see any possibility that people with blood types O and B (who together represent nearly 60 percent of the population of the U.S.) are not being helped by the Ornish program."[76]

D'Adamo believes that the risk of heart disease for type O's is reduced by eating meat.[77] There is, however, no evidence in the world medical literature for this belief. In fact, it is difficult to find supporting evidence anywhere for any of D'Adamo's theories. Like Barry Sears, his books have no footnotes, so there is no way to track sources or substantiate his remarks. And, like Sears, he has never published any supporting research of his own in any accredited medical or scientific journal.

The blood-type diet's explanation for why type O's presumably need meat is that type O's do "well on animal products and protein diets—foods that require more stomach acids for proper digestion." In fact, D'Adamo says that "type O's can efficiently digest meats because they tend to have high stomach acid content."[78]

It is well known, however, that not all men and women with type O blood produce more hydrochloric (stomach) acid; some secrete normal levels and some have less than normal. Further, it is pepsin, not hydrochloric (stomach) acid, that is responsible for meat protein digestion. In people who have large amounts of hydrochloric acid, the stomach environment becomes unusually acidic. An especially acidic stomach actually make pepsin less effective at digesting protein.[79]

D'Adamo's beliefs regarding the diets of early humans, likewise, seem to have no basis in fact. He writes,

"The appearance of our Cro-Magnon ancestors in around 40,000 B.C. propelled the human species to the top of the food chain, making them the most dangerous predators on earth . . . (with) little to fear from any of their animal rivals . . . (and no) natural predators other than themselves. Protein—meat—was their fuel. . . . By 20,000 B.C. Cro-Magnons had . . . decimated the vast herds of large game."[80]

The foundation of D'Adamo's blood-type theory is his belief that Cro-Magnons, who lived 40,000–20,000 years ago, were all type O's and ate mainly meat. Types A, B, and AB came along later, he says, and only they are genetically equipped for a diet that includes grains. There is no evidence anywhere in the scientific literature, however, that suggests Cro-Magnons were mainly or all type O's. Instead, there is considerable evidence that all four blood types existed in the time of the Cro-Magnons.

Were Cro-Magnons the heavy meat eaters D'Adamo portrays? Not according to paleontologist Richard Leakey, who is widely acknowledged as one of the world's foremost experts on the evolution of the human diet. Leakey points out, "You can't tear flesh by hand, you can't tear hide by hand. Our anterior teeth are not suited for tearing flesh or hide. We don't (and Cro-Magnons didn't) have large canine teeth, and we wouldn't have been able to deal with food sources that required those large canines."[81]

In fact, says Leakey, even if Cro-Magnons had large canine teeth, they *still* almost certainly would only rarely have eaten meat. Their diet would have been similar to that of the chimpanzee, our closest genetic relative.

Molecular biologists and geneticists have compared proteins, DNA, and the whole spectrum of biological features and have established very convincingly that humans are closer to chimpanzees than horses are to donkeys. This is remarkable, because horses and donkeys can mate and reproduce, although their offspring, mules, are sterile. A significant difference between humans and chimpanzees, though, is that chimpanzees have large canine teeth that can tear apart their prey, and have more strength and speed than humans. Still, even with these traits, which would be advantages for a meat-eater, chimpanzees, like other primates, eat a mainly vegetarian diet. Dr. Jane Goodall, whose work with chimpanzees represents the longest continuous field study of any living creature in science history, says chimpanzees often go months without eating any meat whatsoever. Indeed, she says, "The total amount of meat consumed by a chimpanzee during a given year will represent only a very small percentage of the overall diet."[82]

D'Adamo's entire theory is based on his assumptions about the blood types and diets of our prehistoric ancestors. Even though his assumptions seem to be mistaken, however, his diet has been embraced by many in the naturopathic community, and some schools of naturopathic medicine have even begun to include this theory in their curriculum. As a result, some naturopaths are now recommending that vegetarians and vegans who are blood type O or B eat meat daily. However, other naturopaths decisively disagree. The founder of naturopathy, Dr. Benedict Lust, called for "the elimination of . . . habits such as . . . meat eating." Similarly, Henry Lindlahr, M.D., whose work has been widely read in naturopathic colleges, defined naturopathy as favoring a "strict vegetarian diet." After a detailed and thorough discussion of the blood-type diet's underpinnings, contemporary naturopaths Dr. Deirdre B. Williams and Dr. John J. McMahon conclude, "The blood type theory of diet doesn't have a leg to stand on."[83]

Unfortunately for naturopathy, the acceptance of the blood-type diet theory by some in that community has served to reinforce the image held by many in the mainstream scientific community of naturopaths as gullible and ignorant. This diet has been denounced by all of the leading scientific organizations, including government health organizations, and all of the major universities and medical journals, that have commented on it. (Noting the many ways D'Adamo has found to make money from his program, one satirical critic called it the "Eat Right for My Tax-Bracket" diet.)

Tufts University Health and Nutrition Letter actually gave the blood-type diet its lowest possible rating: "The author speaks of his 'work' and his 'research' throughout the book but doesn't reference a single study that he has published in a scientific journal. In fact, D'Adamo's 'work' appears to consist entirely of anecdotes he has gathered from his caring for his 'patients' (he's not a physician) and of articles he has published in a non-peer reviewed journal that he himself founded and publishes. Not recommended—Tufts' lowest rating."[84]

Suzanne Havala is a registered dietitian and the primary author of the seminal 1988 and 1993 American Dietetic Association position papers on vegetarian diets. I asked her opinion of the blood-type diet, and she replied,

> "Just because an idea is outside the boxes of conventional thinking doesn't necessarily mean it's false. But I don't know of any reliable research that supports the blood-type diet theory. There really is no scientific data to back it up. I'd advise people to consider it for its entertainment value."[85]

Is THAT SO?

> "*Eat Right For Your Type* is the diet solution to staying healthy, living longer, and achieving your ideal weight."
>
> —Peter D'Adamo[86]
>
> "*Eat Right For Your Type* is not only one of the most preposterous books on the market, but also one of the most frightening. It contains just enough scientific-sounding nonsense, carefully woven into a complex theory, to actually seem convincing to the uninitiated. Based on his and his father's 'research' and observation of patients, D'Adamo has pieced together the outrageous hypothesis that blood type determines which foods an individual should or should not eat. . . . Browsing through what at first glance appears to be a fairly impressive list of references, we found none that seem to support a connection between diet and blood type. . . . Selecting the blood type gene as the same one that governs food and digestive capabilities is a purely arbitrary and we think irresponsible decision. He could just as easily have chosen to link food with eye color—and he would have been no farther off target. . . . This outrageous theory is nothing short of sheer nonsense. Were there any truth in it, it's reasonable to hypothesize that the human race would have died out centuries ago."
>
> —Fredrick J. Stare, M.D., Founder and former Chairman of the Nutrition Department at the Harvard School of Public Health[87]

I am sure that there are many good people who have derived some benefit from the blood-type diet, though I doubt that they have done so for the reasons D'Adamo claims. People who lose weight on this diet do so not because their blood type requires them to eat snails instead of cabbage, but because they have established an intention to do something good for themselves, and are, at least for the time being, eating fewer calories.

Like Sears and Atkins, D'Adamo's diet has been popular and his books have sold millions of copies. But like Sears and Atkins, D'Adamo has done the public a disservice by pulling many people toward animal foods. It may not have been these authors' intention, but many who have read their books have come away with negative opinions about vegetarian diets. This is unfortunate, because every day medical science is learning more about plant-based diets and finding them to have many advantages compared to meat-based diets, contributing to lower rates of almost all of the diseases that plague people today.

And even as one fad diet book after another comes and goes, the list of world champion vegetarian athletes keeps on growing. . . .

WHAT WE KNOW

World champion vegetarian athletes[88] (to name just a few):

Ridgely Abele, winner of eight national championships in karate

Surya Bonaly, Olympic figure skating champion

Peter Burwash, Davis Cup winner and professional tennis star

Andreas Cahling, Swedish champion bodybuilder, Olympic gold medallist in the ski jump

Chris Campbell, Olympic wrestling champion

Nicky Cole, first woman to walk to North Pole

Ruth Heidrich, six-time Ironwoman, USA track and field Master's champion

Keith Holmes, world-champion middleweight boxer

Desmond Howard, professional football star, Heisman trophy winner

Peter Hussing, European super heavy-weight boxing champion

Debbie Lawrence, world record holder, women's 5K racewalk

Sixto Linares, world record holder, 24-hour triathlon

Cheryl Marek and Estelle Gray, world record holders, cross-country tandem cycling

Ingra Manecki, world champion discus thrower

Bill Manetti, power-lifting champion

Ben Mathews, U.S. Master's marathon champion

Dan Millman, world champion gymnast

Martina Navratilova, champion tennis player

Paavo Nurmi, long-distance runner, winner of nine Olympic medals and 20 world records

Bill Pearl, four-time Mr. Universe

Bill Pickering, world record-holding swimmer

Stan Price, world weightlifting record holder, bench press

Murray Rose, swimmer, winner of many Olympic gold medals and world records

Dave Scott, six-time winner of the Ironman triathlon

Art Still, Buffalo Bills and Kansas City Chiefs MVP defensive end, Kansas
  City Chiefs Hall of Fame
Jane Welzel, U.S. National marathon champion
Charlene Wong Williams, Olympic champion figure skater

Mathematical odds that the 28 athletes mentioned would all be type A, the
only type that the blood-type diet says does well on vegetarian diets (assuming these athletes have the same blood type distribution curves as the rest of
the population): 1 in 35,000,000,000

chapter 5   # A Healthy
Plant-Based Diet

I f the low-carbohydrate fad diets aren't reliable paths to health and loss of excess weight, why are so many people drawn to them?

The reason is as simple as it is important. On the standard American diet, many people are overweight and unhealthy, and are willing to try anything that's easy and promises improvement. The conventional American diet is failing people. Full of processed and refined foods, sugar and unhealthy fats, it is not providing people with the experiences of their bodies that they want or need. It is, in fact, a tragedy.

The fad diets have a point when they call for reduced consumption of simple carbohydrates. If the carbohydrates in your diet are mostly white flour and white sugar, it's a good idea to cut down. And for most Americans, sadly, the majority of their carbohydrate intake does indeed come from these sources.

White flour and white sugar provide little nutritional value and squeeze healthier foods out of one's diet. The more sugar and refined grains people eat, the less they eat nutritionally complete foods that provide essential vitamins and other micronutrients.

Researchers have found that a high intake of whole grains, on the other hand, consistently reduces the risk of cancer. Consumption of processed and refined grains such as white flour, on the other hand, increases risk for cancer of the mouth, stomach, colon, larynx, and esophagus.

When researchers writing in the *American Journal of Public Health* reported on the Iowa Women's Health Study, they found "substantially lower risk of mortality, including mortality from cancer, cardiovascular disease, and other causes" for women who eat at least one serving a day of whole grain foods compared to those who eat less.

That's from just one serving of whole grains a day. But sadly, most Americans don't get even that. In fact, 98 percent of the wheat eaten in the United States is eaten as white flour. Only 2 percent is eaten as whole wheat flour.

WHAT WE KNOW

Percentage of nutrients lost when whole wheat flour is refined into white flour:[1]

Protein:	25 percent
Fiber:	95 percent
Calcium, Ca:	56 percent
Iron, Fe:	84 percent
Phosphorus, P:	69 percent
Potassium, K:	74 percent
Zinc, Zn:	76 percent
Copper, Cu:	62 percent
Manganese, Mn:	82 percent
Selenium, Se:	52 percent
Thiamin (Vitamin B-1):	73 percent
Riboflavin (Vitamin B-2):	81 percent
Niacin (Vitamin B-3):	80 percent
Pantothenic acid (Vitamin B-5):	56 percent
Vitamin B-6:	87 percent
Folate:	59 percent
Vitamin E:	95 percent

Of the 25 nutrients that are removed when whole wheat flour is milled into white flour, number of nutrients that are chemically replaced (enriched): 5[2]

Percentage of total dietary energy in most traditional diets, worldwide, historically accounted for by whole grains: 75–80 percent

Percentage of total dietary energy in Standard American Diet accounted for by whole grains: 1 percent

---

As the years go by, our food insanity seems to be starting at younger and younger ages. I'm sure you've noticed that today's children are inundated by commercials for sugary cereals, candy, soda, and other junk food. The average U.S. kid sees 1,000 such ads every week, each of them produced at great expense by sophisticated ad agencies for the single-minded purpose of getting impressionable children to eat these unhealthy foods now and for the rest of their lives.

Meanwhile, more than 5,000 schools in the United States today have contracts with fast-food companies and junk-food manufacturers to provide food for their cafeterias and/or vending machines.[3] Coca-Cola and other soft drink companies are giving millions of dollars to cash-strapped school districts in return for exclusive rights to sell their products in schools. In one such deal, a school district in Colorado actually requires teachers to push Coca-Cola consumption in classrooms whenever sales fall below contractual obligations.[4] This is happening even though excess sugar consumption is linked to obesity, kidney stones, osteoporosis, heart disease, and dental cavities.[5]

Today, the average North American consumes, per day, the rather staggering total of 53 teaspoons of sugar.[6] This amounts to a five-pound bag of sugar every 10 days for each man, woman, and child.

As if such dietary patterns weren't doing enough harm, U.S. companies and their practices are now rapidly spreading across the globe. Baskin-Robbins, for example, now has more ice cream stores in Tokyo than in Los Angeles. And Mexico has now surpassed the United States as the number one per-capita consumer of Coca-Cola.[7] The president of Coca-Cola, Donald R. Keough, practically salivates over the Third World as a market opportunity: "When I think of Indonesia—a country on the Equator with 180 million people, a median age of 18, and with a Moslem ban on alcohol," he says, "I feel I know what heaven looks like."[8]

Heaven, indeed. And here I was thinking that the idea was to provide all people with safe drinking water, good food to eat, decent housing, clean air, educational opportunities, and the chance for meaningful lives.

There are signs of hope, though. Public school children in Berkeley, California, are now learning about healthy eating, and growing much of the school cafeteria's food in school gardens. When Berkeley approved the plan in 1999, and began to make its school cafeterias the first in the nation to offer all-organic meals, responses varied. . . .

Is THAT SO?

"Berkeley, California, [is a] longtime hippie haven and world capital for political correctness. . . . Their politics have long been 'crunchy granola' and now their school lunches will be too."

—*Meat Industry Insight*[9]

"Berkeley, California, is now teaching kids about healthy eating and helping them to grow food organically for the cafeteria in school gardens, as part of a whole effort to improve nutrition and educate our kids and our families about good nutrition."

—Karen Sarlo, spokeswoman for the Berkeley Unified School District[10]

The Meat Industry Enters the Fray

Why, you might ask, would the meat industry be so antagonistic toward a program in which school children grow food organically for their school lunches? Does the industry think kids should be eating nothing but meatloaf? Do they oppose anything that could possibly threaten their hold on the American wallet? Why else would they attack programs that encourage children's health, and seek to reinforce nutritional myths that have time and again been proven wrong?

For example, the U.S. meat industry spends a good deal of time suggesting, and sometimes openly stating, that vegetarian and vegan children have poor growth. The reality, however, is that there are typically no problems in the growth and development of vegetarian and vegan children who eat varied diets with enough calories and adequate intake of vitamin B-12.[11]

The meat industry spends even more time insinuating that iron deficiency anemia is more common in vegetarian children. But here again, the truth is far from what the industry ads would have you believe. Vegetarian children, in fact, show no greater incidence of iron deficiency anemia than any other children.[12]

One of the meat industry's most tenaciously held tenets is that children must eat meat in order to have proper brain development. "Consuming two to three servings a day from the Meat Group," says the National Live Stock and Meat Board, "is important . . . to achieve cognitive function."[13] This is a remarkable statement, especially when compared to the scientific data. According to research published in the *Journal of the American Dietetic Association* and elsewhere, the average I.Q. of U.S. children is 99, while the average I.Q. of vegetarian U.S. children is 116.[14]

Is THAT SO?

"If it weren't for our meat-eating ancestors, the vegetarians wouldn't even be around today to complain about dietary choices with which they disagree. . . . The move away from a purely vegetarian diet triggered the growth of the human intellect."

—National Cattlemen's Beef Association[15]

"Nothing will benefit human health and increase the chances for survival of life on earth as much as the evolution to a vegetarian diet."

—Albert Einstein

The meat industry comes up with some amazing material. Dan Murphy is the editor of *Meat Marketing and Technology*, a magazine dedicated to the U.S./Canadian meat processing industry. In 2000, coaching the industry in how to be more persuasive, he wrote,

"When it comes to . . . the nutritional impact of meat-eating . . . I'm here to tell you that . . . with a little positioning, you can turn the debate into a forum for the industry's point of view. . . . You have to make the point that meat production and meat consumption has been part of every culture . . . throughout history, using examples such as Native Americans, whom these PETA types worship as being spiritually attuned to Nature. . . . They can't slam Native Americans. They're role models for these veggie types on issues like saving the environment. . . . Sure, you can almost smell the cynicism. So what? The whole point is to marginalize the debate. . . ."[16]

I wouldn't want to carry that argument to the Tarahumara Indians, who live in Copper Canyon in north-central Mexico. These Native American people are quite possibly the most physically fit people on Earth. Their level of endurance is, by our standards, stupendous. Their favorite pastime is a kind of kickball game that goes on for many days, in which the men run an average of 200 miles and the women (who also play) run an average of 100 miles.[17]

How much heart disease and cancer occurs among the Tarahumara Indians? Virtually none. The average cholesterol level of Tarahumara Indians is 125.[18]

What do you think is the diet of these astoundingly healthy indigenous people? It is almost entirely corn, beans, vegetables, and fruit.[19]

The more I have learned, the more I have wondered how the meat industry can continue so aggressively to promote meat products when medical science has so consistently found these products to do so much harm. Part of the answer, at least, seems to be that industry leaders and medical researchers have very different points of view. . .

Is THAT SO?

"I speak of faith in McDonald's as if it were a religion. And without meaning any offense to the Holy Trinity, the Koran, or the Torah, that's exactly the way I think of it. I've often said that I believe in God, family, and McDonald's—and in the office, that order is reversed."

—Ray Kroc, McDonald's founder[20]

"When you see the Golden Arches, you're probably on the road to the pearly gates."

—William Castelli, M.D., Director, Framingham Health Study;
National Heart, Lung, and Blood Institute[21]

Trusted Friends?

The meat and dairy industries are nothing if not dedicated to keeping their foods at the center of your plate. In the process of seeking to accomplish this goal, they say and do some remarkable things.

"Sales are decreasing," a recent McDonald's internal memo noted with alarm.[22] According to the company's top marketing executive, Ray Bergold, the answer to the problem was a "campaign to make customers believe that McDonald's is their 'Trusted Friend.'"[23]

And how was this to be accomplished? Through a "My McDonald's" campaign whose goal was to make a customer feel that McDonald's "cares about me" and "knows me." Marketing alliances with the NBA, the Olympics, and the Walt Disney Company were to be developed, all "intended to create positive feelings about McDonald's." Ads aimed at "minivan parents" would convey that taking your children to McDonald's is "an easy way to feel like a good parent."[24]

And here all along I had believed that being a good parent had something to do with providing a healthy environment and loving support for your children—and healthy food, too.

Unfortunately, McDonald's has quite had its way with the diets of America's children. In 2000, the Public Health Institute released a major study that found a third of today's teens could face "chronic and debilitating health problems" such as diabetes, heart disease, and cancer by their early thirties.[25] McDonald's, meanwhile, has built an empire hooking young people on foods high in saturated fat, all while seeking to convince you that it's your trusted friend.

Actually, to me, friendship is the very opposite of the calculating and self-serving manipulations that underlie the McDonald's marketing campaign.

I'm thinking, now, of a dear friend of mine—and a friend of life—whose name is Julia Butterfly Hill. Julia has become fairly well known in recent years as a result of her willingness to live by the courage of her convictions. You may have heard of her.

On December 18, 1999, Julia's feet touched the ground for the first time in more than two years. For that entire time, she had been living 180 feet up in "Luna," a magnificent thousand-year-old redwood tree in

Humboldt County, California. Her action was intended to stop the destructive clear-cutting of our forests, and in particular of our few remaining ancient redwoods.[26]

During her 738 days and nights in Luna, Julia endured relentless battering from El Niño storms, savage helicopter harassment, and repeated sieges by logging company "security guards"—all while living perched on a tiny and woefully unprotected platform eighteen stories off the ground.

When Julia Butterfly Hill began her famous tree-sit, she was only twenty-three years old. She had no idea she would come to be called the Rosa Parks of the environmental movement. She never expected to be honored as one of Good Housekeeping's "Most Admired Women" and George magazine's "20 Most Interesting Women in Politics," to be featured in People magazine's "25 Most Intriguing People of the Year" issue, or to receive hundreds of letters weekly from young people around the world.

She also did not know that she would be viciously condemned by the logging and meat industries. When Julia first climbed Luna she knew only one thing—she had to act, had to do something to halt the destruction of our planetary home. Ten years previously, she had made another decision. She had become a vegetarian. She wrote me recently, describing her journey:

> "The more I learned, the more I transformed my eating habits. The more I transformed my eating habits, the more I learned. I went from being vegetarian to becoming a vegan. There is a societal myth that a life without meat and dairy is difficult, prone to malnutrition, and void of satisfaction and texture. On the contrary, I've found that the healthier my eating habits have become, the more flavors and culinary joys I have discovered. I am now in better physical health than I have ever been, with more stamina and zest for life. In my path of being vegan, my body, mind, heart, and spirit have all healed and grown stronger. And the incredible joy I receive from knowing that I am lessening my impact on this beautiful planet fulfills me in a way that a meat and dairy diet never could, and never will."[27]

The contrast between these two paradigms is telling. On the one hand, we have McDonald's cleverly contriving a sophisticated marketing campaign, and spending staggering sums to convince you that the corporate giant is your trusted friend, while selling food that undermines your health with nearly every bite. On the other, we have Julia Butterfly Hill, living for more than two years perched precariously high in an ancient redwood, enduring assault after assault in her effort to help save our precious world, remaining positive despite it all, praying for the well-being of loggers and everyone else, caring far more for the protection of endangered redwoods and species than for her own comfort.

One meat industry executive recently called Julia Butterfly Hill an "eco-terrorist." Yet she has repeatedly pledged to be nonviolent and renounced any actions that might harm any living thing. I don't think the same can be said for the industries that are plundering the planet for private profit.

Who would you say is the better friend, one who presents a façade of friendship in order to make money selling unhealthy food, or one who risks their life trying to prevent the destruction of our environment?

And while I'm at it, I have another question for you. Do you notice that in the whole effort to make you think of McDonald's as a "trusted friend," the fast food chain says nothing at all about the health realities of the food it sells? Could this be because the corporation, and indeed the entire U.S. meat industry, is finding it harder and harder these days to justify meat consumption on health grounds?

Medical science is consistently finding health advantages for diets that incorporate little or no meat. These advantages, by the way, are being found to hold true across cultures, socioeconomic classes, geographical locations, and to be independent of factors such as smoking and exercise.

The health benefits that medical science is finding for vegetarian, vegan, and other plant-based diets are even more impressive when you realize that most of the vegetarians and vegans being studied in the research are eating a significant amount of white flour, white sugar, and other junk foods. Their diets often include excessive amounts of high-fat and high-salt cheeses, margarine, ice cream, eggs, and butter, not to mention chemicals such as artificial colors, flavors, and preservatives. We live in the society, after all, that has given us Twinkies, Wonder Bread, Cheez-Whiz, and Miracle Whip. The mere fact that a diet is meatless is no guarantee that it's healthful.

At the present time, we can only wonder how great the health outcomes would be for people eating whole foods, high-fiber, plant-based diets. We can only imagine, because such a human experiment has never been undertaken on a large scale. There's one thing we do know, though. You could eat all the dairy products, eggs, fish, chicken, and red meat in an entire grocery store and get not one gram of fiber or complex carbohydrates.

A Healthy Plant-Based Diet

What would a healthy plant-based diet look like?

- It would include lots of fresh vegetables and fruits.
- It would be low in refined and processed foods and sugar.
- It would not include hydrogenated fats and trans-fats (found in many margarines and white flour pastries).
- It would be low in both saturated animal fats and vegetable oils such as safflower, corn, sunflower, and cottonseed oils.
- It would include more water and less soda pop, more baked potatoes and less French fries, and more whole grains and fewer products made from refined flour. (The American Institute for Cancer Research says 40 studies have linked regular consumption of whole grains with a 10 to 60 percent lower risk of certain cancers.)[28]
- When possible, it would feature locally and organically grown foods.
- It would not include msg, artificial preservatives, colors, or other chemical additives.
- For infants, it cannot be said too often, there is no product that can even begin to match the advantages of breast milk.
- For vegans, it's important to include foods that are fortified with vitamin B-12, or supplementary sources of the vitamin. For vegan women who are pregnant or nursing, B-12 supplements are indispensable.

Sometimes people say, well, if a vegan diet is a healthful one, and if it's in keeping with our natural relationship to the Earth, how come vitamin B-12, which is necessary for health, is only found in animal products? It's a good question, and the answer is simple.

Animal products have vitamin B-12 because animals ingest plants and/or drink water that are carrying the microorganisms that produce the vitamin. Vitamin B-12 is constantly being produced throughout the environment by bacteria. If you were living in the wild, as your ancestors did, you'd almost certainly get plenty of B-12 in the water you drank. Nowadays, though, it is usually not safe to drink from rivers, streams, and ponds, as they are often contaminated, and most of us drink water that has been chlorinated. If you were living the way your ancestors did, you'd probably be ingesting B-12 along with the bits of dirt in the little grooves in your carrots, and on the peels of potatoes and other foods that didn't get absolutely clean. But today our soils have been sprayed with chemical fertilizers and pesticides, with the result that they are devoid of the B-12 that once was abundant. Furthermore, our food is today so sanitized that even if there were some B-12 in the dirt in which our veggies grew, we wouldn't get it. Hence the need for vegans to take special care to get B-12. The Recommended Dietary Allowance for vitamin B-12 is incredibly tiny, just 2 micrograms per day. That's 2 millionths of a gram.

Although people often think that getting enough protein is a problem for vegetarians, it actually isn't. Vegetarians typically get plenty of protein. But there is another nutrient that can be an issue—Omega-3 fats. Getting enough of these essential fatty acids is crucial to optimum health, and can in fact be an issue for everyone today. In times past, animal products provided ample Omega-3 fats, but today people are eating meats, dairy products, and eggs that contain far fewer of these needed nutrients. You'd have to eat twenty of today's supermarket eggs to get as much Omega-3s as are provided by a single egg from a free range chicken.[29]

Omega-3s are plentiful in flax seeds and in flax seed oil, in fatty fish such as salmon, herring, mackerel, and sardines, and can be found in lesser amounts in walnuts, hemp seeds, green leafy vegetables, and in canola oil. Flax seed oil is widely used in Europe, though it is only recently starting to become popular in the United States. Flax seed oil has many advantages over fish oil. It is high in a particular type of Omega-3, ALA, which the body needs. And unlike fish oil, flax seed oil can be used in salad dressings, which provides an easy way to ingest significant doses. Furthermore, unlike fish oil, unrefined flax seed oil contains lignan, a plant fiber that is associated with reduced incidence of breast, colon, and prostate cancers.

The human body converts Omega-3 fats into DHA—a nutrient that is needed by all of us, and one that is especially critical for the brain development of fetuses and newborns. There are, however, indications that there can be a great deal of variation among people in how efficiently their bodies convert Omega-3 fats into DHA. For this reason, I strongly advise those pregnant and nursing women who choose not to eat fish to be certain to include ample amounts of flax seed oil (2 teaspoons a day) in their diet, and as well to take supplementary DHA. Fatty fish are high in DHA, which is good, but they are often high in toxic metals and environmental contaminants that are particularly damaging to babies.

There are, of course, many issues and concerns that can arise for people who are considering adopting healthy plant-based diets. For complete practical and down-to-earth advice, I highly recommend the books written by the prominent dietitian Suzanne Havala, including *Being Vegetarian for Dummies*.[30] And I also recommend highly two books written by two other well-known dietitians, Vesanto Melina and Brenda Davis—*Becoming Vegetarian* (co-written with Victoria Harrison) and *Becoming Vegan*.[31]

Of course an optimum diet is not just one that affords us the needed nutrients. It should also provide us with sumptuous feasts. To me, the best diet is one that both keeps us healthy and also gives us pleasure. It should nurture our cells, of course, but it should also nourish our spirits by providing us with a variety of delicious culinary delights and by connecting us to the seasons, to the Earth, and to each other.

In every place and in every age, people have gathered together at meal times. In forests and mountains, in humble abodes and great mansions, beneath star-filled skies and beside hearths, we have given thanks for food. To me, the best diet is one that connects us to our humanity and helps us feel grateful for the gift of life.

Taking a Stand

I have a friend, an impeccable researcher, who reported on a study that involved 90,000 female nurses and was originally published in the *British Medical Journal* in 1998.[32] The nurses entered the study in 1980. By 1994, 861 of the nurses had suffered heart attacks and 394 had died from coronary heart disease. The nurses completed food questionnaires in 1980, 1984, 1986, and 1990. Analysis of the data showed the nurses who consumed 5 ounces or more of nuts per week had a 35 percent lower risk of coronary heart disease and heart attacks than nurses who consumed 1 ounce per month or less. This magnitude of risk reduction was constant regardless of intake of fruits, vegetables, fiber, or dietary fats. It was also found to be independent of smoking, alcohol consumption, exercise, body mass index, and the use of vitamin E and other supplements. My friend, always scrupulously careful not to make claims that aren't entirely supported by the data, wrote, "This study suggests support for the hypothesis that there might be an association between nut consumption and a possible reduction in heart disease risk."[33]

My friend, as you can see, tends to speak in the typically restrained fashion of scientists. I love him dearly, but I think there are times to leave such language behind. I think we know enough now to speak with clarity and conviction about the health benefits of a whole foods, plant-based diet. I believe the current evidence is more than adequate to warrant public policies and personal choices that shift us in this direction.

> "Epidemiologists consistently find an inverse correlation between the percentage of animal foods in the diet and better health." (Andrew Weil, M.D.)[34]

I have great regard for accuracy and intellectual rigor. And I know that no single study in medicine or science is definitive in itself. At the same time, I feel it's critically important not to become bogged down in the ever-so-qualified inertia of the academic. If we are too cautious, we play into the hands of the status quo. And the status quo when it comes to food choices—both in this country and throughout the world—is not healthy. The U.S. Surgeon General's Report on Nutrition and Health says that two-thirds of U.S. mortality is diet-related. Heart disease kills more than 100 people every hour in the United States.[35] At a certain point, one decides that the evidence is sufficiently complete and convincing to warrant action. To my eyes, when it comes to the health advantages of a whole foods, plant-based diet, we have passed that point.

T. Colin Campbell, the Senior Science Advisor to the American Institute for Cancer Research, agrees. Dr. Campbell is also the director of the most comprehensive health survey in world medical history—the China-Cornell-Oxford Project. The New York Times called his study "The 'Grand Prix' . . . the most comprehensive large study ever undertaken of the relationship between diet and the risk of developing disease." At the study's conclusion, Campbell wrote, "We found a highly significant association between the consumption of even small amounts of animal based foods and the increasing prevalence of heart disease, cancer, and similar diseases."

I believe the time has come to take a stand. There will always be more to learn, and there will always be studies that seem to conflict with each other. We can wait for 100 percent certainty, but people will continue to suffer and die by the millions while we split hairs. We can wait for every detail to be corroborated and every controversy to be resolved, but to do so is to abdicate our power to respond to one of the great ethical and social issues of our times.

I know many scientists who prefer to keep a certain distance. They call it remaining objective. They are sticklers for high academic standards but would just as soon not engage too much with the real, pressing problems of the world, where they might get their hands, and their ideas, dirty. The problem is that, meanwhile, the public remains beclouded in confusion—confusion often generated by the very industries who want to keep selling products that are causing harm. (The advertising these industries spend hundreds of millions of dollars on is not, by the way, notably meticulous when it comes to telling the whole truth.)

WHAT WE KNOW

Where most Americans get their information about foods: Advertising

Amount spent annually by Kellogg's to promote Frosted Flakes: $40 million[36]

Amount spent annually by the dairy industry on the "milk mustache" ads: $190 million[37]

Amount spent annually by McDonald's advertising its products: $800 million[38]

Amount spent annually by the National Cancer Institute promoting fruits and vegetables: $1 million[39]

It's been said that for every Ph.D. there is an equal and opposite Ph.D. But the data are clear enough. A cultural shift toward a plant-based, whole foods diet would have enormous benefits. For the vast majority of people, it would mean far healthier lives. It would not only mean less heart disease, fewer cancers, and far less obesity; it would also mean far more vibrant, thriving, energetic, creative people. It would mean there would be less fear of growing old and fewer families broken apart by the premature deaths of loved ones. For immense numbers of people, it would mean less suffering and more joy.

Today, it's shameful and tragic that the United States, alone among the world's fully industrialized nations, does not provide basic health care to all its citizens. The reality, however, is that a widespread cultural shift in a vegetarian direction would save enormous amounts of money in medical costs—enough eventually to cover basic health care for all Americans.

WHAT WE KNOW

Annual medical costs in the United States directly attributable to smoking: $65 billion

Annual medical costs in the United States directly attributable to meat consumption: $60–$120 billion[40]

To many of us, it's good news indeed that there is so much to be gained by a cultural shift toward a plant-based, whole foods diet. There are other individuals and groups, however, who don't like it one bit, specifically the industries who profit when you purchase and consume harmful foods.

You will keep hearing their messages, for they have enormous advertising budgets and massive control over our nation's food and agriculture policies. They will keep telling you that there is controversy over this or that detail, that health experts keep changing their minds, and that the bad reputation meat has gotten is undeserved. There will be those who will make great sums writing books telling the public that they can eat all the pork rinds and sausage they want and lose weight in the bargain. They will say there is no need, no need at all, to reduce your consumption of animal products.

Fortunately, even as they speak, there are quiet, clear, and informed voices among us, voices that point in a decidedly different direction, a direction leading to far lower rates of disease and far more vibrant, healthy, and joy-filled lives.

"The China Health Project, a joint Sino-American undertaking, examined the health effects of changes in the Chinese diet since the economic reform of 1978 and concluded that the recent increases in breast cancer, colorectal cancer, cardiovascular disease and obesity are closely linked to increased meat consumption. Moreover, these disease changes occurred at a level of meat consumption that is only a fraction of the typical American or European intake. . . . Dr. Colin Campbell of Cornell University, who headed the China Health Project, conservatively estimates that excessive meat consumption is responsible for between $60 and $120 billion of health care costs each year in the United States alone. Domestic cash receipts for the meat industry totaled roughly $100 billion in 1997. If Campbell's estimates are correct, it's possible that this industry is a net drain on the American economy." (Brian Halweil, Worldwatch Institute)[41]

chapter 6 **Got BS?**

P eople often ask me questions that relate to dairy products: Don't we need
them to get enough calcium? Isn't it
important and necessary to drink milk?

You'd sure think so if you believed the ubiquitous "milk mustache"
ads that have been appearing just about everywhere in recent years. But
there are a few problems with those ads.

Many African American celebrities have been portrayed in the milk
mustache ads promoting milk to cut the risk of osteoporosis. We've seen
actress Whoopi Goldberg, film director Spike Lee, model Tyra Banks,
basketball players Patrick Ewing and Dennis Rodman, tennis players
Venus and Serena Williams, and many others. These celebrities have a
great deal of influence and no doubt believe that by appearing in these
ads they are doing a public service. What they don't know is that there is
no evidence, according to the Food and Drug Administration (FDA),
that increased calcium intake from milk will lower the risk of osteoporosis for African Americans.[1]

Similarly, many male celebrities—including former President Bill
Clinton, former football star Steve Young, and home run champion
Mark McGwire—have appeared in the milk mustache ads promoting
milk for osteoporosis. Here again, though, we have a problem. The FDA

has found no evidence that increased calcium intake from milk lowers the risk of osteoporosis for males.[2]

Perhaps you've seen talk show host Larry King portrayed in milk mustache ads promoting milk to lower the risk of high blood pressure. What the ads didn't tell you was that the FDA has found no evidence that increased milk intake lowers the risk of high blood pressure.[3]

How about women? Dozens of milk mustache ads tell us that the calcium in milk helps women have stronger bones and avoid osteoporosis. But not according to the 12-year Nurses' Health Study, involving 78,000 women, which found no evidence at all that higher intakes of milk reduced osteoporosis or bone fracture incidence. In fact, the study found that the relative risk of hip fracture for women who drink two glasses or more of milk per day was *1.45 times higher* than for those who drink one glass or less per week.[4]

Well then, what about girls? A study published in 2000 in *Pediatrics*, the medical journal of the American Academy of Pediatrics, tracked for six years a large group of girls ages 12 to 18. Adolescence is a critical period for bone health because the average female gains 40 to 60 percent of her skeletal mass during those years. The researchers concluded, "Calcium intake, which ranged from 500 to 1,500 mg/day . . . was not associated with hip Bone Mineral Density at age 18 years, or with total body bone mineral gain." In other words, consistent with previous studies, none of the girls with low calcium intake had any different bone development than girls with high calcium intake. Contrary to the dairy industry message, getting that extra calcium made no difference. The researchers were aware that their findings contradict the commonly held belief that the road to strong bones is higher calcium consumption. Tom Lloyd of Pennsylvania State University, the coauthor of the study, was frank: "We [had] hypothesized that increased calcium intake would result in better adolescent bone gain. Needless to say, we were surprised to find our hypothesis refuted."[5]

In 2000, the Physicians Committee for Responsible Medicine (PCRM) had had enough and filed a petition with the Federal Trade Commission (FTC) requesting an immediate investigation into the health claims of the milk mustache ads. PCRM asked the FTC to investigate whether the National Fluid Milk Processor Promotion Board and the Milk Industry Foundation had been disseminating scientifically un-substantiated, purposefully deceptive, and harmful advertising.

The physicians' group had been for some time protesting the ads, but what prompted them to file the petition was a new set of milk mustache ads that featured the Latin heartthrob Marc Anthony and that implied that milk could help prevent osteoporosis in Hispanic Americans. What Marc Anthony fans need to know, the doctors said, "is that there is little or no evidence that Hispanic Americans benefit from milk drinking. To add insult to injury, the majority of Hispanic-Americans, like Asian-Americans, African-Americans, and Native-Americans, are lactose intolerant and experience gastrointestinal problems from milk."[6]

What we know

Lactose intolerance among adults of Asian descent: 90–100 percent[7]

Among Native Americans: 95 percent

Among people of African descent: 65–70 percent

Among people of Italian descent: 65–70 percent

Among people of Hispanic descent: 50–60 percent

Among people of Caucasian descent: 10 percent

The president of the Physicians Committee for Responsible Medicine, Neal Barnard, M.D., spoke strongly about the dairy ads. "The dairy industry continues to whitewash the dangers of cow's milk," he said. "The ubiquitous 'milk mustache' campaign makes misleading claims about milk preventing osteoporosis, lowering blood pressure, and enhancing sports performance. Recent studies, including the Harvard Nurses' Health Study, have shown that milk offers no protection against broken bones. And, unlike prescription drug ads, the mustache ads don't reveal the many unwanted 'side-effects' of milk, among them increased risk of prostate and ovarian cancer, diabetes, obesity, and heart disease."

By the way, the milk mustache ads were created for the National Fluid Milk Processors Promotion Board by the ad agency Bozell Worldwide,

Inc. Seeing how effective the ads were, the Distilled Spirits Council subsequently hired Bozell, hoping that their help would increase hard liquor consumption.[8]

I think it's important to look at the claims made by the dairy industry in their ads, because these ads have insinuated themselves into our psyches and affected the way you and I think and act. They've influenced all of us greatly, which is exactly why the dairy industry has been willing to spend several hundred million dollars a year to place them constantly before us.

The Calcium Conspiracy

For years, the dairy industry barraged us with ads telling us that milk is Nature's perfect food. Of course, the ads usually didn't mention that milk is Nature's perfect food for turning a 90-pound calf into a 450-pound cow in one year.

Now we have the Dairy Bureau stating, "It's irresponsible to suggest some physicians recommend against using milk."[9] But in fact many physicians—including well-known authors Frank Oski, M.D. (former Director, Department of Pediatrics, Johns Hopkins University School of Medicine and Physician-in-Chief, Johns Hopkins Children's Center), Benjamin Spock, M.D., Neal Barnard, M.D., John McDougall, M.D., Michael Klaper, M.D., Robert Kradjian, M.D., Charles Attwood, M.D., and many others—have publicly and emphatically recommended against consuming dairy products.[10]

A central point of the dairy ads, of course, is that we need to drink milk products to get enough calcium. "For humans to get the calcium they need from food without consuming milk products," says the Dairy Bureau, "is extremely difficult. One of the reasons is bio-availability. The calcium in many other foods, like most fruits, vegetables and legumes, is poorly absorbed by the human digestive system. That is, it's not 'bio-available.'"[11]

This sounds convincing. But is it true that calcium is better absorbed from milk than from vegetables?

WHAT WE KNOW

Calcium absorption rates[12] (according to the *American Journal of Clinical Nutrition*):

Brussels sprouts	63.8 percent
Mustard greens	57.8 percent
Broccoli	52.6 percent
Turnip greens	51.6 percent
Kale	50 percent
Cow's milk	32 percent

In another dairy advertisement, we're told, "Of course there's calcium in other foods besides milk products. But can we meet our daily calcium needs eating them? With great difficulty. . . . To get the same 300 mg of bio-available calcium [as 1 cup of milk], you'd have to eat either 11 cups of kidney beans, 8 cups of cooked spinach, 2½ cups of sesame seeds, 2 large servings of calcium-processed tofu or 2½ cups of broccoli."

Sounds convincing. But according to the most widely used reference book for food values and nutrients (*Bowes and Church's Food Values of Portions Commonly Used*), it's not even close to true. One cup of milk contains 300 mg of calcium, but only 32 percent (96 mg) of it is bio-available. Contrary to the dairy industry's assertions, you can derive this amount of bio-available calcium from just over ½ cup of firm tofu made with calcium, from 1.5 cups of cooked broccoli, or from ⅓ cup of sesame seeds.[13]

IS THAT SO?

"A low calcium intake in the children of vegans is a cause for major concern."
—Dairy Bureau of Canada[14]

"Beyond weaning age, children and adults of various countries and food cultures subsist on diets differing markedly in their calcium content. These differences in calcium intake . . . have not been demonstrated to have any consequences for nutritional health."
—Health Canada's Nutrition Recommendations[15]

The Dairy Bureau tell us, "Without milk products, calcium intakes in excess of 300 mg/day are difficult to achieve."[16]

This is remarkable, because there is no evidence at all to support such a statement. Actually, many studies have assessed the calcium intake of vegans (vegetarians who consume no dairy products). None of these studies have found average calcium intakes below 300 mg/day. On the contrary, the average calcium intakes in 10 studies of vegans ranged from a low of 437 mg/day to a high of 1,100 mg/day, with an average of 627 mg/day.[17]

While vegans get far more calcium from their diets than the dairy industry would have you believe, they do not usually get the level of calcium that the federal government has set as the daily requirement. But this requirement has been set controversially high, primarily due to the political pressure of the dairy industry. Not only most vegans, but 90 percent of all Americans don't reach it.

It is misleading to assume that all people have the same calcium requirements. A person with a low intake of animal protein and salt might have half the calcium requirements of a person eating a typical North American diet.[18] If you are sedentary, drink cola beverages, eat too much salt, and/or eat significant amounts of animal protein, your bones are going to suffer for it, in which case it might be a good idea to consume the levels of calcium the government—heavily influenced by the dairy industry—recommends. That may help a bit, but don't expect the increased calcium to make up for bad habits. If you are concerned about your health and the strength of your bones, it would be a far better idea to exercise regularly, avoid drinking Coke and Pepsi, eat a moderate amount of salt, and reduce if not stop eating meat and other animal protein. You'll feel better, your bones will be stronger, and your overall health will improve in many other ways, as well.

In fact, these other factors and especially regular exercise are so important for bone strength that many authorities, with sound science behind them, deplore today's hyped-up calcium mania as a harmful distraction. They say, and I believe they are right, that it has diverted attention away from far more important issues.

I continue to be amazed at how often dairy industry ads are off the mark. You've probably seen their ads telling us that consumption of dairy products will build stronger bones in the elderly. But in 1994, the *American Journal of Epidemiology* published a study of elderly women and men that found something quite different. Elderly people with the highest dairy product consumption actually had double the risk of hip fracture compared to those with the lowest consumption.[19]

The National Dairy Council funded a study in which post-menopausal women drank three additional 8-ounce glasses of skim milk (to provide a total of 1,500 mg of calcium daily) compared to the control group of postmenopausal women. The council was not thrilled when the results, published in the *American Journal of Clinical Nutrition*, found that the women who drank the extra milk actually lost more calcium from their bones than the control group of women who did not drink it.[20]

The scientists who conducted the study knew why drinking milk was linked with increased calcium loss.[21] Many studies have shown that the more animal protein we eat, the more calcium we lose.

The calcium-losing effect of animal protein on the human body is not a matter of controversy in scientific circles. Researchers who conducted a recent survey of diet and hip fractures in 33 countries said they found "an absolutely phenomenal correlation" between the ratio of plant to animal foods. The more plant foods people eat (particularly fruits and vegetables), the stronger their bones, and the fewer fractures they experience. The more animal foods people eat, on the other hand, the weaker their bones and the more fractures they experience.[22]

Similarly, in January 2001, the *American Journal of Clinical Nutrition* published a study that reported a dramatic correlation between the ratio of animal to vegetable protein in the diets of elderly women and their rate of bone loss. In this seven-year study funded by the National Institutes of Health, more than 1,000 women, ages 65 to 80, were grouped into three categories: those with a high ratio of animal to vegetable protein, a middle range, and a low range. The women in the high ratio category had three times the rate of bone loss as the women in the low group, and nearly four times the rate of hip fractures.

Might this have been due to other factors than the ratio of animal to vegetable protein? According to the study's lead author, Deborah Sellmeyer, M.D., Director of the Bone Density Clinic at the University of California, San Francisco, Medical Center, researchers found this to be true even after adjusting for age, weight, estrogen use, tobacco use, exercise, calcium intake, and total protein intake. "We adjusted for all the things that could have had an impact on the relationship of high animal protein intake to bone loss and hip fractures," Sellmeyer said. "But we found the relationship was still there."

I don't believe, by the way, that dairy products cause osteoporosis. But the many studies linking intake of animal protein to bone loss, and showing a worse calcium balance with increased dairy consumption, certainly show how unfounded are ads that promote dairy products as the only path to strong bones.

WHAT WE KNOW

Countries with the highest consumption of dairy products: Finland, Sweden, United States, England[23]

Countries with the highest rates of osteoporosis: Finland, Sweden, United States, England[24]

Daily calcium intake for African Americans: More than 1,000 mg

Daily calcium intake for black South Africans: 196 mg[25]

Hip fracture rate for African Americans compared to black South Africans: 9 times greater[26]

Calcium intake in rural China: One-half that of people in the United States[27]

Bone fracture rate in rural China: One-fifth that of people in the United States[28]

Foods that when eaten produce calcium loss through urinary excretion: Animal protein, salt, and coffee

Amount of calcium lost in the urine of a woman after eating a hamburger: 28 milligrams[29]

Amount of calcium lost in the urine of a woman after drinking a cup of coffee: 2 milligrams[30]

Cow's Milk versus Soy Milk

Lately, the dairy industry has been waging war against soy milk, suing the manufacturers of soy beverages for using the word *milk* and claiming that the dairy industry alone has a right to use it. This is ironic, because I believe a case could be made that the dairy industry should not be allowed to use the word *milk* unless they specifically state that they are referring to "cow's milk." For truth in labeling, shouldn't every cow's milk carton say on it, "Cow's milk"? Isn't that actually what it is?

Suzanne Havala is the primary author of the American Dietetic Association's (ADA) 1988 and 1993 position papers on vegetarian diets and is a charter fellow of the ADA, a status granted to fewer than 1 percent of its nearly 70,000 members. She reminds us, "Milk is species specific. Each species' milk is tailor-made for its own kind. So how on Earth did people start drinking milk from cows? Even adult cows don't drink cow's milk. And if we drink cow's milk, why stop there? Why not drink dog's milk? Or bear's milk?"[31]

Bear's milk aside for the moment, in 2000 the National Milk Producers Federation tried to keep soy beverages from being sold alongside cow's milk in the grocery aisles. A spokesperson for the National Milk Producers Federation made it clear why the industry was upset. "It is," he said, "a clear attempt to compete with dairy products."[32]

Heaven forbid.

Meanwhile, the dairy industry is spending ever more hundreds of millions of dollars on ads and other forms of promotion, telling us things about cow's milk and soy milk that, well—let's just say they don't mind stretching the truth a little.

For example, here's what the Dairy Bureau tells us about the nutritional comparison between cow's milk and soy milk: "Unfortified soy beverages contain only half of the phosphorus, 40 percent of the riboflavin, 10 percent of the vitamin A, (and) 3 percent of the calcium . . . found in a serving of cow's milk."[33]

Let's look at this carefully for a moment.

Only half the phosphorus? Brenda Davis is a registered dietitian and Chair of the American Dietetic Association's Vegetarian Practice Group. She is not impressed by the dairy industry claims. "We get plenty of phosphorus in the diet," she says, "and possibly even too much. Providing only half the phosphorus of cow's milk is an advantage, not a disadvantage."[34]

Only 40 percent of the riboflavin? It's true that unfortified soy milks contain only about half as much of this nutrient as cow's milk, but riboflavin is plentiful in nutritional yeast and green leafy vegetables, and is found in nuts, seeds, whole grains, and legumes, so getting enough riboflavin isn't a problem for people who eat a variety of healthy foods. In fact, vegans (who consume no dairy products) consume as much, or nearly as much, of this vitamin as lacto-ovo vegetarians and non-vegetarians.[35] A mere teaspoon of Red Star Nutritional Yeast powder contains as much riboflavin (1.6 mg) as an entire quart of cow's milk.[36]

Only 10 percent of the vitamin A? Too much vitamin A is toxic, so this could be a good thing. Vitamin A deficiency is quite rare among North Americans and Europeans who eat plant-based diets. Furthermore, vitamin A is high in cow's milk only because it's added to it, and there is no reason it could not be added to non-dairy beverages if there was some advantage to doing so.[37]

Only 3 percent of the calcium provided by cow's milk? Where does the dairy industry come up with this stuff? All of the most popular soy beverages sold in the United States provide vastly more calcium than the 3 percent claimed by the Dairy Bureau. Soymoo provides 116 percent as much calcium as cow's milk; Westsoy Plus provides 100 percent as much; Vitasoy Enriched provides 100 percent as much; Pacific Soy Enriched provides 100 percent as much; and Edensoy Extra provides 67 percent as much. Even those soy beverages that have not been enriched provide two to nine times as much calcium as claimed by the Dairy Bureau.

Meanwhile, there are a few more things the dairy industry isn't telling you about the nutritional comparison between cow's milk and soy milk.[38] For example:

- Cow's milk provides more than nine times as much saturated fat as soy beverages, so is far more likely to contribute to heart disease.

- Soy beverages provide more than 10 times as much essential fatty acids as cow's milk, so provide a far healthier quality of fat.

- Soy beverages are cholesterol-free, while cow's milk contains 34 mg of cholesterol per cup, which again means that cow's milk is far worse for your heart and cardiovascular system.

- Soy beverages lower both total and LDL ("bad") cholesterol levels, while cow's milk raises both total and LDL cholesterol levels, providing yet more reasons soy milk is better for your health.[39]

- Soy beverages, unlike cow's milk, provide substantial amounts of substances known as "phytoestrogens" (genestein, daidzen, and so on), which lower both heart disease and cancer risk.

- Men who consume one to two servings of soy milk per day are 70 percent less likely to develop prostate cancer than men who don't.[40]

The dairy industry has fought long and hard to keep soy beverages from being included in the milk group in the Dietary Guidelines for Americans. But in 2000, the Dietary Guidelines Advisory Committee, despite being stacked with members who had received grants from the National Dairy Promotion and Research Board and had been "visiting professors" with the National Dairy Council, recommended that soy beverages be included as an option in the milk group.[41]

WHAT WE KNOW

Antibiotics allowed in U.S. cow's milk: 80[42]

Antibiotics found in soy milk: None

Children with chronic constipation so intractable that it can't be treated successfully by laxatives, who are cured by switching from cow's milk to soy milk: 44 percent[43]

Average American's estimate when asked what percentage of adults worldwide do not drink milk: 1 percent[44]

Actual number of adults worldwide who do not drink milk: 65 percent[45]

The Dairy Industry Feels Threatened

If you suspect that the dairy industry is not entirely pleased with me, you'd be right. But if you think, as I did, that on account of this they would be unable to appreciate my finer points, well, you'd be as wrong as I was.

This was brought home to me a few years after *Diet for a New America* had been published, and the media was calling me "the dairy industry's public enemy number one." This was not the nicest of things to be called, but I rather liked it at first, actually, as it made me feel that somebody, at least, was listening to me.

What happened next was that I started receiving in the mail, anonymously sent, the minutes from the meetings of the executive board of one of the largest dairy organizations in the country. Whoever it was that was sending the minutes to me obviously wanted me to see them, but didn't want me to know who the sender was. The envelopes were always plain, with no return address, and contained no cover letter or explanation.

At first I didn't make much of it, and even thought they might contain erroneous information sent to me with the intent to mislead or confuse me. But the minutes dealt mainly, as board meeting minutes are wont to do, with what I call "adminis-trivia"—the details of running an organization—and only occasionally did they mention topics that were of any interest to me. Hence I concluded that they quite probably were just what they seemed to be, the actual minutes of actual meetings, not something that had been sent to deceive me.

The minutes were, in point of fact, quite boring. Except once. What made the whole thing worthwhile to me was this one occasion when the minutes contained notes from a lengthy discussion that the dairy board had evidently had on the subject of "What are we going to do about John Robbins?"

I didn't know that there was a particular need to do anything about me, actually, and hadn't heard anyone speak like that since my junior high school vice principal, and he was no one I care to remember, I can tell you that. But the venerable members of the dairy board evidently had embarked on a considerable discussion about me and what to do about my work. It was clear, through it all, that they were not only taking me seriously, but were worried to death that the American public might actually listen to what I had to say.

There were a number of ideas on the topic of what to do about me that were recorded in the minutes. And I present their exact words to you, just in case you, like me, had underestimated how perceptive these gentlemen can be. What they said is this: "We've got to do something about John Robbins. People are listening to him. He's handsome, eloquent, charismatic, and believable. What are we going to do about this? We don't want the public to learn what he's talking about."

I had hardly opened the envelope when I was on the phone to my wife, telling her all about it, and particularly about how they had called me "handsome." But putting aside for the moment the topic of my appearance, please notice that they didn't say what I was talking about was untrue, but only that they didn't want the public to learn about it.

As fun as it was to see them fretting about me, it still sometimes strikes me as ironic that I am a threat to the dairy industry. Not only did my father and uncle own the world's largest ice cream company, but my father's father, before him, had run a dairy in Tacoma, Washington. Like lots of kids, I made sure to drink my three glasses of milk a day. I also, dutifully, did my part for the family business by never once letting a day go by without eating a large amount of ice cream. There were days, actually, that I had ice cream for breakfast, lunch, and dinner, although most days I was not nearly that indulgent, mind you, and only had it for two meals plus of course several snacks.

The record will show that I loved every scoop. Indeed, I was literally the poster boy for Baskin-Robbins, in that my father put large photographs of me (and of my sisters and my two Baskin cousins) in all the stores, showing me smiling while happily eating a double-scoop cone.

I didn't realize, being a youngster at the time, that there was anything unusual in this. Doesn't everybody have swimming pools shaped like giant ice cream cones in their back yards? Doesn't everybody have clocks in their houses that, instead of the numbers 1 through 12, have the number 31 in each location? And doesn't everyone name their pet cats and dogs after ice cream flavors?

It is quite possible that my parents would have named me "Jamoca Almond Fudge" rather than "John" but for the fact that the flavor had not yet, when I was born, been invented.

You Never Know What to Expect

Life certainly can take us in amazing directions. A few years after receiving the notice relating the dairy board's interest in me, another thing happened that showed me you never know what to expect. I was giving a talk in Los Angeles. By this time I had had nothing whatever to do with Baskin-Robbins for more than twenty-five years, and, with my father long since retired, I no longer knew a single person who was involved with the company.

It was a fair-sized crowd, so it was not nearly possible for me to be aware of each person, but there was a couple in the back who for some reason drew my attention. She seemed all ears to what I had to say, while he, presumably her husband, seemed guarded at first, with his legs and arms crossed in front of him, although as time went along he seemed to relax and from his body language I began to gather that he was enjoying my presentation.

At one point, someone asked why I had left Baskin-Robbins and the opportunity to live the life of the rich and famous, and I had said simply, "If I hadn't left, I'd probably look in the mirror today and see someone who was fat, rich, and unhappy." It was a flippant remark, I suppose, but I then launched into a discussion of how we each must be true to our integrity and follow the call of our souls, or else, whatever else we might have, we still may end up bereft.

Anyhow, at the end of my talk, people came up to me to ask me to sign their copies of my book, and sure enough the couple in the back were among them. In fact, the man made a beeline straight for me, and, I had the distinct impression even before he spoke that he was a formidable fellow. His voice firm and strong, standing first in line, he announced to me, "You said that if you were today the president of Baskin-Robbins, you'd be fat, rich, and unhappy. Well, I want you to know that I *am* the president of Baskin-Robbins, and I'm not fat, I'm not rich, and I'm not unhappy."

I almost fainted, but somehow managed to hang on, and soon enough was conversing with Glenn and Amy Bacheller: he indeed the president of the company, and she his wife, a nutritionist; both of them, it turns out, vegetarians and major fans of *Diet for a New America*. Amy told me that she was a vegan, while Glenn still ate ice cream, though not at home, and only for professional reasons. She said that she could tell whenever he ate it at the office, because that night he would snore. He nodded, attesting to all she said, and added that he agreed with everything I had said in my lecture.

As it happened, Glenn and Amy became two of our closest friends. Amy served as a director of EarthSave for a number of years, and they both provided substantial guidance and support to the organization. Shortly after our meeting, Glenn left Baskin-Robbins and stopped eating dairy products entirely, later becoming the president of Jamba Juice, a rapidly growing company that sells made-to-order fruit smoothies. He felt great about the move for, while the people at Baskin-Robbins were often wonderful, he had grown tired of working for a company that produced a product that was in conflict with his own values.

And wouldn't you know it, things do change in unexpected ways, because not only did Glenn leave Baskin-Robbins and become one of my closest friends, but my dear father—not one, mind you to be swayed by the latest fad—my father, who prided himself on being a staunch conservative and set as solidly as concrete in his ways, ended up also giving up eating sugar entirely, and becoming, as he put it, "not a card-carrying vegetarian," but closer than I would have ever imagined.

It just shows, you never quite know what will happen. Both Glenn and my father experienced major health improvements, and Glenn, for one, attributes his health improvements to completely eliminating dairy products from his diet, which puts him in the same category as the thousands of people who've written me reporting dramatic health benefits after giving up dairy. Truly, there are a lot of people nowadays who are realizing that dairy products are not what they've been hyped up to be.

And this brings me, at last, to why I criticize the dairy industry. My criticism is not with the people who eat an ice cream cone, or a bowl of yogurt, or enjoy some cheese. My criticism is with the dairy industry for putting out ads that are deceptive and untrue, and that trick people, and do so quite intentionally, into believing that dairy products are necessary for a healthy diet. I don't like to see people misled for commercial purposes. I don't like to see commercials that imply that without dairy products, your bones will surely break. That just isn't true, as the people in most Asian countries can tell you. They have until very recently consumed little or no dairy products, and yet have had a much lower incidence of osteoporosis than people in the United States. The reasons their bones are so much stronger than are Americans' are several, including that they eat more vegetables, get a lot of physical exercise, and don't drink nearly the quantity of cola drinks we do. But a major reason is also that they eat much less animal protein than Americans do, including hardly any dairy products, and their bones are far healthier for it.

Dairy products simply aren't necessary to avoid osteoporosis, indeed may not even be helpful, and this is now recognized by many leading researchers. Walter Willett is Chairman of the Nutrition Department at the Harvard School of Public Health, and co-authored a major study of more than 75,000 American nurses that found that women with the highest calcium consumption from dairy products actually had substantially more fractures than women who drank less milk. Like me, he is not at all pleased with the dairy industries' campaigns to keep us all consuming their products.

Have you noticed that the dairy industry bombards us with ads claiming milk products are necessary to prevent osteoporosis, but never makes such claims on milk cartons? Why do you think the claims aren't on the cartons? Because the Food and Drug Administration (FDA) won't allow them! The ads are subject only to comparatively lax Federal Trade Commission (FTC) regulations, while the cartons are subject to FDA regulations that would require the statements to be backed up with facts.

chapter 7 # Unsafe
On Any Plate

In 1991, amidst enormous media excitement, eight scientists were sealed inside a giant bubble in the middle of the Arizona desert. They intended to remain inside the sealed, glass-enclosed, 3.15-acre bubble for two years.

The bubble, the public was assured, had everything it needed to be its own complete world, and to sustain life for these eight intrepid pioneers. It contained deserts, grasslands, tropical forests, and even a miniature ocean. Four thousand different plant and animal species had been painstakingly chosen and carefully brought in to produce a self-sustaining ecological world. The scientists were accompanied by insects, pollinators, fish, reptiles, and mammals that were selected to maintain ecosystem functions.

The bubble was named Biosphere II—the Earth itself being Biosphere I. It was believed that the ecosystems within Biosphere II were so sophisticated, and so brilliantly designed, that human life could be sustained within it indefinitely. Water would be produced and purified, oxygen generated, carbon dioxide absorbed, wastes recycled, and food produced, using only the energy of the sun. It was seen as "a portent of things to come as we rocket off to the stars."[1]

Things didn't work out quite the way that had been hoped. Despite extraordinary efforts and planning, oxygen levels inside the bubble began to drop to the level found at 17,000-foot elevations, subjecting the people inside to all the problems that come with insufficient oxygen intake. Then nitrogen levels soared, exposing the scientists to possible brain damage. Meanwhile, most of the insects that had been so carefully selected to serve as pollinators died, dooming the plants on which the bionauts relied for food and for air and water purification. Cockroaches, however, proliferated like crazy.

Eventually, the pioneers came out. The failure was not for lack of trying. More than $200 million had been spent on the effort, and the scientists persevered despite extremely severe conditions.

As it turned out, Biosphere II failed because the concrete pad on which the Bubble was erected unexpectedly pulled oxygen out of the air as it dried, and because the mix of soil organisms, bacteria, and other microbes had produced the wrong composition of gases.[2] It was one enormous lesson in humility. And a reminder of how critical to life on this planet are life forms so small that more of them can be found in a teaspoon of soil than there are human beings alive today on the Earth.

David Suzuki is a geneticist and the former host of CBC-TV's *The Nature of Things*. Reflecting on Biosphere II, he says, "We've been trained to look at big creatures as the most noble, the most important, the most pivotal and valuable, with ourselves as the biggest creature of all. We've ignored the relationships all large creatures must have with small ones, like ants, bacteria and fungi, which provide the real fundamentals of survival."[3]

The original inhabitants of Earth were bacteria and other micro-organisms, and for more than half of the time that life has existed on Earth they were the planet's only life forms. Even today, though too small to be visible to our eyes, they remain the dominant organisms on the planet. In fact, their collective biomass is greater than that of all the ancient forests, great herds of mammals (including humans), vast flocks of birds, enormous schools of fish, and countless insects combined.[4]

Micro-organisms are everywhere in the environment, on and in everything that can support life, including our bodies. A square centimeter of human skin harbors 100,000 microbes. The number of bacteria in the gut of each of us is greater than the total number of people who have *ever* lived on Earth. Ten percent of human body weight is composed of bacteria.[5] Each and every human being is, in fact, an aggregate of quadrillions of bacteria.[6]

Most microbes are not harmful, and many play critical roles in human life functions. Without the aid of certain micro-organisms, we could not digest our food and absorb its nutrients. Other microbes help us fight off pathogenic intruders.

But there are a few micro-organisms that can make us sick, and in some cases, even kill us. And some of these—including E. coli 0157:H7, Campylobacter, Salmonella, and Listeria—can enter our bodies through the food we eat.

Food-Borne Disease

It does not come easy to me to speak about the dangers of these microbes, and of food-borne disease. We have enough fear already in our lives. Indeed, I believe we frequently have too much fear for our own good, as evidenced in the obsessive and futile effort to rid our homes and bodies of all bacteria through antimicrobial sprays, disinfectants, and soaps, not to mention antibacterial sponges. These products have a place, and indeed can save lives when rightly used. But we're using them everywhere today, with the result that we're upsetting the microbial balance of our skin and intestines, and creating ever more powerful and resistant pathogens.

We'll never win by trying to exterminate bacteria. They live and thrive in extremes of heat and cold where no other organisms could ever survive. They have been found getting along quite happily in the depths of Antarctic ice, at the bottom of oceans, at the top of Mt. Everest, and in the molten lava of exploding volcanoes. And as the pioneers of Biosphere II learned, they play crucial, if not always noticed, roles in our lives.

In times past, food-borne illness was typically characterized by stomach cramps, vomiting, and diarrhea—symptoms that usually occurred two to six hours after eating contaminated food and were relatively easy to trace to the offending food. But human activities have changed the world immeasurably in recent years. Now many of the pathogens that cause our worst food-borne diseases do not cause symptoms right away. E. coli 0157:H7, for example, usually does not cause illness until three to seven days after a person eats the infected food, making it more difficult to recognize what food might have been the culprit.

Another example of the delayed effect is Listeria, a microbe particularly dangerous to pregnant women. Pregnant women who become infected with Listeria expose their growing babies to damage and death, but these events may never be linked back to the food-borne pathogen, because the disease may take as long as 70 days to manifest itself.

Many other illnesses, including urinary tract diseases in women, can result from food-borne microbes without ever being traced to their origins. Only recently, for example, have we learned that many cases of Crohn's disease may be caused by a micro-organism known as MAP (Mycobacterium avium subspecies paratuberculosis) present in cow's milk and not killed by pasteurization.[7]

Official estimates of annual cases of all types of food-borne illness in the United States run from 20 million to 80 million, but these estimates are probably far lower than the reality, because they rely on the number of cases that are reported and confirmed. Recognizing that most cases are never accurately identified, the CDC's Morris Potter suggests that there may be more than one case per person per year in the United States.[8]

Many cases of food poisoning are inaccurately called "the stomach flu." In fact, the stomach flu does not exist. The flu (influenza) is actually a respiratory disease caused by a virus. What are mistakenly labeled stomach flus are usually intestinal diseases caused by food-borne or water-borne bacteria.

We can only wonder how many children have suffered cramping, vomiting, and diarrhea without realizing that the so-called stomach flu they were experiencing was caused by the food they'd eaten. We can only speculate how much misery people have endured because foods they thought were safe were not.

In December 1998, when 21 deaths from Listeria were associated with Sara Lee products, Sara Lee recalled and destroyed 15 million pounds of Ball Park Franks, Mr. Turkey cold cuts, Hygrade Franks, and other brands of hot dogs and luncheon meats.[9] The year before, Hudson Foods was forced to recall and destroy 25 million pounds of ground beef after the company's hamburger was linked to a major E. coli 0157:H7 outbreak. Three years prior, 225,000 people were poisoned from eating Schwan's ice cream. In 2000, a deadly outbreak of E. coli 0157:H7 was traced to Sizzler Steakhouses in Milwaukee.

Learning of these incidents, many consumers jump to the conclusion that the problem lies with Sara Lee or Hudson or Schwan products, or that they are safe as long as they don't patronize Sizzler restaurants. But the vilification of one company or another leads to complacency regarding the true risks. By branding these companies as the ones to watch out for, consumers implicitly paint a halo over all other meat, dairy, and egg providers. It's easy to scapegoat one individual company and blame it for the problems of an entire industry, but that blinds us to the more widespread dangers. The truth, as epidemiologists at the CDC continually point out, is that, given the way livestock are raised and slaughtered today, there are risks now in virtually all U.S. meats, dairy products, and eggs.

It's actually quite amazing how often it is products of animal origin that cause food-borne illness. Although E. coli 0157:H7 has occasionally been found in raw apple juice and sprouts, and in water contaminated by cattle waste or infected humans, it's most often found in ground beef. In fact, it's so often a problem in ground beef that the serious illness it produces has been called "the hamburger disease."

Following the same pattern, outbreaks of Salmonella have been caused by contaminated tomatoes, mustard cress, bean sprouts, cantaloupe, and watermelon, but far more cases have been caused by eggs and other animal products. Similarly, Campylobacter is occasionally detected on vegetables, but it's widespread on U.S. chickens. Likewise, Listeria has found on coleslaw (when the cabbage was grown in a field fertilized with manure from Listeria-infected animals), but far more often the culprit is soft cheeses and processed meats.

Among plant foods, salad bars are most problematic, because pathogens can breed while the salad sits at warmer-than-refrigerator temperatures, exposed to light and air. Sprouts have the same problem. But the contribution of sprouts and salad bars to food-borne disease is still small compared to that of meats, dairy products, and eggs.

The meat, dairy, and egg industries know their products are the ones most frequently implicated. They say, however, that the problems resulting from these pathogens are not their fault—it's the consumers' responsibility to cook and handle animal foods properly. The companies want, naturally, to shift liability away from themselves. It is certainly helpful for consumers to know how to practice food safety in their kitchens, by washing their hands, chilling leftovers promptly, cooking animal products thoroughly, and avoiding cross-contamination. But countries where animals are treated more humanely and raised in healthier conditions do not have nearly as many problems with food-borne disease.

While chickens in the United States, for example, are frequently infected with Campylobacter and Salmonella, this is not the case in Sweden and Norway. In these countries, livestock are treated more humanely, and given more space, with the result that they are healthier and harbor fewer pathogens. But factory farming, as it has evolved in the United States, is geared for maximum corporate profit, not for animal well-being or for food safety.

In 1998, a letter published in the journal WorldWatch described the trend:

> "First it was E. coli and Salmonella poisoning, then the Mad Cow disease, and now the Hong Kong flu. . . . What do these growing epidemics have in common? They are all transmitted to human consumers through chickens and other animals raised in factory farms. And little wonder. In the filthy, crowded pens, harmless micro-organisms mutate into virulent pathogens. Routine use of antibiotics ensures their resistance to life-saving drugs. It makes one wax nostalgic for the good old days when meat eating was associated only with heart disease, stroke, cancer, diabetes, and atherosclerosis."[10]

No one disputes that the Salmonella, Campylobacter, E. coli, and other bacteria that sicken, cripple, and even kill U.S. consumers stem from factory farms. Yet amazingly, there is currently no requirement in the United States that such farms be tested for these dangerous pathogens. As a result, unsafe meat and eggs are shipped every day to processing plants, where they contaminate clean product and in turn the human food supply.

Meanwhile, the U.S. meat industry has aggressively fought any legislation that would require factory farms to be tested for bacteria that cause food-borne illness, and has repeatedly opposed regulations that would ensure a safer product.

In June 1998, Rep. Nita Lowey (D-NY) proposed an amendment to the agriculture appropriations bill that would have given the USDA the power to assess fines for unsanitary conditions in meatpacking plants. The House Appropriations Committee, however, rejected it by a vote of 25 to 19. A subsequent investigation found that the 25 members who voted against Lowey's motion received six times the campaign contributions from the meat and poultry industries as the 19 who voted for it.[11]

In the years that I have been involved with these issues, I've time and again been saddened to see industries that seem to have become callous to the pain and suffering caused by the way they produce their products. In 1993, for example, after E. coli 0157:H7 from Jack in the Box hamburgers severely poisoned hundreds of American children in the state of Washington, and killed some of them, public pressure was at a peak for changes to be made in meat processing. On November 1 of that year, however, demonstrating a cynicism that is almost beyond belief, the American Meat Institute filed a lawsuit seeking a permanent injunction against the USDA to halt its testing of hamburger for E. coli 0157:H7.

How could they possibly justify such a tactic? Testing, they said, might cause consumers to assume their meat was safe and to ignore the cooking and handling instructions.

Ironically, these are the very instructions the meat industry had until a short time earlier fought long and hard to keep off meat, out of fear that consumers might be alarmed to see such labels.[12]

Public Citizen Speaks

Am I being unfair in attributing a major portion of the responsibility for food-borne disease to the meat industry?

Public Citizen is a nonprofit organization that describes itself as "the consumer's eyes and ears in Washington. With the support of more than 150,000 people, we fight for safer drugs and medical devices, cleaner and safer energy sources, a cleaner environment, fair trade, and a more open and democratic government."

Public Citizen has neither a vegetarian nor an animal rights agenda. Yet, in 2000, the organization stated categorically that the meat industry's factory farms "are responsible for most of the problems with foodborne disease."[13] Public Citizen explained,

> "Many cows are raised in dirty conditions in huge, city-sized feedlots where they become smeared with fecal matter and other filth. In this condition, they are transported to slaughterhouses, where rapid processing takes place. Workers are under pressure to work as quickly as possible, killing and gutting as many as 330 animals per hour. In such an intensive operation, a cow's body cavity is slit open, and if any errors occur in cutting, the intestines can be punctured and feces released. The carcasses are immediately dipped in a cold water bath, which becomes a fecal stew. Later, as the meat is cut up and made into hamburger, the consumer may eat parts of multiple cows in one burger—so if there is contamination in the meat of one carcass, it could be spread to thousands of pounds of meat."

The organization notes that meat inspectors have been severely handicapped in their ability to keep feces-contaminated meat out of the marketplace, first by having their numbers reduced, and second by having their regulatory authority substantially compromised.

In the poultry industry, too, the fervent desire to maximize profits has set the stage for infection and disease. When you cram 50,000 birds into one building, give them feed and water that are contaminated and exposed to mice and rats, give them antibiotics that will make them more vulnerable to disease as strains of bacteria become resistant to the drugs, and then deprive them of food and water for several days before going to slaughter, you create near perfect conditions for pathogens to spread.

The journey to the slaughterhouse isn't exactly clean and tidy, either. Public Citizen points out that the chickens are "transported to slaughterhouses in large trucks, where they are crushed together and become encrusted with feces and urine. At the slaughterhouse, birds are hung, stunned, bled, killed, and scalded, then finally plucked by a large machine with rubber fingers that becomes worn and cracked, harboring pathogens that spread to other birds."

It's not a pleasant sight, but that's not the end of it. The organization continues:

"Individual chickens are gutted by a machine with a metal hook, which often breaks the intestine and contaminates the cavity of the bird. The bird should be removed at this point, but often it is not. The chicken carcass is then rinsed and left in a bath of cold water for one hour, so it will become heavier. Research shows this bath is one of the leading causes of fecal contamination and the spread of pathogens. It is also during this step that water weight is added to the bird. . . . The added water weight provides Tyson Foods Inc., one of the nation's largest poultry companies, with $40 million in extra annual gross profits."[14]

How did the U.S. meat industry respond to Public Citizen's report? Not with a lot of appreciation. Dan Murphy, editor of *Meat Marketing and Technology*, evidently did not feel hampered from having a strong opinion of the report by the detail that he hadn't actually read most of it. He wrote, "The Public Citizen report . . . is some of the worst, most turgid, most blatantly slanted pseudo-science I've ever encountered. Not that I made it past page six. . . . Personally, I'd like to arrange for hundreds of [meat] industry people to order thousands of copies . . . then light a huge bonfire with the reports somewhere in Washington, invite the media, and roast hot dogs over the flames."[15]

After *Diet for a New America* came out, another prominent meat executive wrote, "It's a pity book-burning isn't allowed in this country anymore, because *Diet For A New America* would be my first choice for such a fate."

Sometimes people reveal a lot about themselves by how they respond to criticism.

Food Irradiation

The U.S. meat industry is extremely aware of the problems, and deaths, that can be caused by E. coli 0157:H7 and other pathogens in animal products. The issue of food-borne disease has their attention, if only because of liability concerns and the possibility of lawsuits. So the industry has come up with an answer. But it isn't to correct the filthy factory farm and slaughterhouse conditions that give rise to contamination in the first place. Instead, it's irradiation—the deliberate exposure of food to nuclear radiation in order to kill pathogens.

The cattlemen are enthusiastic about irradiation, but many public health groups are not. They see it as a quick fix for food-borne disease, and dangerous, because although it kills disease-causing bacteria, it doesn't clean up the environment in which bacteria and other microorganisms flourish. Nor does it do anything to clean up the cows who, covered with feces, urine, and pus, become our hamburgers.

The two points of view could hardly be more different. . .

Is THAT SO?

"The National Cattlemen's Beef Association supports the use of food irradiation, and will continue to work to educate consumers on the benefits of irradiation."

—National Cattlemen's Association[16]

"Consumers want safe food, not irradiated filth."

—Center for Science in the Public Interest

While the cattlemen are among the most zealous cheerleaders for food irradiation, they do recognize that the technology has a problem with public acceptance. Accordingly, the cattlemen are fighting to prevent products that have been irradiated from being labeled. And they are lobbying aggressively to get the process renamed either "cold pasteurization," or "electron beam pasteurization."[17] These are nice, healthy-sounding labels, though I wonder how accurate they are, given that food irradiation exposes food to the equivalent of 2.5 million chest X-rays.

You might not want to eat a fast-food burger that had been "nuked." But thanks to the cattlemen's effort, you may already have. On February 22, 2000, the USDA legalized the irradiation of beef and other meat products. Three months later, grocery store chains began selling irradiated meat to consumers. And while a label disclosing that meat products have been irradiated is required when those products are sold in a store, labeling is not required for foods served by restaurants and school lunch programs. Without their knowledge, customers of McDonald's and Burger King, and children eating in school cafeterias, may now be guinea pigs in an experiment with a technology that could be extremely dangerous.[18]

The meat industry, however, says irradiation is safe. . .

Is THAT SO?

"I don't understand all the fuss. Meats are being irradiated to make them safer, to kill E. coli and other harmful bacteria. Consumers should be glad we're doing it. This is an example of how the meat industry gets a bad rap for doing the right thing. If anything, the labels should say 'Treated to promote health.' People should just relax and trust us to know what we're doing. Believe me, irradiated foods are safe to eat."

—Dominique Jenokins, CEO of a major U.S. meat company[19]

"Food irradiation causes a host of unnatural and sometimes unidentifiable chemicals to be formed within the irradiated foods. Our ignorance about these foreign compounds makes it simply a fraud to tell the public that 'we know' irradiated foods would be safe to eat. It is dishonorable to trick people into buying irradiated foods."

—John W. Gofman, M.D., professor emeritus of molecular and cell biology, University of California at Berkeley; professor at the University of California School of Medicine in San Francisco; and founder of the Biomedical Research Division at Lawrence Livermore National Laboratory[20]

Problems from microbial contamination in modern meat are so widespread, so serious, and increasing so rapidly, that many industry leaders would like to see all meats irradiated.

Yet no long-term studies have ever been conducted on the safety of food irradiation. And from short-term studies we know that irradiating food destroys vitamins A, B-1, C, K, and E, and forms new and potentially carcinogenic chemical compounds. Plus there is a very real possibility that it could create mutant bacteria and viruses.

E. Coli 0157:H7—The Hamburger Disease

Despite its dangers, irradiation has been approved for meats, and the primary reason is none other than the notorious *E. coli* 0157:H7. *Escherichia coli* (E. coli) is a huge family of rod-shaped bacteria, most of which peacefully inhabit the intestinal tract and aid in human and animal digestion. Until the 1990s, scientists thought most strains were harmless. But all that changed with the appearance of E. coli 0157:H7.

Instead of existing symbiotically within the human intestine, E. coli 0157:H7 attacks the lining of the colon, exposing blood vessels and causing them to bleed. The first symptoms are usually abdominal cramping and bloody diarrhea.

How common is E. coli 0157:H7 poisoning? Currently, according to the Centers for Disease Control and Prevention (CDC), about 200 people in the United States officially become sick *every day* from E. coli 0157:H7, and several die.[21] In all likelihood, though, these CDC numbers greatly underestimate the reality. William Keene, an Oregon epidemiologist, believes that only 2 percent of E. coli 0157:H7 cases that occur are reported.[22]

To counter the deadly potential of E. coli 0157:H7 bacteria, the meat industry is calling for irradiation of meats, and also for consumers to be sure to fully cook ground beef and other meat products. This makes sense, but also constitutes a tragic irony. While undercooked meat is far more likely to result in E. coli 0157:H7 poisoning, overcooked meat is far more likely to result in cancer.[23]

WHAT WE KNOW

Primary source of E. coli 0157:H7 infections: Hamburgers and other forms of ground beef

Potential consequence of ingestion of deadly E. coli 0157:H7 bacteria in humans: Devastating illness with multiple organ failure and high death rate[24]

Long-term afflictions suffered by many survivors of E. coli 0157:H7 poisoning: Epilepsy, blindness, lung damage, kidney failure[25]

Mary Heersink's twelve-year-old son Damion nearly died from eating undercooked hamburger. She describes the heart-rending story of what happened:

"As soon as my son popped the little morsel (of hamburger) into his mouth, he could tell it was all mushy and raw. He told me he'd been too embarrassed in front of his friends to spit it out. Exactly six days later, all hell breaks loose. It started with bloody diarrhea, then his platelet level dropped. He was hallucinating—he didn't recognize us any more. Then his kidneys shut down and he required dialysis. That required one surgery. Then his lungs became a problem. He was put on a respirator because his lungs were filling up with fluid, and tubes were punched into his chest to drain the fluid off. And then his heart became involved. It enlarged grotesquely. X-rays showed it two-and-a-half times the normal size. Three times the doctors went in and drained off the fluid around his heart. They couldn't believe they got a whole liter each time. . . . That's when they wanted to go in and cut a window in the membrane around his heart. When they got in there, the sac was so shredded and full of pus, they just stripped the whole thing off. . . . (Later) we gave him something to drink. He took a few sips and then he collapsed. He looked at us in total agony, then passed out. What we had watched was that he was perforating his intestines . . . So now his intestines are emptying out into his abdominal cavity. . . . This disease is so destructive and ugly. And then you find out what's causing it—filth in the country's slaughter-houses. I got so furious about it I had to do something."[26]

With every reason to be furious, Mary Heersink joined with the parents of other victims of E. coli 0157:H7 to establish the food safety group Safe Tables Our Priority—STOP. The group provides a hotline for new victims, serves as a clearinghouse for new information, and has pushed for better reporting of E. coli 0157:H7 cases.

How frequently does E. coli 0157:H7 appear in U.S. cattle carcasses? The industry insists it is uncommon. Tom Billy, the administrator of the USDA's Food Safety and Inspection Service, on the other hand, says that E. coli 0157:H7 bacteria can be found in up to 50 percent of U.S. cattle carcasses.[27]

What about the finished product? This, of course, is what's really important. How common is E. coli 0157:H7 bacteria in the beef that is ground into hamburgers? Here again, the industry seems to have its own unique point of view.

IS THAT SO?

"The prevalence [of E. coli 0157:H7] is very low."
—National Cattlemen's Beef Association[28]

"A report by the United States Department of Agriculture estimates that 89 percent of U.S. beef ground into patties contains traces of the deadly E. coli strain."
—Reuters News Service[29]

With the U.S. meat industry regularly downplaying the prevalence of E. coli 0157:H7 in the U.S. meat supply, many Americans do not understand the severity of the problem. Nicols Fox is a researcher and journalist, and author of a widely heralded 1997 book about food-borne disease. She writes:

"Most Americans have heard of the Jack-in-the-Box outbreak. And most probably think of it as an anomaly, a freak accident in an age of unprecedented food safety when the combined forces of government regulation, technological innovation, scientific methods of production and inspection, and industrial accountability guarantee that what we eat will not harm us. They assume that whatever went wrong has been fixed, and that such outbreaks are behind us now. Nothing could be further from the truth. . . . Unless these cases are part of a widespread outbreak that cannot be ignored, the public never hears of them."[30]

It can be disturbing to learn how common food-borne diseases are today, and how serious they are. As I've uncovered the truth, I've at times felt like turning away and putting my attention on something more reassuring and comfortable. But then I've realized how important it is to face what is happening. If we confront the reality, then we can understand it more fully, and do something about it.

I think it's important to talk about these issues, because our safety and that of our families is of paramount importance. It's worth the discomfort of confronting distressing realities if, as in this case, there is light at the end of the tunnel. There are choices we can make to protect ourselves and those in our care, and the more we know, the better equipped we are to make them.

Campylobacter

Although E. coli 0157:H7 is primarily a problem in hamburger and other ground beef products, if there were a contest for the most frequently contaminated food product in the United States, chicken would stand an excellent chance of winning.[31]

The poultry industry does not dispute that the majority of chicken carcasses and parts sold in U.S. supermarkets are contaminated with Campylobacter bacteria. According to CDC numbers, Campylobacter kills more Americans every year than E. coli 0157:H7 and is increasing even more rapidly.

In humans, Campylobacter burrows into the mucosal layer of the intestines and causes a disease marked by sometimes bloody diarrhea, and usually accompanied by fever, body ache, and abdominal pain. Unlike food poisonings that occurred in the past, Campylobacter poisoning normally doesn't cause symptoms until a week after exposure, making it very difficult to track. The disease usually lasts about a week, but in 20 percent of cases, there are relapses, and the disease can become severe, prolonged, and life-threatening.

Roughly 40 percent of the cases of Guillain-Barré syndrome, a life-threatening disorder of progressive paralysis, follow recognized infection with Campylobacter.[32] Since so many cases of food-borne illness are not recognized for what they are, there is a very real possibility that many of the distressing and difficult to diagnose autoimmune disorders of our time are actually the product of such infections.

WHAT WE KNOW

Leading cause of food-borne illness in the United States: Campylobacter

People in the United States who become ill with Campylobacter poisoning every *day:* More than 5,000

Annual Campylobacter-related fatalities in the United States: More than 750[33]

Primary source of Campylobacter bacteria: Contaminated chicken flesh

American chickens sufficiently contaminated with Campylobacter to cause illness: 70 percent[34]

American turkeys sufficiently contaminated with Campylobacter to cause illness: 90 percent[35]

Number of hens in three commercial flocks screened for Campylobacter by University of Wisconsin researchers: 2,300[36]

Number of hens that were *not* infected with Campylobacter: 8[37]

I continue to be amazed to learn how filthy are the poultry products that Americans are being asked to buy and consume. Former USDA microbiologist Gerald Kuester says of today's processed chicken, "(The) final product is no different than if you stuck it in the toilet and ate it."[38] When I first heard this I thought that surely he was exaggerating. I figured he'd gotten carried away with his metaphors.

But I was wrong. In fact, it may be an understatement. A study by the University of Arizona found higher levels of coliform bacteria in the American kitchen than on the rim of the toilet. Food-borne disease authority Nicols Fox says that this contamination seems to arrive "as a bonus on the animal foods people bring into their kitchens. The bathroom is cleaner because people are not washing their chickens in the toilet."[39]

It's incredible to contemplate that the chickens regularly brought home to be cooked and eaten by consumers could really be *that* contaminated. But an article in *Time* magazine confirms that they, indeed, *are* that bad: "The good news about chicken is that thanks to modern processing techniques, it costs only about a third of what it did two decades ago. The bad news is that an uncooked chicken has become one of the most dangerous items in the American home."[40]

Utensils, cutting boards, and human hands that come into contact with meat infected with pathogenic bacteria can spread the germs. In a kitchen where meat is prepared, these microbes can easily spread to salad vegetables. Since these foods are not cooked, the salad eater may become ill. And even cooked foods are placed in bowls, on plates, and eaten with cutlery that has been touched by hands that may have touched the contaminated meat. Thus, unless great care is taken, food-borne disease is liable to be spread in any kitchen that it enters, be it in a home, a restaurant, or a public service institution.

It can be frightening to learn how vulnerable we all are to these pathogens. And it can be infuriating to learn that there is much the industry could do, if it were willing, to reduce the contamination, but doesn't. For example, one of the ways chickens become infected with Campylobacter is through contaminated litter (the bedding material on the floor of the chicken house). The litter might be rice hulls, or wood shavings, or some similar material, but whatever is used soon becomes mixed with chicken manure. In Europe, the litter is scooped out and replaced between every flock, which is a matter of weeks. In the United States, on the other hand, it is often left in place for one or two years.[41]

I asked one chicken producer why, in view of the Campylobacter problem and the illnesses it causes, he didn't clean out the litter more often. His answer was not reassuring:

"We're very concerned about Campylobacter contamination in our chickens today," he replied. "And we're real sorry for the people who get sick and their families. Believe me, we bend over backward to produce a clean product."

"Yes," I said, "but why don't you clean out the litter more often?"

"Oh, there'd be costs to that."

Similarly, the prevalence of E. coli 0157:H7 is hundreds of times greater in cattle who are kept in feedlots and fed grain (not their natural diet) than in cattle allowed to graze, but this hasn't slowed the beef industry's zeal for grain-fed beef.

One industry executive told me, "We're quite anxious about E. coli and are doing everything in our power to deal with it."

"How about letting the animals out to pasture?" I asked.

"It's not going to happen," he answered. "Because it would lower profits."

Hearing the industry speak this way, I find myself reminded of something Leo Tolstoy once said: "I sit on a man's back . . . making him carry me, and yet assure myself and others that I am very sorry for him and wish to ease his lot by any means possible, except getting off his back."

Salmonella

U.S. chickens today are contaminated not only with Campylobacter. They are also regularly contaminated with Salmonella. Informed estimates of how many American chickens are contaminated by Salmonella range from 20 to 80 percent.[42] Symptoms of Salmonella poisoning include abdominal cramps, fever, headache, nausea, vomiting, and diarrhea. Attacks are most serious for infants, pregnant women, older people, and people who are already sick or have immune system disorders.

Salmonella has been recognized as a major problem in U.S. chickens since at least 1987, when *60 Minutes* did a major exposé and found over half the birds they purchased in U.S. supermarkets to be contaminated with the pathogen. Less well known is that Salmonella is actually a problem in all animal foods in the United States today. Mitchell Cohen, M.D., is with the Centers for Disease Control and Prevention. He says, "We have had outbreaks of Salmonella (in the United States) related to almost every food of animal origin: poultry, beef, pork, eggs, milk, and milk products."[43]

And the microbe, it turns out, is especially a problem in today's eggs. . .

WHAT WE KNOW

Americans sickened from eating Salmonella-tainted eggs every year: More than 650,000[44]

Americans killed from eating Salmonella-tainted eggs every year: 600[45]

Increase in Salmonella poisoning from raw or undercooked eggs between 1976 and 1986: 600 percent[46]

In the first *Rocky* movie, the fighter trained for his title match by breaking raw eggs into a glass and then drinking them. If that character were real and did that today, it's doubtful he'd make it to the ring without massive illness. The Centers for Disease Control and Prevention now strongly advises consumers "to avoid recipes using raw eggs."[47] Many egg-based foods that were regularly consumed in the past are actually now considered by the CDC to be too unsafe to eat, due to the Salmonella contamination of eggs. These include soft-boiled eggs, poached eggs, sunny side-up eggs, mousses of all descriptions, Caesar salad, homemade eggnog, lemon meringue pie, Hollandaise sauce, raw cookie dough, and several classic types of cake frosting.[48]

As so often happens, however, industry and public health groups have different opinions. . .

IS THAT SO?

"We don't want Congress to get carried away just because somebody somewhere happens to get sick. The problems with eggs and Salmonella have been overblown."

—Franklin Sharris, spokesperson for a leading U.S. egg company[49]

"Year after year the egg industry goes to [Congress] to try to turn back public health improvements. Eggs remain at the top of the list of foods that are causing food-borne outbreaks."

—Center for Science in the Public Interest[50]

Listeria

Listeria is another of the food-borne pathogens that has emerged only in the last few decades. It is not to be taken lightly. Ninety-two percent of people who become infected require hospitalization.[51] And 20 percent die.[52]

Listeria thrives on the inside walls of refrigerators, where it can grow from just a few cells to millions in a matter of weeks.[53] And it is particularly dangerous to pregnant women and the growing babies they carry. In pregnant women, the pathogen often causes meningitis or bacteremia, and then miscarriage, as the bacteria enters the bloodstream and then the uterus. Infants who survive may have brain damage or cerebral palsy.

Because of the danger posed by Listeria, the Center for Science in the Public Interest advises pregnant women to avoid the foods most likely to carry it—soft cheeses, rare meat and poultry, foods containing raw eggs, raw shellfish, ready-to-eat hot dogs and luncheon meats (unless heated to steaming), and unpasteurized juices.[54]

So frequently are these products contaminated with Listeria, and so dangerous is the germ, that in 2000, numerous public interest groups— including the Center for Science in the Public Interest, Safe Tables Our Priority, the American Public Health Association, the Consumer Federation of America, the National Consumers League, and the Government Accountability Project—called for regulations that would require ready-to-eat hot dogs and deli meat packages to carry labels warning the public that they may be contaminated with Listeria.[55]

It probably won't come as a complete surprise to you by now to learn how the American Meat Institute responded. Displaying something besides the utmost concern for the health of the American public, they pledged their resolute opposition to any such warning labels.[56]

The consumer groups also called for mandatory testing of these products to see if they are infected with Listeria. The American Meat Institute also, predictably, opposed such testing. A Meat Institute spokeswoman declared, "We don't agree with end-product testing as a way of measuring food safety."[57]

The Safest Meat Supply in the World?

The U.S. meat and egg industries say repeatedly that "we have the safest meat and poultry supply in the world." Steve Bjerklie, editor of *Meat and Poultry*, writes that you hear this repeated "like a mantra . . . over and over, at convention after convention, meeting after meeting . . . by industry speaker after industry speaker. . . . You hear it at every industry convention."[58]

But Bjerklie, who has also served as the editor of *Meat Processing* magazine, knows this statement is not true. In fact, he says, the U.S.

meat supply is nowhere near as safe as claimed. Other countries are doing far better. He writes,

> "The Netherlands E. coli 0157:H7 testing program makes USDA's look like quality control at the 'Laverne and Shirley' brewery . . . The USDA supposedly conducted a worldwide search of E. coli 0157:H7-related information, but somehow the Department missed the epidemiological reports, which is a little like missing Egypt in a search for ancient civilizations. . . . The European Union's much-maligned 'hormone ban,' is usually described in the United States as a politically motivated trade barrier to protect Europe's interventionist beef programs . . . [but] published concerns [indicate] that hormones and antibiotics [used routinely in U.S. livestock but not in Europe's] might make livestock susceptible to infections."[59]

Despite the number of times that the meat and poultry industry in the United States repeat that we have the safest meat and poultry supply in the world, the facts suggest otherwise.

WHAT WE KNOW

Leading cause of kidney failure in U.S. and Canadian children: Hemolytic Uremic Syndrome[60]

Cases of Hemolytic Uremic Syndrome that are caused by E. coli 0157:H7: 85 percent[61]

Annual Hemolytic Uremic Syndrome cases in the Netherlands: 25[62]

Annual Hemolytic Uremic Syndrome cases in the United States: 7,500[63]

Annual Salmonella cases in Sweden: 1 for every 10,000 people[64]

Annual Salmonella cases in the United States: 1 for every 200 people[65]

Chickens infected with Campylobacter in Norway: 10 percent

Chickens infected with Campylobacter in the United States: 70 percent

It's not easy to listen to the U.S. meat industry continually repeat that we have the safest meat supply in the world when the truth is so very different. Nor is it easy to hear them telling us that the answer is irradiation, blaming the public for not cooking meats sufficiently, and even implying that consumers should wash their hands, plates, and cutlery with chemical disinfectants before each meal.

Sure, good clean-up and careful cooking helps, but ultimately I don't think people want to eat food that has been contaminated with Salmonella, E. coli 0157:H7, Campylobacter, Listeria, or any of the other food-borne infectious pathogens, and I don't think people want food that has been nuked.

I think people want wholesome food that doesn't have to be treated as if it's contagious.

chapter 8

Policing the
Pathogens

In the eight years from 1989 through 1996, a total of 32 millions pounds of contaminated meats were recalled—an average of 4 million pounds per year.[1] In the last few years, though, the amount of U.S. meat that's been recalled because of contamination has skyrocketed. It's become common now for single recalls to involve 10 million pounds of tainted meat. In 1997, 25 million pounds of contaminated ground beef were involved in one recall by Hudson Foods. In 1999, the Michigan firm Thorn Apple Valley broke that record by recalling 30 million pounds of hot dogs. In one instance in 2000, Cargill Turkey Products recalled 17 million pounds of turkey products believed to be contaminated with the deadly bacteria Listeria.[2]

You may hear of such huge recalls and conclude that the system is working and that infected product is being caught and pulled back before it can reach the consumer. But unfortunately this is not what is actually happening. USDA records show that much of the contaminated meat is never successfully pulled out of circulation.[3]

For example, in 1999 a Minnesota firm recalled 170,780 pounds of ground beef, but only 2,818 pounds were actually recovered. A Nebraska firm recalled 82,929 pounds of beef but recovered only 10,601 pounds.[4] What, you might ask, happens to the millions of pounds of meat known to be contaminated that are recalled but not recovered? It gets eaten, presumably, by unsuspecting consumers.[5]

Numerous consumer groups are calling for the Secretary of Agriculture to be granted the authority to issue mandatory recalls of meat. Federal agencies have the power to recall toys, tires, and other items that might be hazardous, but not meat. Why not? Because of adamant opposition from the meat industry. . .

Is THAT SO?

"We have too many recalls already and it's costing the industry money. There are people out there who want to make Americans afraid of their food. It's not reasonable to give in to fear-mongers and alarmists."
—Sam Abramson, CEO, Springfield Meats[6]

"Is it reasonable that if a consumer undercooks a hamburger that their three-year-old dies?"
—Dr. Patricia Griffin, Centers for Disease Control and Prevention[7]

"Cattle producers continue to be actively involved in assuring that beef products are safe and wholesome for consumers."
—National Cattlemen's Beef Association[8]

"Nearly every food consumers buy in supermarkets and order in restaurants can be eaten with certainty for its safety—except for meat and poultry products."
—Steve Bjerklie, Executive Editor, *Meat Processing* magazine[9]

Safety Last

With recalls not being very successful, the USDA has had to do something to respond to the repeated outbreaks of food-borne disease carried by meat and poultry products. In 1996, the USDA introduced a new meat inspection system called HACCP (Hazard Analysis of Critical Control Points). There are differing viewpoints of its efficacy. . .

Is THAT SO?

"HACCP is tight, it puts us totally on top of things. It's the complete answer to food-borne illness. With it in place, the American consumer can once again rest assured that everything possible is being done, and that we have the safest meat supply in the world, bar none."

—Sam Abramson, CEO, Springfield Meats[10]

"(The meat industry says) HACCP is the best thing since apple pie and Chevrolet . . . but the inspectors are reporting back that HACCP is a joke. . . . The agency is giving away the shop. . . . They have handcuffed the inspectors. . . . Under HACCP today, inspectors are no longer inspecting. Industry is inspecting itself; inspectors are basically doing paperwork. . . . As an analogy, imagine that as a driver you must write yourself a ticket every time you exceed the speed limit because you're breaking the law. Some plants cheat; others won't cheat until they're forced to in a competitive environment. . . . The labels are misleading the public. The label should declare that the product has been contaminated with fecal material. . . . When I started as a (meat) inspector, I looked at 13 animals a minute. Today, nationwide, line speeds are up to 140 to 160 carcasses per minute. It's not humanly possible for meat inspectors to do what they're required to do, which is to protect the consumer."

—Delmer Jones, President of the U.S. Meat Inspection Union[11]

The Center for Public Integrity is a nonprofit, nonpartisan research organization that publishes investigative studies that serve as reference materials for journalists, academicians, and policymakers. In 1998, the Center produced a study about the growing threat of food contamination. After interviewing meat inspectors about the new meat inspection system called HACCP, the Center noted, "Many food inspectors refer to HACCP as 'Have a Cup of Coffee and Pray,' because it allows industry to largely inspect itself."[12]

That was in 1998. I wish I could tell you things have improved since then. But that is, regrettably, not the case. So great is the industry's control over federal policy that in 2000, the federal agency overseeing food inspection began imposing new rules, actually reclassifying as safe for human consumption animal carcasses with cancers, tumors, and open sores.

It was a pretty upsetting turn of events. And the outcry from consumer groups, as you might imagine, was immediate. They loudly protested the move to reclassify tumors and open sores as aesthetic problems, thus permitting the meat to obtain the government's purple seal of approval as a wholesome product.[13]

In late 2000, the Government Accountability Project (GAP) surveyed 6 percent of U.S. food inspectors. Felicia Nastor, food safety director for GAP, described what was learned:

> "Federal inspectors check paperwork, not food, and are prohibited from removing feces and other contaminants before products are stamped with the purple USDA seal of approval."

The inspectors said they regularly could take no action against animal feces, vomit, and metal shards in meat.[14]

Even today's watered-down regulations are sometimes challenging to enforce. In 2000, three state and federal meat inspectors requested that a sausage factory near San Francisco raise the temperature of its meat while preparing sausage, but they ran into considerable resistance from the sausage factory owner, a former candidate for mayor. The owner actually shot and killed the three inspectors.[15]

Antibiotic-Resistant Bacteria

It is ironic, and sad, that even as the meat, dairy, and egg industries in the United States are increasingly producing products that carry pathogenic bacteria and cause food-borne disease, industry practices are also undermining the very medicines we need to treat them.

Antibiotics have saved millions of lives, and their discovery ranks with the great medical achievements of history. But even Sir Alexander Fleming, the man who first discovered penicillin, warned that overuse of the drug would lead to bacterial resistance. Unfortunately, his warning was not heeded. When he spoke, no *Staphylococcus aureus* were resistant to penicillin. Today, more than 95 percent worldwide are resistant.[16]

Jeffrey Fisher, M.D., is a pathologist and consultant to the World

Health Organization. He says, "The pendulum has incredibly begun to swing back to the 1930s. Hospitals are in jeopardy of once again being overwhelmed with untreatable infectious diseases such as pneumonia, tuberculosis, meningitis, typhoid fever and dysentery."[17]

We are trapped in a vicious cycle. The levels of antibiotic resistant bacteria are accelerating rapidly. Trying to cope, hospitals are using higher doses and employing ever more antibiotics, particularly the broad-spectrum types. The amount of antibiotics used by hospitals in the United States is today 100 times greater than it was 35 years ago.[18] And yet, even with such enormous use in hospitals, the Union of Concerned Scientists announced in 2001 that antibiotics in factory farms account for the overwhelming majority of all antibiotic use in the country.

The scientific consensus regarding antibiotic-resistant bacteria has been gathering strength for many years. It's now widely recognized that the routine use of antibiotics in factory farms has eroded the ability of these medicines to cure human illness. In the United States, antibiotics have for many years been routinely mixed into the daily feed of healthy livestock to encourage weight gain. This practice, along with overuse in human medicine, has led to increased resistance among bacteria and to multi–drug-resistant bacteria, jeopardizing human health and causing diseases that are difficult or impossible to cure.

In 1989, the Institute of Medicine, a division of the National Academy of Sciences, stated that the use of antibiotics in factory farms was responsible for antibiotic resistance in bacteria and was seriously undermining the ability of these agents to protect human health.[19] Three years later, the Institute of Medicine stated that multi–drug-resistant bacteria had now become a serious medical concern, causing diseases that were difficult or impossible to cure. The Institute of Medicine laid the problem squarely on the doorstep of animal factories.[20]

In 1997, the World Health Organization called for a ban on the routine feeding of antibiotics to livestock.[21] A year later, the journal *Science* called the meat industry "the driving force behind the development of antibiotic resistance in certain species of bacteria that cause human disease."[22] Later in 1998, the Centers for Disease Control (CDC) blamed the serious emergence of Salmonella bacteria resistant to no less than five different antibiotics on the use of antibiotics in livestock.[23]

By then, many nations, including the United Kingdom, the Netherlands, Sweden, Finland, Denmark, Canada, Germany, and many other European countries had banned the routine feeding of antibiotics to livestock. In the United States, bills had been introduced in Congress to follow suit, but lobbying by the meat industry had successfully prevented these bills from becoming law.

In 1999, a study in the *New England Journal of Medicine* reported that infections in humans by antibiotic-resistant bacteria had increased nearly eightfold between 1992 and 1997.[24] Part of the increase was traced to foreign travel, and part of the increase was linked to the use of antibiotics in chickens. Even the increase due to foreign travel may have been caused by the use of antibiotics in chicken in countries such as Mexico, where the use of antibiotics in poultry had quadrupled in recent years.[25] The CDC placed a major portion of the blame for this dramatic rise in infections on the routine use of antibiotics in livestock production.

Well, said some meat industry leaders, even if pathogenic bacteria do develop resistance to certain antibiotics, there will be other, stronger antibiotics to handle the problem.

Events, however, have not supported such optimism.

"Recent studies show that bacteria in chickens are resistant to fluoroquinolones, the most recently approved class of antibiotics and one that scientists had been hoping would remain effective for a long time." (*New York Times*, 1999)[26]

It has only been since 1995 that fluoroquinolones began to be used in United States poultry production. Before then, fluoroquinolone resistance was unknown in the United States, except for people who had traveled to one of the few countries that permitted their use in animal agriculture or had previously taken the drugs for illness.[27] But since then, resistant strains have been emerging at an alarming rate in the United States in both poultry and humans.[28]

In 1999, an outbreak of fatal fluoroquinolone-resistant Salmonella infections in Denmark was traced to meat from infected pigs. Dr. Stuart Levy, director of the Center for Adaptation Genetics and Drug Resistance at Tufts University, commented, "Fluoroquinolones have become the drug of last resort for these infections. . . . We're beginning to lose these drugs. Where do we go from here?"[29]

"Perhaps to vancomycin," said one meat industry executive.[30] Vancomycin is a particularly potent antimicrobial that is often considered the last-chance weapon in dealing with infections involving multi–resistant-bacterial strains. But a "super bug" recently discovered in Great Britain has not only become resistant to the antibiotic vancomycin, it has learned to use it as food. It actually lives and grows off the antibiotic.[31]

What we know

Antibiotics administered to people in the United States annually to treat diseases: 3 million pounds[32]

Antibiotics administered to livestock in the United States annually for purposes other than treating disease: 24.6 million pounds[33]

Antibiotics administered to livestock in Denmark annually for purposes other than treating disease: None[34]

Adverse effects on animal health as a result of Denmark's reduction in antibiotics administered to livestock: None[35]

Adverse effects on producers' income as a result of Denmark's reduction in antibiotics administered to livestock: None[36]

Prevalence of antibiotic-resistant bacteria in chickens in Denmark prior to ban on the routine use of antibiotics in chickens: 82 percent[37]

Prevalence three years after the ban: 12 percent[38]

The U.S. meat industry continues to defend its routine use of antibiotics, while public health agencies see things differently. . .

Is THAT SO?

"Antibiotic use in animal agriculture makes a very small contribution to the resistance issue."
—National Cattlemen's Beef Association[39]

"Public health is united in the conclusion. There is no controversy about where antibiotic resistance in food-borne pathogens comes from ... (It) is due to the heavy use of antibiotics in livestock."
—Dr. Frederick J. Angulo, epidemiologist in the food-borne and diarrheal disease branch of the Centers for Disease Control and Prevention[40]

What new microbes will emerge to beset us in the coming years? It is impossible to know, but there are four things that, based on past experience, we can predict with virtual certainty.

First, newly emerging food-borne disease pathogens often find their way into the human body via animal foods.

Second, our ability to treat bacterial infections will be increasingly compromised due to antibiotic resistance.

Third, as these problems develop, the meat, dairy, and egg industries will do their best to deflect attention and downplay their responsibility.

And fourth, the surest way to protect ourselves and our loved ones will be to move away from dependence on animal products.

Hormones in U.S. Meat

Antibiotics are not the only pharmaceutical substance routinely used in U.S. beef production though banned just about everywhere else. Currently, U.S. beef cattle are routinely implanted with sex hormones, including Zeranol, trenbolone acetate, progesterone, testosterone, and/or estradiol. These steroid hormones are used to make the cattle gain more weight, much as bodybuilders and weightlifters sometimes take steroids to become bigger, even though doing so jeopardizes their health.

How widespread is the use of hormones in U.S. beef production? More than 90 percent of U.S. beef cattle today receive hormone implants, and in the larger feedlots the figure is 100 percent.[41]

The U.S. cattlemen repeatedly say such use of hormones is safe. But since 1995, the European Union has completely prohibited treating any farm animal with sex hormones to promote growth, for the reason that these sex hormones are known to cause several human cancers and types of reproductive dysfunction.[42]

Is THAT SO?

"The use of hormone implants results in the efficient production of beef that is safe. . . . Hormones in beef from implanted steers have no physiological significance whatsoever."

—National Cattlemen's Beef Association[43]

"The hormone 17 beta-oestradiol (widely used in U.S. beef production) has to be considered as a complete carcinogen. It exerts both tumor initiating and tumor promoting effects. In plain language this means that even small additional doses of residues of this hormone in meat, arising from its use as a growth promoter in cattle, has an inherent risk of causing cancer."

—Report by the European Union's Scientific Committee on Veterinary Measures[44]

How do you think the U.S. meat industry has responded to the European Union's adamant refusal to import U.S. hormone-treated beef? Not politely. It has used tariffs to try to ram U.S. beef down Europe's throat.[45]

After the European Union banned the sale of hormone-treated meat within European Union countries, the United States complained to the World Trade Organization (WTO). The WTO's three-lawyer panel ruled that the European Union was required to pay the United States $150 million per year as compensation for lost profit. They issued this ruling despite a lengthy report by independent scientists showing that some hormones added to U.S. meat are "complete carcinogens"—capable of causing cancer by themselves.[46]

To the European Union, the health risks from the hormones in U.S. beef are so great that they are willing to pay $150 million a year if necessary rather than allow U.S. beef to cross their borders.

You may believe that if you eat U.S. "hormone-free" beef you will be safe from the dangers of hormone-implanted beef. But I wouldn't be too sure. In 1999, when the European Union spot-checked meat samples from the Hormone Free Cattle program run jointly by the U.S. beef industry and the USDA, they found that 12 percent of the U.S. "hormone-free" cattle had in fact been treated with sex hormones.[47]

Similarly, when the Swiss government checked U.S. beef that was supposedly free of hormones in 1999, they found 7 percent of the U.S. "hormone-free" cattle had in fact been treated with sex hormones.[48]

The U.S. cattle industry continues to defend its use of synthetic hormones as completely safe. In 2000, Sam Abramson, CEO of Springfield Meats, expressed his understanding of why the Europeans see things differently: "They're just paranoid over there because they've had problems with mad cow disease."[49]

Apparently, the distinction between paranoia and prudence is too subtle for some. But he had one thing right. The Europeans, and particularly the British, have had severe problems with Mad Cow disease.

Mad Cows and Mad Cowboys

Mad Cow disease is a member of a family of diseases called transmissible spongiform encephalopathies, or TSEs, seen in various animal species including humans, sheep, cows, mink, deer, and cats. TSEs are known by different names in different animals—for example, Creutzfeld-Jacob Disease (CJD) in humans, scrapie in sheep, chronic wasting syndrome in deer and elk, and bovine spongiform encephalopathy or BSE in cows. Whatever animal is afflicted, however, the diseases have similar characteristics. They attack the central nervous system, causing disintegration of the brain; they have a long incubation period (measured in years if not decades) between the time when infection first occurs and the appearance of symptoms; they are always fatal; and they are transmitted by the eating of animals or animal parts, especially brains and spinal cords.[50]

The new cases of the human form of this disease are called new variant Creutzfeld-Jacob Disease (nvCJD).[51] The primary prognosis for humans infected with nvCJD could not be more serious—progressive destruction of brain cells, leading to dementia and death. The mortality rate for the disease is considered to be 100 percent.

"It is, by all accounts, a horrific way to die. First come mood swings and numbness, then hallucinations, uncontrolled body movements and finally a progressive dementia that destroys the mind as thoroughly as Alzheimer's disease—except that this illness can strike at any age. No wonder Europe is terrified of . . . mad cow disease. The illness started attacking British cattle in the mid-1980s. Then it crossed the species barrier; a human version of the disease has killed more than 80 Britons since 1995. Then it leaped across the Irish Sea and the English Channel, afflicting cows in 12 European nations. Last week Italy confirmed its first cases. Late last year, it hit Spain and Germany. Earlier this month, the German ministers of health and agriculture resigned in disgrace when their assurances that German beef was safe proved false. A handful of human deaths have been reported in France and Ireland—so far."
—*Time*, 2001[52]

More than 167,000 British dairy cattle died from the bovine form of this disease, popularly known as Mad Cow disease, between 1985 and 1995.[53] During this entire time, British health officials adamantly maintained that there was nothing unsafe about eating British beef. Even as evidence mounted to the contrary, the government held stubbornly to this position. Then, in 1996, a panel of government scientists told the British Parliament that the "most likely explanation" for new cases of Creutzfeld-Jacob Disease, the human form of Mad Cow disease, was that BSE had moved from cows to people. By that time, more than 1 million infected cows had been consumed in Britain.[54] In the next few years, more than 2.5 million British dairy cattle infected with mad cow disease were killed and incinerated at extremely high temperatures in an attempt to eradicate the disease.

The U.S. meat industry was, of course, following events in Britain. Steve Bjerklie, Executive Editor of *Meat Processing* magazine, lamented, "Meat is a lush medium for pathogenic bacteria and germs; it can harbor parasites, toxic chemicals, and metal contaminants. And now it can bring death by brain-rot."

How many people will come down with the disease from having eaten British beef is literally incalculable, because people typically are infected with nvCJD for 10 to 30 years before symptoms appear. In

2000, the *New Scientist* published a report from the Wellcome Centre for the Epidemiology of Infectious Diseases in Oxford, saying the death toll could eventually run as high as 500,000.[55]

In 1999, the U.S. Food and Drug Administration and Canadian health authorities told blood centers to refuse blood donations from people who had spent six or more cumulative months in England during the past 17 years, because anyone who had spent substantial time in England during this period might be infected with the human form of the disease, which can be transmitted through blood.[56] The Red Cross, despite a constant need for blood, instituted a similar policy.

In 2000 and 2001, European concern over Mad Cow disease rose to new heights. It began when researchers at the Department of Infectious Disease Epidemiology at London's Imperial School of Medicine estimated that between 4,700 and 9,800 French cattle had become infected with Mad Cow disease, and up to 100 of those had entered the human food chain.[57] Then, when it became clear that the disease had spread into Spain and Germany, the European Union called for the destruction of up to another 2 million cattle.[58] In a remarkable twist, given that the problem originated in England, the British began banning French beef.

By 2001, Germany was joining France and Ireland in killing many hundreds of thousands more cattle suspected of carrying the disease, and the European Union was spending more than $1 billion purchasing and destroying such animals. Throughout Europe, beef consumption was plummeting, dropping by half in some countries, including Germany. People in Germany, France, and Belgium were outraged at politicians who had claimed that local livestock were Mad Cow disease-free, and were chasing them out of office. The French government was prosecuting a farmer who sold an infected cow to a supermarket chain. And at least one insurer was offering discounts to vegetarians.

Why was there so much fuss when the death toll was still comparatively small? Because there is no way of knowing how many animals may be harboring Mad Cow disease, or how many people may be incubating the human form of the disease and passing it on to others through infected blood, organ donations, or contaminated surgical instruments (the infectious agent survives all standard sterilization techniques).

The disease is not only mysterious but unstoppable. It murders by driving its victims insane, literally turning their brains into something that looks like Swiss cheese. Yet the *London Times* reported in 2001 that Britain's largest processor of animal carcasses unfit for human consumption, Doncaster-based Prosper de Mulder, had mistakenly exported animal feed containing protein from ruminant livestock to as many as 70 countries, including Israel, Japan, Kenya, Lebanon, Malta, Saudia Arabia, Singapore, South Korea, Sri Lanka, Taiwan, and Thailand.[59] No nation on Earth, it seemed, was safe.

Many Americans first learned of Mad Cow disease in 1996, when Oprah Winfrey did a show exposing the problem. Her featured guest was my close friend and current EarthSave president, former cattle-rancher-turned-vegan Howard Lyman. What Oprah and Howard said on the program provoked the U.S. beef industry first to pull $600,000 in advertising from Oprah's network, and then to sue her and Howard Lyman for $20 million.[60]

What did Oprah do to prompt such a reaction? After learning that cattle byproducts were being used in cattle feed and that the American beef industry, in turning the cow—a natural herbivore—into a cannibal, was doing just what Britain had done for so many years, Oprah said, "That has just stopped me cold from eating another burger."

Howard Lyman said that the disease could exist or be discovered in the United States, and that "we are following exactly the same path that they followed in England (using cattle byproducts in cattle feed)."

This did not exactly please feedlot owner and multimillionaire Paul Engler or his company, Cactus Feeders. They hired a powerhouse team of attorneys to file a lawsuit demanding $20 million in damages and punitive fines. "Get in there and blow the hell out of somebody," Engler said.[61]

The lawsuit, filed in Amarillo, Texas, a month after the program aired, asserted that Oprah allowed "anti-meat activists to present biased, unsubstantiated and irresponsible claims against beef, not only damaging the beef industry but also placing a tremendous amount of unwarranted fear in the public." The behavior of Oprah Winfrey and Howard Lyman, stated the lawsuit, "goes beyond all possible bounds of decency and is utterly intolerable in a civilized community."[62]

After evaluating the cattlemen's case, however, the U.S. Fifth Circuit Court saw things differently. Said the judges, "Stripped to its essentials, the cattlemen's complaint is that the [Oprah] show did not present the Mad Cow issue in the light most favorable to United States beef."

Were Lyman's statements off base? Hardly. "Lyman's opinions," said the Court, "were based on truthful, established fact."[63] In fact, the Court pointed out that the opinions for which Howard Lyman and Oprah Winfrey were sued were virtually identical to the conclusions the FDA reached nine months later.

While time has shown Oprah Winfrey and Howard Lyman to have been correct in their stand, it has not been as kind to the statements made at the time of the trial by National Cattlemen's Beef Association product safety director James Reagan. He said that there was no evidence linking eating meat in Great Britain with developing the human form of the disease.[64] Today, the scientific consensus is so strong that even the National Cattlemen's Beef Association acknowledges that "nvCJD likely developed as a result of people consuming products contaminated with central nervous system tissue from cattle infected with BSE."[65]

At the conclusion of the trial, Oprah Winfrey stood on the courthouse steps and made two statements. The first was widely reported in the mainstream media. She said, "The first amendment not only lives, it rocks." But she also made another statement that was not nearly as widely reported. What she said was this:

"I'm still never going to eat another burger."

What we know

Statement made by Gary Weber that was edited out of the Oprah show, but that the cattlemen felt was important and should have remained: "The cattle industry adopted a voluntary ban on 'recycling' felled cattle as feed."

Reality: The "voluntary" ban was initiated just before the show, and had no impact whatsoever on industry feeding practices; agricultural extension agents and feed salesmen confirmed that the practice of feeding rendered cattle back to cattle continued and may even have increased after the voluntary ban was declared.[66]

Another statement made by Gary Weber that was edited out of the *Oprah* show, that the cattlemen felt was important and should have remained: "What is fed to cattle . . . has been cooked at temperatures high enough to sterilize it."

Reality: The infectious agent of Mad Cow disease remains infectious even after exposure for an hour to a temperature of 680 degrees—enough to melt lead—and can withstand antibiotics, boiling water, bleach, formaldehyde, and a variety of solvents, detergents, and enzymes known to destroy most known bacteria and viruses.[67]

Sixteen months after the *Oprah* show, the FDA formally banned the practice of feeding cow meat and bone meal back to cows. But the practice of feeding pigs and chickens the bones, brains, meat scraps, feathers, and feces of their own species remained legal and widespread in the United States as this book went to press.

And the U.S. meat industry was still adamantly asserting that Mad Cow disease did not exist in the United States, so there was little reason to worry about the safety of U.S. meat. They could be right, but there are some disturbing realities.

In 2001, the FDA reported that hundreds of U.S. livestock feed producers were systematically violating the very regulations meant to keep Mad Cow disease out of the country. After inspecting feed mills and rendering plants, the FDA concluded that the rules intended to keep American livestock from eating slaughtered animal parts linked to the deadly brain disease were regularly flouted.[68]

According to the FDA, only two-thirds of licensed feed mills are ever inspected, and more than 20 percent of these mills do not follow FDA rules designed to keep Mad Cow disease at bay. "Worse," noted a prominent meat industry journal, "there are about 8,000 feed mills that aren't even licensed at all, and less than one-half of those have ever had an FDA inspection. . . . USDA likes to tout the fact that 'thousands' of suspect cattle have had brain tissues examined post-mortem to ensure that no signs of the degeneration common to Mad Cow disease are present, and none have ever been found. That sounds impressive, until you stop to consider that millions of cattle are slaughtered *every week*."[69]

In reality, out of 900 million U.S. cattle slaughtered in the last decade, the USDA only tested 12,000 for Mad Cow disease—roughly one in every 75,000 cattle.[70] Meanwhile, the stakes are extremely high. One infected animal whose remains are "rendered," powdered and mixed into feed, could potentially infect thousands of other animals, and the thousands of people who eat them.

Meanwhile, the method of air-injected stunning used in most U.S. packing plants potentially drives central nervous system tissue from the brain into the bloodstream of cattle.

The U.S. beef industry continually expresses confidence in the nation's firewall, and says there is little risk to consumers. But as Newsweek noted in a March 12, 2001, cover story on Mad Cow disease, "In truth, however, America's safeguards and surveillance efforts are far weaker than most people realize."

The expected rate of occurrence of CJD (the human variation of Mad Cow disease) has been 1 in 1 million people. Up until the advent of Mad Cow disease, CJD was, literally, a "one-in-a-million" disease. Yet in one U.S. study, when people diagnosed with Alzheimer's disease (whose symptoms can be difficult to distinguish from CJD) were examined after death, 5.5 percent of the presumed Alzheimer's victims were found actually to have CJD.[71] And in a study at Yale University, when people diagnosed with Alzheimer's disease were examined after death it was found that 13 percent of the presumed Alzheimer's victims actually had CJD.[72]

Four million Americans are currently diagnosed with Alzheimer's.[73]

PART **II**

Our Food,
Our Fellow
Creatures

chapter 9 **The Pig Farmer**

One day in Iowa I met a particular gentleman—and I use that term, *gentleman,* frankly, only because I am trying to be polite, for that is certainly not how I saw him at the time. He owned and ran what he called a "pork production facility." I, on the other hand, would have called it a pig Auschwitz.

The conditions were brutal. The pigs were confined in cages that were barely larger than their own bodies, with the cages stacked on top of each other in tiers, three high. The sides and the bottoms of the cages were steel slats, so that excrement from the animals in the upper and middle tiers dropped through the slats on to the animals below.

The aforementioned owner of this nightmare weighed, I am sure, at least 240 pounds, but what was even more impressive about his appearance was that he seemed to be made out of concrete. His movements had all the fluidity and grace of a brick wall.

What made him even less appealing was that his language seemed to consist mainly of grunts, many of which sounded alike to me, and none of which were particularly pleasant to hear. Seeing how rigid he was and sensing the overall quality of his presence, I—rather brilliantly, I thought—concluded that his difficulties had not arisen merely because he hadn't had time, that particular morning, to finish his entire daily yoga routine.

But I wasn't about to divulge my opinions of him or his operation, for I was undercover, visiting slaughterhouses and feedlots to learn what I could about modern meat production. There were no bumper stickers on my car, and my clothes and hairstyle were carefully chosen to give no indication that I might have philosophical leanings other than those that were common in the area. I told the farmer matter of factly that I was a researcher writing about animal agriculture, and asked if he'd mind speaking with me for a few minutes so that I might have the benefit of his knowledge. In response, he grunted a few words that I could not decipher, but that I gathered meant I could ask him questions and he would show me around.

I was at this point not very happy about the situation, and this feeling did not improve when we entered one of the warehouses that housed his pigs. In fact, my distress increased, for I was immediately struck by what I can only call an overpowering olfactory experience. The place reeked like you would not believe of ammonia, hydrogen sulfide, and other noxious gases that were the products of the animals' wastes. These, unfortunately, seemed to have been piling up inside the building for far too long a time.

As nauseating as the stench was for me, I wondered what it must be like for the animals. The cells that detect scent are known as ethmoidal cells. Pigs, like dogs, have nearly 200 times the concentration of these cells in their noses as humans do. In a natural setting, they are able, while rooting around in the dirt, to detect the scent of an edible root through the earth itself.

Given any kind of a chance, they will never soil their own nests, for they are actually quite clean animals, despite the reputation we have unfairly given them. But here they had no contact with the earth, and their noses were beset by the unceasing odor of their own urine and feces multiplied a thousand times by the accumulated wastes of the other pigs unfortunate enough to be caged in that warehouse. I was in the building only for a few minutes, and the longer I remained in there, the more desperately I wanted to leave. But the pigs were prisoners there, barely able to take a single step, forced to endure this stench, and almost completely immobile, 24 hours a day, seven days a week, and with no time off, I can assure you, for holidays.

The man who ran the place was—I'll give him this—kind enough to answer my questions, which were mainly about the drugs he used to handle problems such as African Swine Fever, cholera, trichinosis, and other swine diseases that are fairly common in factory pigs today. But my sentiments about him and his farm were not becoming any warmer. It didn't help when, in response to a particularly loud squealing from one of the pigs, he delivered a sudden and threatening kick to the bars of its cage, causing a loud "clang" to reverberate through the warehouse and leading to screaming from many of the pigs.

Because it was becoming increasingly difficult to hide my distress, it crossed my mind that I should tell him what I thought of the conditions in which he kept his pigs, but then I thought better of it. This was a man, it was obvious, with whom there was no point in arguing.

After maybe 15 minutes, I'd had enough and was preparing to leave, and I felt sure he was glad to be about to be rid of me. But then something happened, something that changed my life, forever—and, as it turns out, his too. It began when his wife came out from the farmhouse and cordially invited me to stay for dinner.

The pig farmer grimaced when his wife spoke, but he dutifully turned to me and announced, "The wife would like you to stay for dinner." He always called her "the wife," by the way, which led me to deduce that he was not, apparently, on the leading edge of feminist thought in the country today.

I don't know whether you have ever done something without having a clue why, and to this day I couldn't tell you what prompted me to do it, but I said Yes, I'd be delighted. And stay for dinner I did, though I didn't eat the pork they served. The excuse I gave was that my doctor was worried about my cholesterol. I didn't say that I was a vegetarian, nor that my cholesterol was 125.

I was trying to be a polite and appropriate dinner guest. I didn't want to say anything that might lead to any kind of disagreement. The couple (and their two sons, who were also at the table) were, I could see, being nice to me, giving me dinner and all, and it was gradually becoming clear to me that, along with all the rest of it, they could be, in their way, somewhat decent people. I asked myself, if they were in my town, traveling, and I had chanced to meet them, would I have invited them to dinner? Not likely, I knew, not likely at all. Yet here they were, being as hospitable to me as they could. Yes, I had to admit it. Much as I detested how the pigs were treated, this pig farmer wasn't actually the reincarnation of Adolph Hitler. At least not at the moment.

Of course, I still knew that if we were to scratch the surface we'd no doubt find ourselves in great conflict, and because that was not a direction in which I wanted to go, as the meal went along I sought to keep things on an even and constant keel. Perhaps they sensed it too, for among us, we managed to see that the conversation remained, consistently and resolutely, shallow.

We talked about the weather, about the Little League games in which their two sons played, and then, of course, about how the weather might affect the Little League games. We were actually doing rather well at keeping the conversation superficial and far from any topic around which conflict might occur. Or so I thought. But then suddenly, out of nowhere, the man pointed at me forcefully with his finger, and snarled in a voice that I must say truly frightened me, "Sometimes I wish you animal rights people would just drop dead."

How on Earth he knew I had any affinity to animal rights I will never know—I had painstakingly avoided any mention of any such thing—but I do know that my stomach tightened immediately into a knot. To make matters worse, at that moment his two sons leapt from the table, tore into the den, slammed the door behind them, and turned the TV on loud, presumably preparing to drown out what was to follow. At the same instant, his wife nervously picked up some dishes and scurried into the kitchen. As I watched the door close behind her and heard the water begin running, I had a sinking sensation. They had, there was no mistaking it, left me alone with him.

I was, to put it bluntly, terrified. Under the circumstances, a wrong move now could be disastrous. Trying to center myself, I tried to find some semblance of inner calm by watching my breath, but this I could not do, and for a very simple reason. There wasn't any to watch.

"What are they saying that's so upsetting to you?" I said finally, pronouncing the words carefully and distinctly, trying not to show my terror. I was trying very hard at that moment to disassociate myself from the animal rights movement, a force in our society of which he, evidently, was not overly fond.

"They accuse me of mistreating my stock," he growled.

"Why would they say a thing like that?" I answered, knowing full well, of course, why they would, but thinking mostly about my own survival. His reply, to my surprise, while angry, was actually quite articulate. He told me precisely what animal rights groups were saying about operations like his, and exactly why they were opposed to his way of doing things. Then, without pausing, he launched into a tirade about how he didn't like being called cruel, and they didn't know anything about the business he was in, and why couldn't they mind their own business.

As he spoke it, the knot in my stomach was relaxing, because it was becoming clear, and I was glad of it, that he meant me no harm, but just needed to vent. Part of his frustration, it seemed, was that even though he didn't like doing some of the things he did to the animals — cooping them up in such small cages, using so many drugs, taking the babies away from their mothers so quickly after their births — he didn't see that he had any choice. He would be at a disadvantage and unable to compete economically if he didn't do things that way. This is how it's done today, he told me, and he had to do it too. He didn't like it, but he liked even less being blamed for doing what he had to do in order to feed his family.

As it happened, I had just the week before been at a much larger hog operation, where I learned that it was part of their business strategy to try to put people like him out of business by going full-tilt into the mass production of assembly-line pigs, so that small farmers wouldn't be able to keep up. What I had heard corroborated everything he was saying.

Almost despite myself, I began to grasp the poignancy of this man's human predicament. I was in his home because he and his wife had invited me to be there. And looking around, it was obvious that they were having a hard time making ends meet. Things were threadbare. This family was on the edge.

Raising pigs, apparently, was the only way the farmer knew how to make a living, so he did it even though, as was becoming evident the more we talked, he didn't like one bit the direction hog farming was going. At times, as he spoke about how much he hated the modern factory methods of pork production, he reminded me of the very animal rights people who a few minutes before he said he wished would drop dead.

As the conversation progressed, I actually began to develop some sense of respect for this man whom I had earlier judged so harshly. There was decency in him. There was something within him that meant well. But as I began to sense a spirit of goodness in him, I could only wonder all the more how he could treat his pigs the way he did. Little did I know that I was about to find out. . .

We are talking along, when suddenly he looks troubled. He slumps over, his head in his hands. He looks broken, and there is a sense of something awful having happened.

Has he had a heart attack? A stroke? I'm finding it hard to breathe, and hard to think clearly. "What's happening?" I ask.

It takes him awhile to answer, but finally he does. I am relieved that he is able to speak, although what he says hardly brings any clarity to the situation. "It doesn't matter," he says, "and I don't want to talk about it." As he speaks, he makes a motion with his hand, as if he were pushing something away.

For the next several minutes we continue to converse, but I'm quite uneasy. Things seem incomplete and confusing. Something dark has entered the room, and I don't know what it is or how to deal with it.

Then, as we are speaking, it happens again. Once again a look of despondency comes over him. Sitting there, I know I'm in the presence of something bleak and oppressive. I try to be present with what's happening, but it's not easy. Again I'm finding it hard to breathe.

Finally, he looks at me, and I notice his eyes are teary. "You're right," he says. I, of course, always like to be told that I am right, but in this instance I don't have the slightest idea what he's talking about.

He continues. "No animal," he says, "should be treated like that. Especially hogs. Do you know that they're intelligent animals? They're even friendly, if you treat 'em right. But I don't."

There are tears welling up in his eyes. And he tells me that he has just had a memory come back of something that happened in his childhood, something he hasn't thought of for many years. It's come back in stages, he says.

He grew up, he tells me, on a small farm in rural Missouri, the old-fashioned kind where animals ran around, with barnyards and pastures, and where they all had names. I learn, too, that he was an only child, the son of a powerful father who ran things with an iron fist. With no brothers or sisters, he often felt lonely, but found companionship among the animals on the farm, particularly several dogs, who were as friends to him. And, he tells me, and this I am quite surprised to hear, he had a pet pig.

As he proceeds to tell me about this pig, it is as if he is becoming a different person. Before he had spoken primarily in a monotone; but now his voice grows lively. His body language, which until this point seemed to speak primarily of long suffering, now becomes animated. There is something fresh taking place.

In the summer, he tells me, he would sleep in the barn. It was cooler there than in the house, and the pig would come over and sleep alongside him, asking fondly to have her belly rubbed, which he was glad to do.

There was a pond on their property, he goes on, and he liked to swim in it when the weather was hot, but one of the dogs would get excited when he did, and would ruin things. The dog would jump into the water and swim up on top of him, scratching him with her paws and making things miserable for him. He was about to give up on swimming, but then, as fate would have it, the pig, of all people, stepped in and saved the day.

Evidently the pig could swim, for she would plop herself into the water, swim out where the dog was bothering the boy, and insert herself between them. She'd stay between the dog and the boy, and keep the dog at bay. She was, as best I could make out, functioning in the situation something like a lifeguard, or in this case, perhaps more of a life-pig.

I'm listening to this hog farmer tell me these stories about his pet pig, and I'm thoroughly enjoying both myself and him, and rather astounded at how things are transpiring, when once again, it happens. Once again a look of defeat sweeps across this man's face, and once again I sense the presence of something very sad. Something in him, I know, is struggling to make its way toward life through anguish and pain, but I don't know what it is or how, indeed, to help him.

"What happened to your pig?" I ask.

He sighs, and it's as though the whole world's pain is contained in that sigh. Then, slowly, he speaks. "My father made me butcher it."

"Did you?" I ask.

"I ran away, but I couldn't hide. They found me."

"What happened?"

"My father gave me a choice."

"What was that?"

"He told me, 'You either slaughter that animal or you're no longer my son.'"

Some choice, I think, feeling the weight of how fathers have so often trained their sons not to care, to be what they call brave and strong, but what so often turns out to be callous and closed-hearted.

"So I did it," he says, and now his tears begin to flow, making their way down his cheeks. I am touched and humbled. This man, whom I had judged to be without human feeling, is weeping in front of me, a stranger. This man, whom I had seen as callous and even heartless, is actually someone who cares, and deeply. How wrong, how profoundly and terribly wrong I had been.

In the minutes that follow, it becomes clear to me what has been happening. The pig farmer has remembered something that was so painful, that was such a profound trauma, that he had not been able to cope with it when it had happened. Something had shut down, then. It was just too much to bear.

Somewhere in his young, formative psyche he made a resolution never to be that hurt again, never to be that vulnerable again. And he built a wall around the place where the pain had occurred, which was the place where his love and attachment to that pig was located, which was his heart. And now here he was, slaughtering pigs for a living—still, I imagined, seeking his father's approval. God, what we men will do, I thought, to get our fathers' acceptance.

I had thought he was a cold and closed human being, but now I saw the truth. His rigidity was not a result of a lack of feeling, as I had thought it was, but quite the opposite: it was a sign of how sensitive he was underneath. For if he had not been so sensitive, he would not have been that hurt, and he would not have needed to put up so massive a wall. The tension in his body that was so apparent to me upon first meeting him, the body armor that he carried, bespoke how hurt he had been, and how much capacity for feeling he carried still, beneath it all.

I had judged him, and done so, to be honest, mercilessly. But for the rest of the evening I sat with him, humbled, and grateful for whatever it was in him that had been strong enough to force this long-buried and deeply painful memory to the surface. And glad, too, that I had not stayed stuck in my judgments of him, for if I had, I would not have provided an environment in which his remembering could have occurred.

We talked that night, for hours, about many things. I was, after all that had happened, concerned for him. The gap between his feelings and his lifestyle seemed so tragically vast. What could he do? This was all he knew. He did not have a high school diploma. He was only partially literate. Who would hire him if he tried to do something else? Who would invest in him and train him, at his age?

When finally, I left that evening, these questions were very much on my mind, and I had no answers to them. Somewhat flippantly, I tried to joke about it. "Maybe," I said, "you'll grow broccoli or something." He stared at me, clearly not comprehending what I might be talking about. It occurred to me, briefly, that he might possibly not know what broccoli was.

We parted that night as friends, and though we rarely see each other now, we have remained friends as the years have passed. I carry him in my heart and think of him, in fact, as a hero. Because, as you will soon see, impressed as I was by the courage it had taken for him to allow such painful memories to come to the surface, I had not yet seen the extent of his bravery.

When I wrote *Diet for a New America,* I quoted him and summarized what he had told me, but I was quite brief and did not mention his name. I thought that, living as he did among other pig farmers in Iowa, it would not be to his benefit to be associated with me.

When the book came out, I sent him a copy, saying I hoped he was comfortable with how I wrote of the evening we had shared, and directing him to the pages on which my discussion of our time together was to be found.

Several weeks later, I received a letter from him. "Dear Mr. Robbins," it began. "Thank you for the book. When I saw it, I got a migraine headache."

Now as an author, you do want to have an impact on your readers. This, however, was not what I had had in mind.

He went on, though, to explain that the headaches had gotten so bad that, as he put it, "the wife" had suggested to him he should perhaps read the book. She thought there might be some kind of connection between the headaches and the book. He told me that this hadn't made much sense to him, but he had done it because "the wife" was often right about these things.

"You write good," he told me, and I can tell you that his three words of his meant more to me than when the *New York Times* praised the book profusely. He then went on to say that reading the book was very hard for him, because the light it shone on what he was doing made it clear to him that it was wrong to continue. The headaches, meanwhile, had been getting worse, until, he told me, that very morning, when he had finished the book, having stayed up all night reading, he went into the bathroom, and looked into the mirror. "I decided, right then," he said, "that I would sell my herd and get out of this business. I don't know what I will do, though. Maybe I will, like you said, grow broccoli."

As it happened, he did sell his operation in Iowa and move back to Missouri, where he bought a small farm. And there he is today, running something of a model farm. He grows vegetables organically—including, I am sure, broccoli—that he sells at a local farmer's market. He's got pigs, all right, but only about 10, and he doesn't cage them, nor does he kill them. Instead, he's got a contract with local schools; they bring kids out in buses on field trips to his farm, for his "Pet-a-pig" program. He shows them how intelligent pigs are and how friendly they can be if you treat them right, which he now does. He's arranged it so the kids, each one of them, gets a chance to give a pig a belly rub. He's become nearly a vegetarian himself, has lost most of his excess weight, and his health has improved substantially. And, thank goodness, he's actually doing better financially than he was before.

Do you see why I carry this man with me in my heart? Do you see why he is such a hero to me? He dared to leap, to risk everything, to leave what was killing his spirit even though he didn't know what was next. He left behind a way of life that he knew was wrong, and he found one that he knows is right.

When I look at many of the things happening in our world, I sometimes fear we won't make it. But when I remember this man and the power of his spirit, and when I remember that there are many others whose hearts beat to the same quickening pulse, I think we will.

I can get tricked into thinking there aren't enough of us to turn the tide, but then I remember how wrong I was about the pig farmer when I first met him, and I realize that there are heroes afoot everywhere. Only I can't recognize them because I think they are supposed to look or act a certain way. How blinded I can be by my own beliefs.

The man is one of my heroes because he reminds me that we can depart from the cages we build for ourselves and for each other, and become something much better. He is one of my heroes because he reminds me of what I hope someday to become.

When I first met him, I would not have thought it possible that I would ever say the things I am saying here. But this only goes to show how amazing life can be, and how you never really know what to expect. The pig farmer has become, for me, a reminder never to underestimate the power of the human heart.

I consider myself privileged to have spent that day with him, and grateful that I was allowed to be a catalyst for the unfolding of his spirit. I know my presence served him in some way, but I also know, and know full well, that I received far more than I gave.

To me, this is grace—to have the veils lifted from our eyes so that we can recognize and serve the goodness in each other. Others may wish for great riches or for ecstatic journeys to mystical planes, but to me, this is the magic, and the implacable grandeur, of human life.

chapter 10

Old McDonald Had a Factory

I can still see it. The opening and closing ceremonies of the Olympic games, until recently, included the release of hundreds of white doves. These beautiful birds ascending into the sky produced a dramatic sight.

But we don't do that anymore. Why? Because it dawned on us that while the ritual provided us with entertainment and a sense of wonder, it was cruel. What we were actually seeing were birds who had been trucked in, crowded underground, and then propelled upward, and who were terrified, confused, and disorganized. What we were seeing were birds who were exhausted and panicked, and who, trying to fend for themselves in strange surroundings, would perish as a result of the theatrical display. At the Korean games, many of the frightened and disoriented doves actually flew into the Olympic flame, with the result that the millions watching were treated to the less than inspiring spectacle of seeing the birds burned alive.

There are still many places, including Disneyland, where dove releases persist. But as people have started to be more aware of what really takes place, the practice has become for many people as unappealing as cock-fighting, bull-fighting, dog-fighting, or any other form of "entertainment" in which animals are mutilated or killed.

Before I knew better, I liked watching the doves be released. I never thought of the actual birds, or what happened to them. I assumed they just flew free. But once you know, you can never forget.

So often I've been blind.

I remember, when I was a child, thinking that fur coats were fabulous. I never imagined that fur-bearing animals trapped in the wild inevitably suffer slow, agonizing deaths. Or that when we purchase the products of fur farms, we support massive animal pain and death. But slowly it dawned on me that, as beautiful as furs are, they look a lot better on their original owners (the foxes, minks, and other animals from whom they were taken). When I see someone wearing a fur now, I don't see a fashion statement, I see ignorance of the pain that is involved, and I see cruelty.

When I was a child, I would go to a friend's house where there were deer heads on the walls. I thought they were cool. But comedian Ellen DeGeneres has a point when she says, "You ask people why they have deer heads on the wall. They always say, 'Because it's such a beautiful animal.' There you go. I think my mother's attractive, but I have photographs of her."

I remember thinking ivory was incredible. I thought wearing an ivory bracelet gave you some connection to the elephants, and maybe even let you carry some of their awesome power. I didn't want anyone to limit my freedom and tell me I shouldn't buy or use ivory. But now I know there's nothing positive about the merchandising of extinction.

We're learning that there's nothing cool about cruelty, but sometimes we still have to rethink our attitudes. I used to think it was great to see dogs and cats have litters. The puppies and kittens were so adorable. But then I learned how great is our cat and dog overpopulation problem. Seventy thousand puppies and kittens are born every day in the United States, and only 15,000 of them will ever be adopted as pets. Twenty million cats and dogs are killed each year at U.S. animal shelters because there are no homes for them. Now I think "Neuter is cuter."

It's amazing to me how good I was at *not* seeing animal suffering, even when, or maybe particularly when, my own actions were causing pain. I didn't want to see it. I wanted to keep my eyes closed, lest I be troubled by the pain and feelings of helplessness that such awareness can bring.

This is another of the reasons the pig farmer is one of my heroes. He broke through the wall of denial. He saw that what he was doing with his life was causing animals to suffer, and he decided, even though he did not know how he would manage to feed his family, to stop and find a better way. Armed only with the depth of his feeling that what he had long been doing was contrary to his own spirit and to the well-being of life, he did the one thing that many of us find the hardest to do, and the one thing that integrity always requires. He brought his life into alignment with his heart.

What gave him the strength to do this? I believe it was not only that his childhood feelings reemerged with such force. This was important, but it took something else, too. I believe he drew strength, whether he knew it or not, from the changes that are sweeping across our society in the way we treat animals.

An awareness is dawning. We no longer allow entrepreneurs to trade in protected and endangered species. Every day more people are deciding not to purchase or wear furs, and not to condone trophy hunting. More and more frequently, people are asking whether it's really necessary to test oven cleaners and floor waxes by dripping them into the eyes of rabbits. And whether schoolchildren should be forced to dissect animals when there are more sophisticated learning techniques that yield more knowledge with less suffering.

You see the changes in many places. You see people refusing to buy shampoos or other body care products from companies that test on animals, and instead buying cosmetics and other household products that are made without cruelty.

We're learning to see what we didn't see before, and then, when we have the courage, creating the changes that make our lives congruent with what we know. Every day, you see people adopting animals from local pounds or shelters instead of puppy mills (which are really puppy hells). Every year, you see people coming to understand the responsibilities of having pets and treating their beloved animal companions as friends for life.

Once you start to notice the surging interest in compassion toward animals, you find it's everywhere. You see people working to create wildlife sanctuaries and to preserve natural habitat for wild animals. You see people choosing not to consume tunafish that isn't dolphin-safe, and others refusing to buy tunafish because they don't want to kill the tuna (magnificent creatures who may be the most powerful swimmers in the ocean, reaching speeds of up to 70 miles an hour). You see people starting to take crimes against animals seriously.

We're helping each other to become mature, and to accept the responsibility that allows us to be fully human. We're looking at our actions, and trying, when we can, to change those that are causing other beings to suffer.

This is what makes my heart sing—people making their lives into statements of compassion. I celebrate it with all my might. And yet there remains one area where most of us, whether we know it or not, still contribute quite directly to the unnecessary exploitation of animals. It is an area where, to this point, most of us haven't yet looked at the impact of our choices. And it is, strangely enough, the very area in our lives where most of us have the greatest direct contact with animals.

It's an area the pig farmer knows quite a lot about.

Not Humanity at Its Finest

Since ancient times, the industries and people who raise animals for meat, milk, and eggs were obligated to make sure that the basic needs of the animals in their care were met. If many animals fell sick or suffered from lack of food, water, or protection, the productivity of the operation suffered, as well as the animals. Livestock operators had a vested interest in the well-being of the animals they raised. They did well only if the animals did well.

It made sense, historically, for farmers to place animals in environments as harmonious to them as possible, and to protect the animals from predators, weather extremes, drought, and famine. The image of the biblical shepherd leading his animals to green pastures suggests how long this way of life persisted.

Much changed, with the advent of intensive factory farming. Modern technology has made possible a shift in the time-honored responsibility livestock producers had for the welfare of their animals. Starting in the last half of the twentieth century, it began to be not only pos-

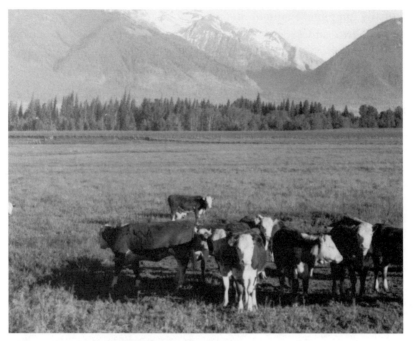

For centuries, farm animals have grazed in pastures.

sible, but economically advantageous, to raise animals in conditions that are completely unnatural and unhealthy and that frustrate virtually all of their urges and instincts.

Although extreme crowding of animals greatly increases the rates of the animals' illnesses and deaths, it nevertheless also raises profits. Even when more than 20 percent of pigs and chickens die prematurely in today's intensive husbandry systems, for instance, producers find their profits increased by such practices.

The overcrowding that's typical today would once have been unthinkable, because animals kept in such conditions would have been decimated by diseases. But now, with antibiotics mixed into every meal, with the widespread use of hormones, drugs, and biocides, enough of the animals can be kept alive so that overcrowding becomes cost-effective. Although nearly all of the animals get sick, and many die prematurely, the overall economic efficiency of the system is maximized.

It might seem obvious that animals born with bones and muscles are meant to move. But modern animal factories have found it pays to virtually immobilize animals in crates and cages. And although animals clearly have distinct social needs, factory farms now find it in their financial interest to raise billions of animals in conditions that so completely disregard these needs as to violate the animals' biological natures.

Chickens, for example, are highly social animals. In any kind of natural setting, be it a farmyard or the wild, they develop a social hierarchy, often known as a "pecking order." Every bird yields, at the food trough and elsewhere, to those above it in rank, and takes precedence over those below. The social order is extremely important to these birds. Ac-

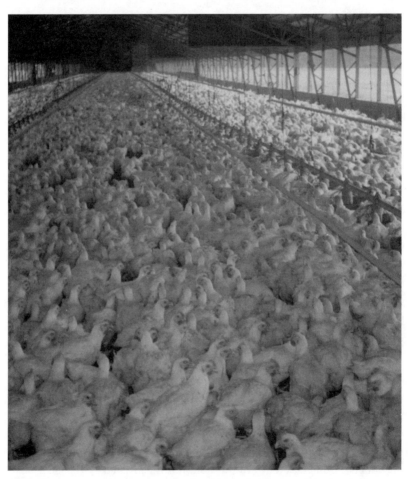

Today, "broiler" chickens are crammed by the tens of thousands into a single building.

cording to studies published in the *New Scientist*, chickens can maintain a stable pecking order, with each bird knowing all the others individually and aware of its place among them, in flocks with up to 90 chickens.[1] With more than 90 birds, however, things can get out of hand. In any kind of natural setting, flocks would never get that large. But in the warehouses where today's chickens are fattened for meat, flocks tend to be a larger than the 90-bird limit. How much larger? There are as many as 30,000 or more "broiler" chickens crowded together inside one building.

Layer hens, meanwhile, are crammed together in cages so tiny that they do not have enough space even to begin to lift a single wing. The amount of space the birds are given for their entire lives is less than they would have if you stuffed several of them into a file drawer. One building will frequently house 100,000 hens packed together under such conditions.

The industries behind all this, however, tell the public that it's all being done for the animals' own good. Immobilizing animals for their entire lives, they say, is done for the sake of the animals themselves. . .

IS THAT SO?

"Animal behavior is as varied as human behavior. In some cases, animals are restrained to avoid injuring themselves, other animals, or the farmer. All forms of restraint are designed for the welfare of the animal as well as efficiency of production."

—Animal Industry Foundation[2]

"One of the best things modern animal agriculture has going for it is that most people . . . haven't a clue how animals are raised and processed. . . . If most urban meat-eaters were to visit an industrial broiler house, to see how the birds are raised, and could see the birds being 'harvested' and then being 'processed' in a poultry processing plant, some, perhaps many of them, would swear off eating chicken and perhaps all meat. For modern animal agriculture, the less the consumer knows about what's happening before the meat hits the plate, the better."

—Peter R. Cheeke, Professor of Animal Science, Oregon State University; Editorial Board Member, *Journal of Animal Science*[3]

Pigs are highly sociable and active creatures, who will in a natural setting travel 30 miles a day grazing, rooting, and interacting with their environment. In the evening, groups of pigs will prepare a communal nest from branches and grass, in which they will spend the night together.[4]

In today's pig factories, however, pregnant sows are isolated and locked in individual narrow metal crates that are barely larger than the pigs' bodies. Unable to take a single step or turn around, they are restrained in this un-bedded, cement-floor crate for months at a time, subject to what the industry calls "full confinement" virtually all their lives. Some crates are so narrow that the animal is literally boxed in, almost completely immobilized, so that simply standing up or lying down

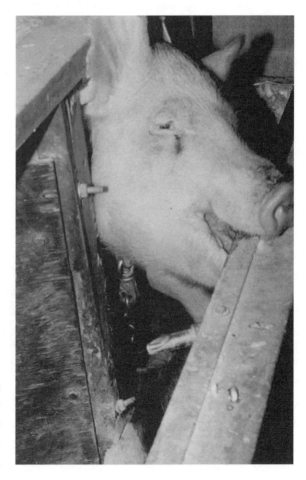

Pigs are almost completely immobilized in cages barely larger than their bodies.

require strenuous effort. Often, the sows are tied to the floor by a short chain or strap around their necks. Thus, these naturally gregarious and active animals are deprived of all social contact and all possibility of natural physical movement.[5]

Meanwhile, the industry tells the public it wouldn't think of mistreating these animals. . . .

Is that so?

"Animal welfare is the cornerstone of good animal husbandry. . . . Confinement rearing has its precedents. Schools are examples of 'confinement rearing' of children which, if handled properly, are effective."
—National Live Stock and Meat Board[6]

"U.S. society is extremely naïve about the nature of [animal] agricultural production. . . . In fact, if the public knew more about the way in which agricultural animal production infringes on animal welfare, the outcry would be louder. . . . If the public knew, for instance, that some swine [pigs] raised in total confinement literally never see the light of day, it would be more, not less, hostile to current agriculture."
—Bernard Rollin, Colorado State University expert on animal farming, author of more than 150 papers and 10 books on ethics and animal science[7]

The Veil Begins to Lift

If a substantial percentage of the public became aware of how farm animals are treated today, there would be changes. But the meat, dairy, and egg industries have sought to perpetuate the myth that the animals are perfectly content. The Perdue chicken company, for example, has boasted of raising "happy chickens." Meat packages are sometimes decorated with pictures of happy animals peacefully cavorting in idyllic conditions. The Carnation Company has presented ads portraying "contented cows." Egg cartons often carry drawings of joyful hens, dancing under the blessings of a smiling sun.

That's for the public. Industry journals, however, reveal a slightly different picture.

"What we are really trying to do is to modify the animal's environment for maximum profit. . . . Forget the pig is an animal. Treat him just like a machine in a factory." (Hog Farm Management)[8]

In Great Britain, the veil began to be lifted, and public consciousness began to be raised as early as the late 1960s, when Ruth Harrison's book *Animal Machines* introduced the public to industrialized agriculture. The book mobilized social concern to the point that the British government appointed a royal commission to investigate. In confinement farming, Harrison warned, "cruelty is acknowledged only where profitability ceases."[9]

In the United States, popular understanding of the realities of modern meat production was first sparked in the late 1970s, when Peter Singer wrote the seminal *Animal Liberation*, followed in 1980 by the classic book *Animal Factories*, co-written with Jim Mason. In the late 1980s, *Diet for a New America* brought the issue to the attention of a great number of people, and contributed to the wider cultural awareness of how our livestock are treated. Noting the human health consequences to factory farming, I wrote . . .

"Increasingly, in the last few decades, the animals raised for meat, dairy products and eggs in the United States have been subjected to ever more deplorable conditions. Merely to keep the poor creatures alive under these circumstances, even more chemicals have had to be used, and increasingly, hormones, pesticides, antibiotics and other chemicals and drugs end up in foods derived from animals." (Diet for a New America)[10]

How do you think the cattlemen countered this charge? Responding to this statement, they wrote,

"An analogy would be to say that 'increasingly, in the last few decades, humans have been subjected to ever more deplorable conditions as they moved from rural homes (with no running water, no plumbing, no electricity and no indoor toilet) into urban homes (with central air and heat, telephones, electricity, plumbing, running water, and indoor toilets). It's true that more chemicals are used now than then, for humans and farm animals, but not merely to keep them alive (but) because they improve living conditions." (National Cattlemen's Association's response to *Diet for a New America*)[11]

The U.S. meat and dairy industries have sometimes responded to the growing public awareness of the animal suffering in factory farms by trying to deny that there is any problem. . .

Is THAT SO?

"Don't worry about farm animals. Today's farmers treat their livestock with the same caring concern as ordinary people treat their pets."
— Robert "Butch" Johnson, poultry producer[12]

"Agribusiness companies tell us that animals in factory farms are 'as well cared for as their own pet dog or cat.' Nothing could be further from the truth. The life of an animal in a factory farm is characterized by acute deprivation, stress, and disease. Hundreds of millions of animals are forced to live in cages or crates just barely larger than their own bodies. While one species may be caged alone without any social contact, another species may be crowded so tightly together that they fall prey to stress-induced cannibalism. Cannibalism is particularly prevalent in the cramped confinement of hogs and laying hens. Unable to groom, stretch their legs, or even turn around, the victims of factory farms exist in a relentless state of distress."
— Humane Farming Association[13]

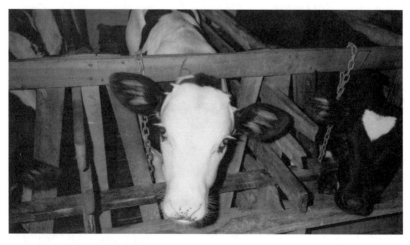

Many farm animals are chained in individual cages so small they cannot take a single step in their entire lives.

In the 1980s, in Sweden, children's author Astrid Lindgren, who was appalled by the treatment of animals in confinement systems, was leading a campaign that resulted in Swedish legislation that greatly restricts confinement agriculture and mandates that the rearing of animals be suited to the animals' natures. The law was passed by the Swedish Parliament virtually unopposed in 1987, and produced stunning benefits to public health as well as to animal welfare by greatly reducing the incidence of food-borne disease. By 1995, the editor of the U.S. journal *Meat and Poultry* was writing that, while there are more than 1 million cases of Salmonella poisoning in the United States annually, in Sweden the number had dropped to a mere 800.[14]

During the 1990s, laws prohibiting confinement rearing of pigs and cage rearing of poultry were passed in several other European countries. Meanwhile there were many groups in the United States working to educate ever more people about the actual conditions in which modern livestock are raised, and to strengthen the demand that changes be made to reduce the animals' suffering. But industry groups, often speaking through the Animal Industry Foundation, were opposing them at every turn.

WHAT WE KNOW

Organizations advocating the factory farming of livestock: Animal Industry Foundation, and their board of trustees, which includes the American Veal Association, National Cattlemen's Beef Association, National Chicken Council, National Milk Producers Council, National Pork Producers Council, National Turkey Federation, United Egg Producers, U.S. Poultry and Egg Association, American Feed Industry Association, and many others

Nonprofit groups dedicated to educating the public about the realities of factory farming: People for the Ethical Treatment of Animals (PETA), Humane Farming Association (HFA), Farm Sanctuary, Compassion in World Farming, Farm Animals Concern Trust (FACT), Farm Animal Reform Movement (FARM), United Poultry Concerns, GRACE Factory Farm Project, Friends of Animals, Animal Welfare Institute, Humane Society of the United States (HSUS), Animal Rights International, EarthSave, and many others

Ever eager to discredit anyone who openly discusses the way animals are treated in today's factory farms, some in the livestock industry say that those speaking out on behalf of animals don't know what they're talking about. . .

Is THAT SO?

"There are a lot of loud-mouthed activists out there who want everyone to think modern meat is produced on terrible factory farms where animals are mistreated. So boo-hoo. Most of these self-styled experts wouldn't know which part of a cow to milk."
—*The Beef-Eater's Guide to Modern Meat*[15]

"A common perception of livestock people is that animal rights activists don't understand the livestock industry (they don't 'get it,' in current terminology) because of their urban backgrounds. . . . The activists do 'get it,' they know what is going on, and they don't like it."
—Peter R. Cheeke, Professor of Animal Science, Oregon State University; Editorial Board Member, *Journal of Animal Science*[16]

Did Somebody Say McLibel?

In 1999, McDonald's was nominated for the prestigious Business Ethics Award, given by the judges at *Business Ethics* magazine. But the magazine decided not to grant the award to McDonald's. An open letter from the judges to McDonald's, published in the November/December 1999 issue of *Business Ethics*, explained why:

"We must express concern about slaughterhouse cruelty by McDonald's suppliers. . . . Federal standards require that 100 percent of cows be fully stunned before they are skinned, but (according to) . . . a McDonald's training video . . . it's acceptable if five cows in every 100 are conscious while skinned and dismembered. It's inhumane to allow animals to suffer in this manner. And the real error rate may be far more than 5 percent. . . . In the case of chickens, USDA recommendations say they should have at least 2 square feet of space, yet McDonald's suppliers allow only .55 square feet—not enough space for a chicken to spread one wing. In addition, birds are bred to grow so large, their legs can't bear the weight, and they suffer painful leg deformities. Surely it's not asking too much to change policies, so that these animals are granted a modicum of comfort. The problems cited here go beyond McDonald's. But McDonald's is the nation's largest purchaser of beef, and the second largest purchaser of poultry. It has clout. And as CEO Jack Greenburg himself said, McDonald's wants 'to take industry leadership in animal welfare.' If McDonald's required changes, suppliers would comply."

McDonald's has repeatedly claimed in public announcements that it's the industry leader in animal welfare. But the editors of *Business Ethics* were aware of the extraordinary "McLibel" trial in Great Britain, in which McDonald's sued five unemployed activists who had distributed a pamphlet finding fault with many of its practices. Two of the activists, Helen Steel and Dave Morris, with virtually no financial backing, proceeded to take on one of the world's largest multinational corporations in what became the longest running libel suit in British legal history. McDonald's fought bitterly, spending more than $16 million in legal fees.[17] But in 1997, when Chief Justice Roger Bell of the British High Court in London returned his lengthy findings, he said it had been proven that the animals that became McDonald's products were treated cruelly, and McDonald's was "culpably responsible" for this cruelty.[18] McDonald's subsequently appealed, but an Appeals Court judge agreed with the conclusions of the Chief Justice.

On the matter of chickens, Chief Justice Bell said, "Keeping large numbers of chickens in close confinement inevitably leads to disease. . . . The high density is intentional and unnecessary. . . . In my judgement it's cruel."

Cruel it may be, but more than 99 percent of U.S. eggs and poultry products come from birds kept in such conditions.

Among the many other factory farm practices Justice Bell deplored are the stalls in which pregnant and nursing pigs are kept for months at a time in a space so small the animals cannot even turn around. The judge wrote that "pigs are intelligent and sociable animals and I have no doubt that keeping pigs in dry sow stalls for extended periods is cruel."

Although this practice is now illegal in Great Britain and Sweden, and although the European Parliament has urged a complete ban on it throughout the European Economic Community, it continues to be routine procedure in the United States. In fact, 90 percent of U.S. pigs are raised in confinement, their behavioral and psychological needs totally thwarted, their survival in such conditions made possible only by the use of drugs, hormones, mutilations, and antibiotics.

McDonald's and the others in the meat, dairy, and egg industries repeatedly say that they do what they do in order to bring down the price of food. Making the kinds of changes that animal protection advocates would like, they say, would simply be too costly. But Justice Bell concluded that many cruel farming practices could be easily altered at minimal cost. "There was no evidence," he said, "that the cost would be increased significantly."

Today, the very practices that Chief Justice Bell found to be demonstrably cruel—and some that are far more severe—continue unabated in the United States. The reason? For one thing, the Federal Humane Slaughter Act requires that all animals (excluding birds) be stunned properly prior to slaughter, but the law carries no penalties and is rarely enforced. For another, 30 U.S. states specifically exempt "customary" or "normal" farming practices from the legal definition of animal cruelty. In other words, if the industry as a whole is doing it, then by definition it can't be outlawed. According to attorney David Wolfson, "In effect, state legislatures have granted agribusiness a legal license to treat farm animals as they wish."[19]

PETA Enters the Fray

After the McLibel trial, in 1997 the U.S.-based People for the Ethical Treatment of Animals (PETA) quietly contacted Mike Quinlan (then CEO of McDonald's), and asked, in light of the judgments made by the British Chief Justice, whether the corporation would be willing to take several specific steps to reduce unnecessary animal suffering.[20] If the corporation would show a genuine willingness to address the practices that the Chief Justice had found to be cruel, PETA said, they stood ready and eager to help.

PETA offered to publicly acknowledge McDonald's leadership in reducing animal suffering and cruelty, if the company would follow through on its stated commitment to animal welfare. As well, PETA offered to give McDonald's a free two-page promotional spread in its member magazine, which goes to more than 600,000 people, if the company would test-market a veggie burger nationwide.[21] This seemed reasonable, in that McDonald's restaurants in many European countries offer vegetarian burgers and vegetarian nuggets, and the market for veggie burgers in the United States has been expanding rapidly in recent years. But rather than refer these offers to someone with the authority to change policies and procedures, McDonald's assigned the entire issue of animal welfare and its discussions with PETA to the head of its public relations department.

For two years, PETA engaged in a series of frustrating discussions and negotiations with McDonald's. While these discussions were taking place, the industry continued its campaign to convince the public that industry practices, even those that might to the "inexperienced" observer seem cruel, were actually done for the animals' own good, and that anyone who said otherwise simply did not understand animal welfare.

> "To the inexperienced viewer, some routine farm handling practices necessary to the welfare and health of the animal and the insurance of quality food may appear brutal, just as some life-saving human surgical and medical practices may seem brutal to the casual observer. All of these practices are done . . . to ensure the welfare of the animal." (Animal Industry Foundation)[22]

Temple Grandin is McDonald's livestock handling consultant, and the author of the American Meat Institute's *Recommended Animal Handling Guidelines for Meat Packers*, plus more than 300 articles in both scientific journals and livestock periodicals on animal handling, welfare, and facility design. She also designed the systems in place in the meat plants in which nearly half the cattle in North America are handled. When asked for her input in the discussions underway between McDonald's and PETA, Dr. Grandin indicated that the corporation could with virtually no effort require suppliers to hire two stunners, thus markedly decreasing the number of animals who are skinned and dismembered while still conscious[23]—but the company chose not to do so.

Dr. Grandin also noted that the current way chickens are caught for slaughter causes a high incidence of broken wings and legs, and pointed out that in Britain there are incentive plans in place that are effective in reducing the injury and trauma to chickens.[24] But despite telling the Associated Press that "if Dr. Grandin sees a problem, we correct it," McDonald's again did nothing to improve the situation.[25]

Another McDonald's consultant told the corporation that it would be possible for McDonald's to obtain a reliable supply of cows and pigs that had been more humanely raised—if McDonald's would commit to purchasing them.[26] But the company's response was only to state, as it had done so often, that it's already the leader in animal welfare issues.

Finally, on August 12, 1999, PETA had had enough. In a letter to McDonald's new CEO expressing the organization's frustration, PETA wrote, "Two years of negotiations with McDonald's have proved that you care not one whit about the animals who are raised and killed for your restaurants. We are disappointed and saddened that McDonald's public pronouncements about commitment to animal welfare are nothing more than so much public relations. To date, McDonald's has not even attempted to require slaughterhouses to meet humane standards of slaughter as defined by the USDA."[27]

It was only after the breakdown of two years of frustrating negotiations that PETA in the fall of 1999 launched its international "McCruelty to go" campaign. Graphic billboards and newspaper advertisements—reading "Do you want fries with that? McCruelty to go," above a picture of a slaughtered cow's head—were created to inform consumers about McDonald's failure to implement basic reforms. Despite continual pronouncements from McDonald's about their commitment to animal welfare, PETA noted, the corporation was still serving the flesh and eggs of animals whose lives were characterized by abject misery, and the hamburger chain still had no mechanism in place to penalize slaughterhouses that consistently skin and dismember conscious animals.

Eleven months later, after PETA had conducted more than 400 demonstrations in 23 countries, McDonald's finally budged. In late August 2000, the giant company announced an effort to make improvements in the lives of chickens raised for its restaurants. McDonald's

Corporation sent letters to the suppliers providing the company with 1.5 billion eggs yearly, outlining new regulations for raising hens.

The new guidelines called for chickens to have more space than they did previously (from an average of seven to eight hens per 18-inch-by-20-inch cage to a maximum of five), and for the elimination of "forced molting" (the starving of hens in order to increase egg production). At the same time, McDonald's called for chickens to be caught by more humane methods prior to slaughter, and started auditing slaughter-houses. And for the first time in its history, McDonald's threatened to cut off suppliers who were not in compliance with humane slaughter guidelines. Applauding these steps, PETA declared a one-year moratorium on the campaign against the company.

These were significant steps, and they were important. But Ronald McDonald was still some distance from deserving a halo over his bright orange wig. None of the proposed changes, even if fully implemented, would bring the company up to the basic standards that were already in place in Europe.

Not ones to rest on their laurels, PETA publicly thanked McDonald's, and proceeded in 2001 to launch a campaign to compel Burger King to institute the same improvements McDonald's now had in place. It took more than 1,000 protests at Burger King restaurants, but the fast food chain eventually agreed to demands by PETA to improve slaughterhouse and factory farm conditions for animals. The new standards, agreed to in the summer of 2001, actually went several steps beyond those pledged by McDonald's.

When PETA next turned its focus on Wendy's, the dominoes continued to fall. Two months later, that fast food chain announced it would substantially improve its animal welfare standards.

It appeared that the suffering of the animals destined for America's dinner plates was finally coming to be taken seriously.

In something of an understatement, PETA's Bruce Friedrich commented, "We in the U.S. still have a long way to go."

chapter 11 # Misery on the Menu

Have you ever known an animal and been enriched as a human being through that relationship? Many of us have known dogs, cats, or other animals to be true friends, and even, in some cases, members of our families.

I wonder why it is, though, that we call some animals "pets," and lavish our love and care on them, and then turn around and call other animals "dinner," and allow them to be treated as if they had no feelings or needs of their own.

The Veal Calf

The animal whose treatment has come most to symbolize what's wrong with modern animal factories is the veal calf. From his first day to his last, the life of a "milk-fed" veal calf is one of deprivation, disease, and loneliness. Taken away from his mother shortly after birth, he is chained at the neck into a tiny stall measuring only 22 inches wide and 58 inches long. The veal calf would actually have more space if, instead of chaining him

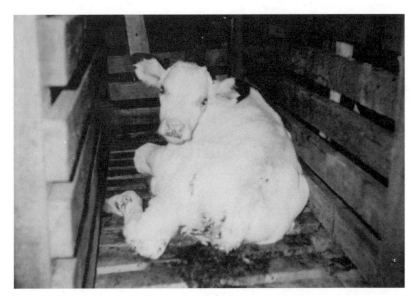

Newborn male calves born to dairy cows are caged in individual stalls. They remain in these stalls, never leaving, until they are slaughtered for veal.

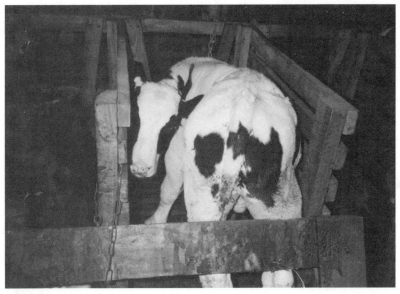

As the months go by and the veal calves grow, they become virtually wedged into their stalls.

in such a stall, you stuffed him into the trunk of a subcompact car and kept him there for his entire life.

Unable to take a single step, unable even to lie down in his natural sleeping posture, he will remain in this stall for four months until he is slaughtered. In many veal barns, the animals are kept in total darkness except for two short feeding times a day.

It's not just animal advocates who find this deploreable. Many ranchers and others in the meat industry privately recognize the cruelty involved in veal production. Bernard Rollin is a Colorado State University expert on animal farming and author of more than 150 papers and 10 books on ethics and animal science. He says,

> "The average person sees white veal as a decadent product, analogous to the *pate de foie gras* produced by force-feeding geese whose feet have been nailed to a board. . . . Some years ago, I had been asked by the Colorado commissioner of agriculture to participate in a seminar on the issues of animal rights and animal welfare for the leaders of Colorado agriculture. Among the speakers was a drug company executive representing the Animal Industry Foundation. . . . He began his presentation by showing a short video called *The Other Side of the Fence*, produced by the American Society for the Prevention of Cruelty to Animals. The video is highly critical of white veal production, arguing that just as human babies have needs, so do calves. Though we try to meet the needs of babies, we do not in the case of calves raised for veal. His stated purpose in showing the tape was to demonstrate the sophisticated level of propaganda directed by animal groups against animal agriculture, in order to galvanize the audience into opposing such activity. A few hours later, I sat with the head of the Colorado Farm Bureau and the president of the Colorado Cattlemen's Association. I asked them for their reaction to the film. The Cattlemen's Association president replied: 'It brought tears to my eyes. There is no cause to raise animals that way. . . . We don't have to torture them. If I had to raise animals that way, I'd get the hell out of the business.' The others at the table concurred. This was not an isolated incident. . . . Indeed, if I were to transcribe the remarks generally made by ranchers about veal into a transcript, one would probably assume from the text that one was reading the opinions of extreme animal rightists."[1]

Several years ago, the Farm Animals Concern Trust (FACT), an organization trying to improve the lot of today's veal calves, produced a brochure making the following charges against the veal industry:

"Veal calves are:

- Denied sufficient mother's milk

- Trucked to auctions when only a day or two old

- Commingled with sick and dying animals

- Sold to veal factories where they are chained for life in individual crates only 22 inches wide

- Fed government surplus skim milk

- Denied solid food to chew on

- Made anemic

- Kept in the dark

- Plagued by respiratory and intestinal disease

- Unable to lie down normally

- Deprived of any bedding

- Unable to walk at all"

A veal producer got hold of the brochure but didn't know how to counter the charges it made. So he sent it to the editor of the industry's journal and requested an effective rebuttal from the industry experts. The editor of *The Vealer USA*, Charles A. Hirschy, answered, "Thank you for the information about FACT. We've read the information and regret that we are unable to counter their statements."

In statements intended for the public, however, the industry often tells a different tale. . .

"Veal calves are generally kept in individual stalls to provide individual attention, improve general health, separate aggressive young bulls from each other, minimize or eliminate injury to the animals and the farmer, and to aid in feeding efficiency and veterinary care. . . . The farmer would be compromising his own economic welfare if calves weren't kept healthy." (Animal Industry Foundation)[2]

Apparently, there are those in the U.S. meat industry who would prefer that the public not become aware that veal production is cruel. In "Our Farmers Care," the Wisconsin Agri-Business Foundation tells us, "Most veal calves are kept in individual stalls similar to a baby's crib."[3] It's almost enough to have you imagining soft cushions, pink bows, and lullabies playing in the background.

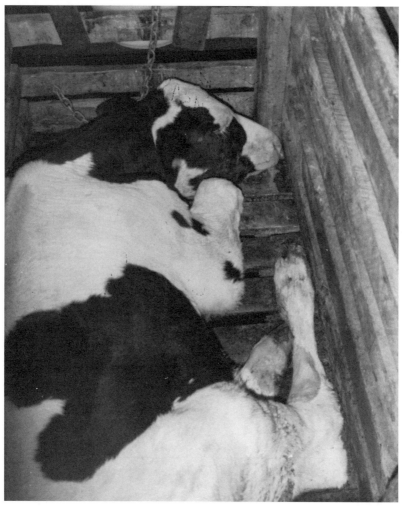

Chained at the neck and barely able to move, veal calves' muscles never develop. Later, their flesh will be prized as tender veal.

The National Cattlemen's Beef Association Veal Committee joins in, telling the public, "Veal farmers have nothing to gain by doing anything other than what is best for the health and well-being of their calves."[4]

Actually, veal farmers have a few other motives. Veal calves are made anemic, for example, to keep their flesh pale. Lighter flesh fetches a higher price because people think lighter-colored meats are healthier. Similarly, in order to keep their flesh tender, veal calves are not allowed to take a single step in their four-month lives. Animals that never move develop no muscle tone, causing their muscles to atrophy and producing "gourmet" veal.

Another aspect of U.S. veal production that has drawn the ire of consumers is the practice of taking baby calves away from their mothers almost immediately after birth. In a publication titled "The Truth about Veal," the National Cattlemen's Beef Association defends this practice, asserting, "This [taking the baby calf away from its mother in its first hours] allows the dairy cow to 'go back to work' producing milk for human consumption. This practice also provides health benefits to both cow and the calf."[5]

What these "health benefits" might conceivably be is not explained. In reality, the calves are too young to walk, so the industry has to find means to move them. Typically, these newborns are thrown and dragged. Often, in the process, they are trampled.

The cruelty of veal crates and anemic diets for calves has been widely recognized in the United Kingdom, where these practices have been banned.[6] They remain, however, standard operating procedure in the veal industry in the United States. While the sale of day-old calves is illegal in Great Britain, and was banned in much of Europe by the end of the 1990s, it is routine in U.S. veal production.

WHAT WE KNOW

Length of time that baby calves will suckle from their mothers in a natural situation: 8 months

Age at which U.S. dairy calves are routinely taken from their mothers and transported to veal stalls: Less than 24 hours

U.S. dairy calves taken from their mothers within 24 hours of birth: 90 percent[7]

Year *Diet for a New America* was published, with its exposé of veal calf treatment: 1987

Years the Humane Farming Association and the Humane Society of the United States launched anti-veal campaigns, respectively: 1986 and 1987

Veal calves raised in the United States in 1987: 3.2 million[8]

Veal calves raised in the United States in 1999: 1.2 million[9]

When I wrote *Diet for a New America*, very few people in the United States were aware of how cruelly calves were treated in the production of U.S. veal. Since then, as I've watched veal consumption in this country drop by a staggering 62.5 percent, I've been greatly heartened. This change has occurred because of an awakening sense of compassion for these animals, and a dawning comprehension of the conditions they are forced to endure.

The dramatic reduction in veal consumption in the United States over the last decade testifies eloquently that once they see what is happening, people in the United States will not tolerate animals being treated with this kind of cruelty. Increasingly, people are taking seriously the lives and deaths of the animals raised for food, and are unwilling to support industries that profit from treating living beings with utter disdain for even their most basic needs. The reduction in veal consumption bespeaks that people are seeing through the reassuring platitudes of corporate agribusiness. People do not want misery on their menus.

Just as ivory, furs, and trophy hunting have lost credibility in the last few decades, so too has veal. The U.S. meat industry, of course, is anything but pleased. What the industry most fears, though, is not the demise of the veal industry. What the industry most fears is that increasing numbers of people will come to understand that, as much cruelty as exists in U.S. veal production, there is actually every bit as much misery in the ways that several other food animals are now routinely raised.

Chickens, for instance.

The Golden Egg

When I asked one poultry producer whether he was worried about the increasing public concern for farm animal welfare, he told me, "They're just stupid birds."[10]

This attitude underlies the way chickens are treated in the poultry industry today. "They're just stupid birds," so there's no limit on how cruelly you can treat them. People with a little more sensitivity, however, look at it differently.

Bernard Rollin, the Colorado State University expert on animal farming, notes that,

> "Contrary to what one may hear from the industry, chickens are not mindless, simple automata but are complex behaviorally, do quite well in learning, show a rich social organization, and have a diverse repertoire of calls. Anyone who has kept barnyard chickens also recognizes their significant differences in personality. . . . There are few more vivid and classic bucolic images than chickens pecking contentedly in a barnyard. . . . Conversely, few images in agriculture are more grating to common sense than chickens squeezed into small cages."[11]

In U.S. egg production, seven or eight hens are typically crammed in each 18-inch-by-20-inch cage (McDonald's pledged in late 2000 to reduce this to five per cage). This provides individual birds with less space than they need simply to lie down. As far as spreading their wings, forget it. The wingspan of a chicken is about 30 inches. There'd barely be room for a hen to spread her wings *if* the cage were twice as big, and *if* she were alone in it.

In Germany, the United Kingdom, Sweden, and Switzerland, however, it became illegal in the 1990s to keep chickens in cages.[12] In the United States, sadly, the practice is not only still legal, but standard. The industry tells us that this is not a problem.

> "Chickens are naturally a flocking animal, so the question of the space they need is irrelevant." (Pamphlet put out by Frank Perdue, one of the largest confinement chicken producers in the United States)[13]

Similarly, a McDonald's senior vice president testified during the McLibel trial that chickens in these cages are "pretty comfortable."

The truth is a little different. When chickens are crowded together this tightly, their innate sense of a pecking order is obliterated. As a result, they become violent and sometimes peck each other to death. The industry responds with a procedure commonly called "debeaking," although some in the industry prefer to call it "beak trimming." The process consists of routinely cutting off one-third of each bird's beak so that they won't kill each other in their frustration at being crammed into tiny cages with no possible outlet for their innate drives and instincts.

Although McDonald's implied in 2000 that the company was banning debeaking, this was not the case. The company was actually only calling for the debeaking procedure to be done more carefully, so that the hens could still be able to eat. If implemented this would be an improvement, because the procedure often leaves the birds so mutilated that they cannot eat properly. Some starve to death because they cannot eat at all.

But McDonald's proposed changes still did little to reduce the conditions that drive the chickens so mad that they attack each other viciously in the first place. The industry is happy with what it euphemistically calls "beak trimming" because it renders the birds incapable of doing much harm to company property — in this case, the other birds.

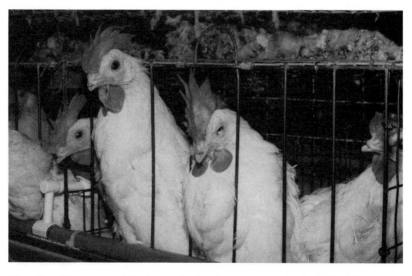

More than 99 percent of the hens who lay the eggs eaten in the United States are debeaked and kept in cages where the excrement from the birds in the upper tiers collects above them, often falling through onto their heads.

Another problem the industry runs into is that the bird's toes and claws often become permanently entangled in the wire on which they're forced to stand. The producers typically handle this difficulty by simply cutting off the birds' toes and claws.

Of course, the industry would have you believe that all this is done for the animals' own good.

> "Egg-laying hens may have their beaks trimmed . . . to avoid injury to each other as a result of the bird's natural cannibalistic tendencies. Claws may be trimmed to avoid injury. . . . All these practices . . . ensure the required results are achieved in the most humane, efficient manner." (Animal Industry Foundation)[14]

What's not said is that chickens' "cannibalistic tendencies" arise only when they are crammed together in totally unnatural conditions.

In an ad for Paramount Chicken, a smiling Pearl Bailey tells us the company looks after their chickens "just like a mother hen." This is a remarkable statement. How many mother hens have ever been known to cut the beaks, toes, and claws off their chicks and force them to live under such oppressive conditions that they are driven to peck each other to death?

When egg production declines, the hens are often subjected to a process called "forced molting," in which they are starved and denied water. This shocks the hens into losing their feathers. Those that survive start a new laying cycle.

WHAT WE KNOW

U.S. hens subjected to forced molting in 2000: 75 percent[15]

Length of time birds subjected to forced molting are given no food (starved): 10–14 days[16]

Length of time birds subjected to forced molting are given no water: 3 days[17]

Bird's body weight lost during forced molting: One-quarter[18]

As this book goes to press, forced molting continues to be regularly employed in U.S. egg production, even though it has been banned in

Great Britain since 1987, and has been linked to Salmonella contamination of eggs. When subjected to the process, hens' immune systems are weakened, making them more vulnerable to Salmonella bacteria, which they are then more likely to pass on to people through their eggs.[19]

The industry has one point of view on the subject of forced molting, while public officials have quite another. . .

Is that so?

"We feel wounded. We feel like we're doing a phenomenal job producing a wonderful product at a wonderful price, but we're being presented as monsters."
—Paul Bahan, a major California egg producer, speaking on why forced molting should be allowed to continue[20]

"This (forced molting) is a very significant public health issue. I was first shocked by the practice because of the horrible cruelty, but the health issues really demand attention."
—California Assemblyman Ted Lempert, who has sponsored a bill to outlaw forced molting[21]

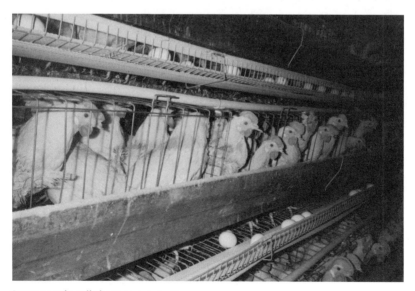

Some people call them concentration camp eggs.

Naturally, the hens who lay the eggs we eat give birth to males as well as females. But there is very little use for roosters in the egg business. So what do you think happens to the males, immediately after they hatch from their eggs? These little guys can't grow up to be egg layers, so the industry, having no use for them, simply throws them into garbage bags to suffocate, or hurls them live into a giant meat grinder, then feeds them back to chickens or other livestock.

More baby male chicks are disposed of in this way in the United States, annually, than there are people in the country. It is standard operating procedure. At least I've never heard the industry justify this particular practice as being done "for the chicks' own good."

Brave New Chicken

I remember a radio interview I did in Columbia, South Carolina. It was a call-in show, and we took a call from a fellow who wanted to know whether I, myself, was a vegetarian.

"Yes," I said gently, sensing this news might be somewhat difficult for him to absorb. I was right about that, because he was not pleased.

"But are you a *real* vegetarian?" he asked, unbelieving.

"Yes," I said, not really knowing exactly what a "real" vegetarian might be, but more or less assuming that whatever it was, I was it.

"I mean," he probed further, his voice growing indignant, "are you a *total* vegetarian?"

At this point I began to imagine that he must be asking whether I consumed any dairy products or eggs. Since I didn't, I answered, "Yes, I'm a total vegetarian." But this still didn't satisfy him.

"I mean," he insisted, "are you a *total and complete* vegetarian?"

Now I'm from California, and I'm sitting in this radio station in South Carolina, and I'm realizing we're dealing with a culture gap. In some circles, people who consume honey are not considered complete vegetarians, because honey is made by bees. I didn't think that was what he was asking about, but by this point I just wasn't sure at all. However, since I was by most standards a "total and complete vegetarian," I said, "Yes, I am."

This was simply too much for the caller. He raised his voice considerably, and, utterly aghast, shouted, "Do you mean to tell me that you don't even eat *chicken?*"

Many people do eat chicken, of course, and lots of it. In the United States today, the raising of chickens for meat (called "broilers") is a mammoth and growing industry. Eight billion broiler chickens are killed for food in the United States each year, a number larger than the entire human population of the planet.[22]

Traditionally, it took a broiler 21 weeks to reach 4-pound market weight. But today, with the birds having been systematically bred for obesity, it takes only seven weeks for them to reach the same weight.[23]

There is a not-so-slight problem with all this. Those broilers used for breeding must be kept under severe food restriction—otherwise they rapidly become too obese to reproduce.

> "If a seven pound human baby grew at the same rate that today's turkeys (and broiler chickens) grow, when the baby reached 18 weeks of age it would weigh 1,500 pounds." (Lancaster Farming)[24]

There's more profit in obese chickens, which is of course why this is done. But from the point of view of the birds, there are a few difficulties.

> "Broilers now grow so rapidly that the heart and lungs are not developed well enough to support the remainder of the body, resulting in congestive heart failure and tremendous death losses." (*Feedstuffs* magazine)[25]

As broilers rapidly become extremely obese, severe vitamin and mineral deficiencies are common, leading to many serious diseases—including blindness, kidney damage, bone and muscle weakness, brain damage, paralysis, internal bleeding, anemia, disturbed sexual development, and deformed beaks and joints.

The more I've learned about how farm animals are treated in U.S. meat production today, the harder it has become for me to listen to industry claims that they treat these animals like members of their own family. All I can say is, if that's true, God help their families.

WHAT WE KNOW

Mass of breast tissue of eight-week old chicken today compared with 25 years ago: 7 times greater[26]

Broiler chickens that are so obese by the age of 6 weeks that they can no longer walk: 90 percent

Each year at Thanksgiving, the U.S. president and vice president pardon a turkey and a vice turkey. This is a nice gesture, but after the turkeys are sent to a small farm, they die from heart attacks or lung collapse within months because their hearts and lungs can't support the bulk.[27]

Turkeys today grow so fast that they find it impossible to mate naturally. They simply cannot get close enough to physically manage. As a result, all 300 million turkeys born annually in the United States are the result of an act of artificial insemination.

(How, you may wonder, is this done? Suffice it to say that there are people, some of whom have Ph.D.s, who have become adept at handling male turkeys in just the right way. The procedure is called—with delicacy but without anatomical accuracy—"abdominal massage." After the semen is thus collected, and then mixed with a myriad of chemicals, there are other "experts" whose job it is to inject the material into the females, using an implement that looks, rather ironically, remarkably like a turkey baster.[28])

What about Free Range and Natural?

As public awareness has grown of the conditions chickens and turkeys are forced to endure in U.S. egg and poultry production, many manufacturers have sought to distance themselves, at least in the public mind, from these practices. This would be fine if they also did something to change the actual conditions. Regrettably, only a few of them do.

Many consumers understandably look to health food stores and "natural" brands for better eggs and poultry products, hoping that if they buy chicken and eggs from a health food store, they will be assured of not eating the misery of factory farms.

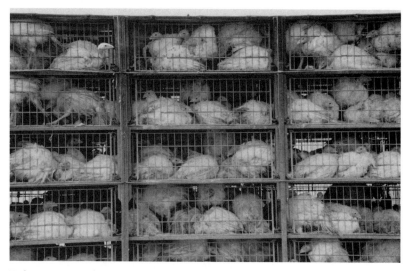

Turkey accommodations aren't exactly spacious.

You've probably seen eggs labeled *vegetarian, natural, hormone-free, organic, cage-free,* and similar terms. Unless the label specifically says "cage-free," however, it's almost certain that the eggs come from caged birds. How about the term "free range"? Allen Shainsky is the developer of "Rocky the Range Chicken," the best-selling "free range" chicken in the western United States. He comments, "Free range doesn't mean anything. . . . Conventional chicken can use (the word) 'natural'. . . . Right now anyone can say almost anything on a label about their chicken. They're just hoodwinking the public."[29]

Steve Bjerklie was the editor of *Meat and Poultry* magazine for fifteen years. His endorsement of so-called natural poultry products is also less than whole-hearted: "When it comes to the words 'natural,' 'organic,' and 'free range' . . . federal law is and always was toothless. It doesn't guarantee a thing. . . . Poultry companies use 'free range' strictly as a marketing gimmick. Legally, the phrase means nothing. There is no law or regulation defining 'free range.' . . . 'Natural' is another meaningless term. . . . By USDA's standards a Burger King Whopper is natural."[30]

Egglands Best and Vegetarian Harvest are two brands of eggs that are nationally available and are labeled "vegetarian." But both of these brands come from caged hens.[31] All the term *vegetarian* means in this case is that the birds were not fed meat. It means nothing about how they were housed or treated.

Similarly, advertisements for Happy Hen Organic Fertile Brown Eggs in Pennsylvania say that the hens run free "in a natural setting," and are "humanely housed in healthy, open-sided housing, for daily sunning— something Happy Hens really enjoy."[32]

In 2000, however, an article in *Poultry Press* revealed that more than 7,000 birds are housed in each Happy Hen barn; the wall-to-wall birds are severely debeaked; and individual hens have even less space than the abysmal industry standard.[33]

Tyson Foods, the world's largest poultry producer, brags in its ads that its products are "hormone free." But "hormone-free" labels likewise mean nothing when it comes to chicken meat and eggs. Although hormones are nearly universal in U.S. beef production, no hormones are currently approved for use with poultry.

Presently, the only certain way not to partake of the misery that pervades factory farm eggs and poultry is to avoid commercial chicken and eggs altogether. As more of us move in this direction, fewer birds will be forced to endure such cruelty. And it will be another step forward in the transformation that began with veal calves, in which increasing numbers of people are saying to animal agriculture, "If you won't treat animals with respect and care, then we won't buy your products."

We are in the midst today of a cultural shift of epic proportions. There is something growing, something taking shape deep within us, preparing to be born. It is the statement that no living creature should be forced to endure such tortured conditions. It is the declaration that all living creatures deserve basic respect. It is a proclamation of the interdependence of all life.

Every day, more people are opposing the most abusive forms of factory farming. They are appalled by veal production, they are beginning to learn about what is done to chickens. And since the late 1990s, with the advent of the enormously popular and Golden Globe-winning movie *Babe*, they are beginning to realize something of the plight of pigs. . .

What about Babe?

The actor who played Farmer Hoggett and starred in the movie *Babe* is James Cromwell. As a result of what he learned about meat production in the course of making the movie, he made a decision—to eat no more animal products. He explains, "If anyone ever realized what was involved in factory farming they would never touch meat again. I was so moved by the intelligence, sense of fun, and personalities of the animals I worked with on *Babe* that by the end of the film I was a vegan. . . . I now don't eat anyone who would run, hop, fly, or swim away if she could."

The National Pork Producers Council is disturbed by this turn of events. James Cromwell is only an actor, they'd like us to think, and doesn't understand how things are done. They tell us their version of how hogs are raised, and it's different from the one described by James Cromwell and other animal advocates . . .

Is THAT SO?

"The farmers who raise hogs (they call themselves pork producers) have always recognized their moral obligation to provide humane care for their animals. . . . Every producer enjoys having healthy and contented pigs."
— National Pork Producers Council[34]

"PETA recently obtained undercover videotape of a North Carolina hog factory. The videotape depicts sows being beaten into and out of their crates with metal rods, disabled sows being kicked, stomped on, and dragged, sows killed by blows to the head with wrenches and cinder blocks, sows having their throats cut while still fully conscious, and sows being skinned alive and having their legs removed while still alive and moaning. . . . Because 'product uniformity' takes precedence over all else, thousands of pigs that don't make weight are killed. These animals are picked up by the hind legs and bashed head first into the concrete floor. Some companies call the process 'thumping.' Smithfield Farms (the nation's largest hog producer) calls it 'PACing'—the company's acronym for 'Pound Against Concrete.' . . . The dead pigs are delivered to rendering plants, where they are ground up and fed back to live pigs, cattle, and other animals."
— Humane Farming Association[35]

As I've learned what's actually done to pigs today, sometimes I've had simply to cry. It can be so painful to see how these sentient creatures are treated, particularly when you remember that they are, as the pig farmer who changed his life so dramatically told me, "intelligent, and friendly if you treat them right."

It really changes the way you look at pork chops and bacon.

When I visited Poplar Spring Animal Sanctuary in Poolesville, Maryland, in 2000, I found myself amazed by the friendliness of the dozens of pigs who live there. These pigs regularly—and quite happily, I might add—get their tummies tickled by the many children who come by to play with them and to experience pigs in a healthy environment, which Poplar Spring definitely is. But I was told that these very same animals, when they arrived there a year before after being rescued from a factory farm, were so terrified of people that any time a human being approached them, they would scream in absolute panic.

It's not hard to understand why, given how pigs are routinely treated in commercial pork production in the United States. Much as the egg industry has taken to cutting off part of birds' beaks and chopping off their toes in order to remedy problems caused by overcrowding, the pork industry has its equivalent. When pigs are packed together and don't have enough space, they become violent, sometimes biting each other's tails and rumps, and even becoming cannibalistic. The industry's response is simply to cut off most of the pigs' tails (a procedure called "tail-docking") and chip off part of the animals' teeth. Like the debeaking of chickens, these mutilations don't make the animals any less frustrated or aggressive, but they do prevent the pigs from doing as much harm to company property—in this case, the other pigs.

In Great Britain, Switzerland, and Sweden, tail-docking of pigs is illegal without anesthetic.[36] In the United States, however, anesthesia is almost never used.

The industry would have you believe that they don't overcrowd the animals, because to do so would harm their profits. They say this repeatedly to the public. But their own journals say something else.

"Over-Crowding Pigs Pays—If It's Managed Properly" (National Hog Farmer)[37]

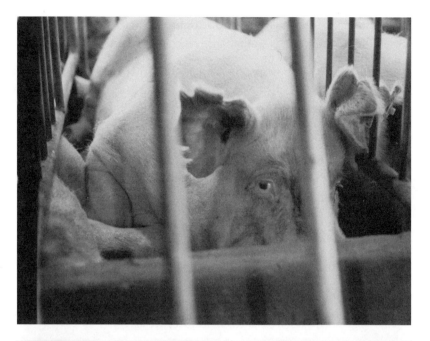

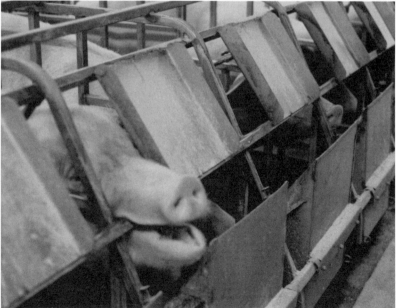

The cages in which pigs are confined barely allow any movement at all.

The public is often told that the reason pigs and other animals are housed the way they are is so that farmers can take better care of them.

> "Animals are kept in barns and similar housing . . . to protect the health and welfare of the animal. . . . Housing also . . . makes it easier for farmers to care for both healthy and sick animals." (Animal Industry Foundation)[38]

I guess it depends on what you mean by *care*. According to the *Wall Street Journal*, the total amount of human attention given to the average factory-farmed pig in four months adds up to exactly 12 minutes.[39]

WHAT WE KNOW

U.S. pigs raised for meat: 90 million[40]

U.S. pigs raised in total confinement factories where they never see the light of day until being trucked to slaughter: 65 million[41]

British pigs raised in total confinement factories: None

Reason: The practice is banned by the Pig Husbandry Law of 1991[42]

U.S. pigs who have pneumonia at time of slaughter: 70 percent[43]

Celebrities for Sanity

James Cromwell is not the only famous actor who has forsworn animal products as a result of learning how the animals are treated. One of my dear friends, while he was alive, was the young actor River Phoenix. His mother, Heart Phoenix, is among my closest friends, and I consider myself fortunate to have known and worked with them both. River and I had many conversations about these issues, and I can tell you he was as devoted an advocate as I have ever known of treating animals with respect and of only eating foods that have been produced without cruelty. After he died, the actor Christian Slater, who replaced him in the movie he was making at the time, donated $75,000 in River's honor to Earth-Save, the nonprofit organization I founded.

I spoke about River, recently, with another young Hollywood star, Alicia Silverstone, world famous for her leading roles in the movies *Clueless, Batman and Robin,* and many others. A few years ago, *Rolling Stone* magazine called her the most popular teenager in the world. I found it ironic that she, whose photo may be on the walls of more teenagers' rooms than just about anyone alive, hoped when she was much younger that she would grow up to marry River.

That she didn't do, of course, but what impressed me the most about her is that she, like River, is a vegan with a tremendous commitment to animals and an unwillingness to sit back and enjoy her good fortune while there is so much needless suffering in the world. She is most definitely not "clueless" about animal suffering.

The meat industry often mocks celebrities who use their exposure to speak out for animals. Ed Begley, Jr., Linda Blair, and Kevin Nealon have put themselves on the line time and time again for animals and for vegetarian causes and have been harshly criticized for it. Edward Asner, Elizabeth Berkley, Kevin Eubanks, Jennie Garth, Woody Harrelson, Marilu Henner, Chrissie Hynde, Casey Kasem, Paul McCartney, Stella McCartney, Rue McClanahan, Alexandra Paul, Alice Walker, and Dennis Weaver are among the many other celebrities who have taken public stands advocating a vegetarian path and been besmirched for their efforts. Pamela Anderson, Bea Arthur, Alec Baldwin, Brigitte Bardot, Kim Basinger, Sandra Bernhard, Pierce Brosnan, Sid Caesar, Doris Day, Ellen DeGeneres, Rhonda Fleming, Tippi Hedren, Bill Maher, Steven Seagal, Hilary Swank, and Loretta Swift are some of the Hollywood stars who have stood up for animals and been attacked as a result.

The U.S. meat industry says these people are publicity hounds, that they are insincere, and that they don't know what they're talking about. But as we've seen time and again, this is an industry that will always do what it can, and not let itself be overly hampered by the truth in the process, to discredit those who challenge it.

To my eyes, these celebrities are using their status to advance the cause of compassion, and they deserve our respect and gratitude for their courage. While some of them may not know all the fine points of each issue, they've got the essential thing right: If we don't include other animals in our circle of compassion, if we permit them to be treated with any degree of cruelty simply because it lowers the price per pound, we are, ourselves, less human in the bargain.

Isn't it odd that we admire star athletes who get paid $20 million to endorse shoes, while other people get paid 20 cents an hour to make them? Isn't it refreshing when celebrities use their name recognition not for financial gain but to promote the greater good of our world?

I applaud Alicia Silverstone, as I applaud James Cromwell and the many other celebrities who put themselves on the line for compassion. We need more people like that, at every level of notoriety.

I am grateful to each of us who stands up to create a more caring and loving world.

chapter 12 # Eating with Conscience

I t's never easy to awaken from the spell that industries weave to shield themselves from public accountability. It's especially hard when it would require us to question our own actions. I never thought much of it when I saw McDonald's TV ads in which the clown Ronald McDonald tells kids that hamburgers grow in hamburger patches.

As if they were flowers.

When I first saw these ads, some years ago, I more or less assumed they were an innocent fantasy, like Santa Claus. I didn't realize they were a sophisticated marketing strategy that managed to obscure the reality that hamburgers are, in fact, ground-up cows.

At Baskin-Robbins, when I was there, there were murals in most stores depicting dairy cows grazing contentedly in beautiful pastures. These murals were huge, extending most of the length of the stores. As I made milkshakes and banana splits for people, I never would have dreamed that the lives of dairy cows were anything but idyllic. So bring on the Rocky Road.

I wish that were true.

But today, there are 10 million dairy cows in the United States, and half are housed in some type of factory system.[1] What's worse, increasing numbers of U.S. dairy cows, particularly in the Midwest and Northeast, are being placed in tie stalls where they are tied in one place, unable to move, for long periods of time.[2]

All this stands in dramatic contrast to the situation in Sweden, by the way, where legislation aimed at respecting the rights of animals has granted cows the right to graze in perpetuity.[3]

Dairy cows in the United States today do not have it easy. The natural lifespan for dairy cows is 20 to 25 years. But under modern conditions, these animals are lucky to make it to age four.

In a natural situation, cows produce enough milk to feed one or two calves. But in today's dairy factories, they actually produce 20 times that amount.[4]

Not that long ago, it took four months for a dairy cow to produce her own weight in milk. Now, some dairy cows produce their own weight in milk in three weeks. And cows who have been injected with bovine growth hormone can produce their own weight in milk in as little as 10 days.

As a result of this, half of the dairy cows in the United States have mastitis (painful udder infections).[5]

A few years ago, *World Farming Newsletter* printed a short article that tells us something of the special relationship between a cow and her calf.

> "Blackie, a two-year-old heifer, broke away from the farm she had been sold to, and, walking seven miles through strange country, homed in on the new farm that her calf had been taken to. The story started when the heifer and her calf were sold separately in Hatherleigh market in Devon. The mother was sent to Bob Woolacott's farm near Okehampton where she was bedded down for the night with a supply of hay and water. But her maternal instinct led her to break out of the farmyard, and over a hedge into a country lane. Next morning she was found seven miles away reunited and suckling her calf at Arthur Sleeman's farm at Sampford Courtenay. Mr. Sleeman was able to identify Blackie as the mother by the auction-labels still stuck on their rumps."[6]

I wouldn't have thought that a cow could manage such a feat. But Dr. Rupert Sheldrake, an eminent natural scientist, checked the details of this story by interviewing the people involved, and what he found corroborated the story.[7]

A similar report was published in *Soviet Weekly*:

> "Caucasian farmer Magomed Ramazhanov was a little surprised when one of his cows went in search of her calf, sold earlier to a farmer in a neighboring district. Originally fearing that the creature had been killed by wild predators, Magomed eventually found his mild-mannered milker reunited with her offspring—30 miles from home."[8]

The bonds of the connection between mammalian mothers and their offspring are profound. This is true of all mammals, not just humans.

For many people, it is heartwarming to see how strong are the bonds that exist between a mother cow and her calves. But this beauty is shadowed for me with sadness. For I also see the heartache that ensues when this bond is ruptured, as it is every day in modern dairies. Separating calves from their mothers at or very near birth is traumatic for both. If a cow were allowed to nurse her calves, there would be enough left for us to take some.

This is how milk has been obtained throughout history. But today, the dairy industry has a better way. They take it all. They don't share it with the calves for whom it is intended. And they make money off the otherwise "useless" male calves by selling them for veal. This way, they say, we get cheap milk.

Sometimes the price of cheap is very, very high.

What We Feed the Animals We Eat

The issue of what the animals who are destined for America's dinner plates are fed is a touchy one within the animal products industry. It is widely accepted that the kinds of diets provided to livestock have dramatic implications for human health. Accordingly, the industry wants you to feel very good about what their animals eat.

Is that so?

"The average U.S. farm animal, from the standpoint of nutrition, eats better than the average U.S. citizen. . . . The farmer who owns the livestock or poultry has an economic incentive to provide animals with exactly the indicated amount of necessary nutrients for animal health. The result is a healthier animal."

—Animal Industry Foundation[9]

"Current FDA regulations allow dead pigs and dead horses to be rendered into cattle feed, along with dead poultry. The regulations not only allow cattle to be fed dead poultry, they allow poultry to be fed dead cattle. Americans who spent more than six months in the United Kingdom during the 1980s are now forbidden to donate blood, in order to prevent the spread of BSE [Mad Cow Disease]'s human variant. But cattle blood is still put into the feed given to American cattle."

— Eric Schlosser, Fast Food Nation, 2001[10]

The meat, dairy, and egg industries in the United States are remarkably creative in what they feed livestock today. Always looking to save money, they've come up with some ingenious ideas to supplement the grain and soybeans the animals are fed.

Recycled chicken manure, for example, is routinely incorporated into the diets of U.S. chickens. (Is it a coincidence that 90 percent of U.S. chickens are now infected with leukosis—chicken cancer—at the time of slaughter?) By the same token, raw poultry and pig manure are routinely fed to U.S. pigs. And the water they are given is often only the liquid wastes draining from manure pits. (Three-quarters of U.S. pigs are infected with pneumonia at the time of slaughter.)[11]

Meanwhile, dried poultry waste and sewage sludge are routinely fed to U.S. cattle (supplementing the basic diet of grain and soybeans).[12] In 1997, in the wake of the British epidemic of Mad Cow disease, the U.S. Food and Drug Administration (FDA) finally banned the practice of feeding cow meat and bone meal back to cows. But pigs and chickens are still routinely fed the bones, brains, meat scraps, feathers, and feces of their own species.

There are many people who love their pets, and would be appalled at the idea of eating cats and dogs. They are glad these animals are not part of the human food chain in our culture. But is that confidence warranted? Tens of millions of unclaimed cats and dogs are euthanized every year by shelters and veterinarians, who then must dispose of these bodies, many of which are picked up by rendering plants. Much of the livestock feed in the United States today is made with rendered ingredients. Thus commercial meat, dairy, and egg products often come from animals whose diet included the ground-up remains of cats and dogs, including the euthanasia drugs injected into their bodies.

It's enough to make you understand why Oprah Winfrey said she would never eat another burger.

Just Ma, Pa, and a Few Animals?

You might be getting the impression by now that the U.S. meat industry is dominated by agribusiness operations whose level of concern for animals is just about nonexsistent. The industry, however, would like you you to believe otherwise. . .

> "It's a myth that farming in the U.S. is controlled by large corporations which care about profits and not about animal welfare." (Animal Industry Foundation)[13]

WHAT WE KNOW

U.S. poultry production controlled by the eight largest chicken processors in 1978: 25.3 percent[14]

In 1998: 61.5 percent[15]

Net worth of chicken producer Donald Tyson: $1.2 billion[16]

Average hourly wage of Tyson poultry processing plant worker: $5.27[17]

Only entities producing more chicken than Tyson Foods: The countries of China and Brazil[18]

U.S. turkey market controlled by the six largest processors: 50 percent[19]

U.S. beef market controlled by the four largest beef-packers: 81 percent[20]

U.S. hog slaughter controlled by four corporations: 50 percent[21]

In North Carolina there is a particular hog producer whose net worth in 1997 was more than $1 billion.[22] His name is Wendell Murphy.

Wendell Murphy accumulated much of his fortune while serving three terms in the North Carolina State House and two in the Senate. During that time, he was responsible for dozens of laws benefiting hog agribusiness, including bills that exempted the industry from sales tax, inspection fees, property taxes on feed, and zoning laws.[23]

Donella Meadows was a systems analyst, author, director of the Sustainability Institute, and professor of environmental studies at Dartmouth College. Writing in 2000, she described the impact Wendell Murphy had in his home state:

> "While Wendell Murphy served ten years in North Carolina's General Assembly, regulatory control of large pig farms was taken from counties and relegated to the state. The state then exempted them from liability for environmental or health damage. Then it decided they needn't pay gas, sales or property tax, either. As the number of hogs in North Carolina rose from 2 million to 13 million, surpassing the human population, the number of hog farms dropped from 21,000 to 7,000."[24]

One of the most noticeable ways in which family farming differs from factory farming is that in the former, animals are often given names—such as Bessie the Cow or Babe the Pig—that recognize the animals as the unique individuals they are. Large-scale agribusiness, on the other hand, has sought to obscure as much as possible the reality that animals are even involved in the process. Hence the names routinely used for animals in U.S. food production—"food-producing units," "protein harvesters," "converting machines," "crops," "grain-consuming animal units," "bio-machines," and "egg machines."

World's Largest Meat Packer Caught Red-Handed

In the end, of course, however they've been raised and whatever they've been called, the animals are killed. Most of us consider that an unfortunate but necessary reality if we are going to eat meat, and are willing to make the bargain. But nearly all of us would want the slaughter to be done humanely. This would seem to be the bare minimum of compassion needed for the creatures whose flesh we consume.

And this is the intent of the Federal Humane Slaughter Act—to see to it that animals are stunned before being slaughtered, so that they are not conscious while being killed. Unfortunately, though, the Federal Humane Slaughter Act is so full of loopholes that it doesn't apply to over 90 percent of U.S. animals (including all poultry) destined for human consumption.[25]

In 2000, the San Francisco-based Humane Farming Association, long in the forefront of the effort to end the cruelty of factory farming, set in motion events that were unprecedented in the history of animal protection in the United States.[26] As a result of the group's efforts, IBP, the world's largest meat packing company, faced potential criminal and civil charges for violations of state and federal law. As well, the scandal brought widespread attention to the way in which billions of farm animals are slaughtered.

The Humane Farming Association had captured on videotape what the group called "some of the most heartbreaking and outrageous evidence of animal abuse imaginable." And the group had sworn affidavits from seventeen of IBP's own workers that provided further documentation, confirming that at the IBP plant in Wallula, Washington, animals had long been systematically treated with almost unimaginable cruelty.

The videotapes, which were aired in spring 2000 by KING-5 TV in Seattle, an NBC affiliate, and in early 2001 by *NBC News/Dateline*, were difficult to watch, but they accurately portrayed the reality. The tapes showed struggling cows hoisted upside down and butchered while still alive. Fully conscious cows were shown being skinned alive, their legs cut off while struggling for freedom. Cows were shown being hit repeatedly with stunning devices that didn't work. Other cows were tormented and repeatedly shocked with electric prods. And workers were shown shoving an electric prod into a cow's mouth.

How could something this awful happen? And not in some small-time plant, but in a major plant owned and operated by the nation's and the world's largest meat packer?

Most people believe that the law requires animals to be dead before being cut into pieces, but this is not the case. According to the Humane Slaughter Act, animals who are covered by the Act must be "insensible to pain" before being chained and cut up. This, in theory, is accomplished through use of an electric shock, called "stunning." The Humane Farming Association tapes showed, however, that often the stunning was not successful.

How often? In one signed affidavit, a slaughterhouse employee said, "I estimate that 30 percent of the cows are not properly knocked (stunned with the electric prod). . . . I can tell that these cows are alive because they're holding their heads up and a lot of times they make noise."[27]

He was one of the seventeen IBP plant employees who risked their jobs and their families' security by signing affidavits reporting cruel conditions at the plant. One stated, "Cows can get ten minutes down the line and still be alive. All the hide is stripped out down to the neck (by then)."[28] Another added, "Workers can open the legs, the stomach, the neck, cut off the feet while the cow is still breathing. . . . I would estimate that one out of ten cows is still alive when it's bled and skinned."[29]

"I've seen thousands and thousands of cows go through the slaughter process alive," said one plant worker. "If I see a live animal," said another, "I cannot stop the line. Because the supervisor has told us that you have to work on [cut up] a cow that's alive."[30]

As a result of the public outcry generated by the widespread media coverage, Governor Gary Locke of Washington initiated a full-scale investigation. When the NBC News affiliate showed the videotape, the station noted, "This is the first time in U.S. history that a Governor anywhere has called for a full investigation of slaughterhouse practices."[31]

This was also the first time thousands of federal meat inspectors had ever joined with an animal protection organization in calling for a criminal investigation of a meat company. The National Joint Council of Food Inspection Locals, the union representing the more than 6,000 USDA inspectors, joined with the Humane Farming Association in seeking charges against IBP.

A week after the videotape was shown by Seattle's NBC affiliate, a team from the Washington State Department of Agriculture conducted a spot check of the IBP plant, and reported they found no abuses. They were, however, detained outside the plant for more than an hour while IBP officials "checked the credentials" of the inspectors. This would, of course, have given plant officials plenty of time to "prepare the plant" for the inspection.

IBP strongly denied the accusations made by the Humane Farming Association. How, then, did the corporation explain the videotaped footage? By implying that disgruntled employees may have intentionally hoisted live cattle to make the company look bad. IBP officials said they intended to investigate the possibility that the workers may have "mishandled the cattle for the camera's benefit."[32]

Joining IBP in the counterattack was Rosemary Mucklow, Executive Director of the National Meat Association. "I seriously doubt," she said, "that what was alleged actually happened."[33]

Dr. Temple Grandin, widely considered the nation's foremost authority on the handling of livestock in slaughterhouses, was flown in by IBP on a corporate jet. But her comments did not exactly exonerate the company. "There's definitely some bad stuff on that tape," she said. "I'm not defending IBP. There was a live cow hung upside down from the chain and another on the ground in the stunning box. These are definitely bad things."[34]

In a written response, IBP sought to downplay the significance of the videotape. "It is a known biological fact that an animal can continue to make involuntary movements after it has died. The untrained observer may misinterpret this as a sign of life."[35]

Workers, on the other hand, testified that they had been "kicked by frantic animals moving along the conveyor."

One IBP executive said it was unfair to blame the company, because the problems shown in the videotape and confirmed in the workers' affidavits were industrywide. In this, unfortunately, he was accurate. Ed Van Winkle is a former slaughterhouse manager for John Morrell & Company, another of the largest meat packers in the United States. Speaking of how slaughterhouses handle animals who are too injured to walk (and those who are unwilling to cooperate), he used words that are painfully graphic:

"The preferred method of handling a cripple is to beat him to death with a lead pipe. . . . If you get a hog in a chute that's had the shit prodded out of him, and has a heart attack or refuses to move, you take a meat hook and hook it into his bunghole [anus] . . . and a lot of times the meat hook rips out of the bunghole. I've seen thighs completely ripped open."[36]

It is very difficult to hear such a description, because the amount of pain is so great. It's easier to think that slaughterhouses are simply efficient factories that turn dumb livestock into sterile, cellophane-wrapped food in the meat display case.

That's what the industry would like you to think.

If you've been to Los Angeles, you may have driven by the high walls of Farmer John's Slaughterhouse and Meatpacking Plant. They are adorned by enormous paintings of beautiful countryside scenes. You see blue skies, fluffy clouds, rivers, trees, picturesque meadows and fields—and lots of very happy farm animals. The facility's windows are painted over with these scenes, so you can't see what actually goes on inside.

What we know

Number of cows and calves slaughtered every 24 hours in the United States: 90,000[37]

Number of chickens slaughtered every minute in the United States: 14,000[38]

Food animals (not counting fish and other aquatic creatures) slaughtered per year in the United States: 10 billion

Bernard Rollin, the Colorado State University expert on animal farming, says it is not only consumers who don't really know what goes on inside slaughterhouses. The same is true, he says, for cattle ranchers, most of whom ship their animals to slaughterhouses but have never actually been inside one. "Few ranchers have ever seen their animals slaughtered," he says. "Even fewer wish to."[39]

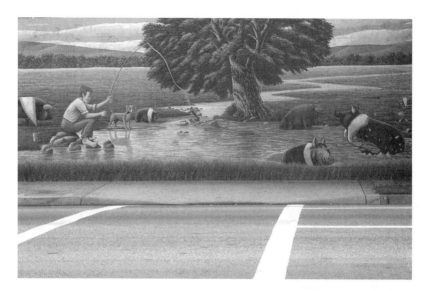

This is one of many paintings on the outside walls of Farmer John's slaughterhouse and Meatpacking Plant in Los Angeles. It all looks so happy for the animals.

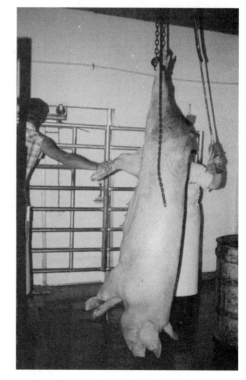

Inside, however, it's a little different. In some U.S. slaughterhouses today, animals are actually skinned and cut up while still alive.

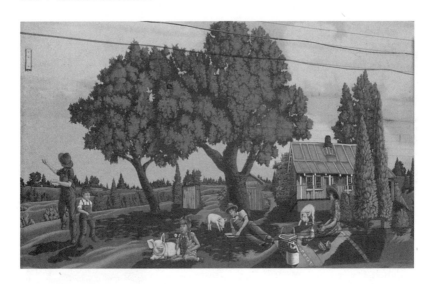

This is another of the many immense paintings on the walls of the Farmer John slaughterhouse in Los Angeles portraying farm animals that are happy as can be. The telephone and power lines that are visible give some sense of the painting's size. Some of these paintings are as tall as airplane hangars. Collectively, they cover more than 35,000 square feet.

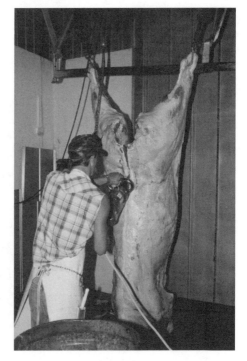

Unfortunately, they could hardly be more misrepresentative of what really goes on inside.

The Battle Continues

The industry might prefer it otherwise, but with each passing day more and more Americans are realizing the extent of animal suffering involved in modern meat production. In 1987, when I published *Diet for a New America*, hardly anyone had any idea what "factory farming" meant, much less had an opinion on the subject. But in 1995, a poll conducted by Opinion Research Corporation found that 95 percent of Americans disapproved of confinement methods used in the production of eggs, veal, and pork.

The U.S. animal agriculture industry has not been pleased to see the public's growing resistance to inhumane farming practices. In response, it has increased its advertising budgets and its propaganda campaigns. And in an act that gives new meaning to the word *sickening*, it has also sought to strip legal protection from farm animals.

Prior to 1990, twelve states had laws that exempted farm animals from legislation protecting animals from cruelty. In these states, sadly, farm animals could legally be subjected to any manner of cruelty, as long as the practices were considered "normal," "accepted," "common," or "customary" farming practices. During the 1990s, bowing to pressure from the animal industries, 18 more states enacted such laws.[40] As a result of these statutes, farm animals in more than half the states now have no legal protection from institutionalized cruelty.

The rationale behind these laws, which exempt farm animals from even the most rudimentary form of legal protection, is that any practice that is the prevailing norm in modern farming or slaughter practices should be deemed acceptable and should not be criticized or banned. It would be hard to construct a system better designed to protect the status quo or to ensure that no progress could ever be made on behalf of animal protection.

It was this very approach that McDonald's attorneys presented in the McLibel trial. They argued that the company should not be considered cruel because what it did was the industry norm. The judge, however, did not agree. He ruled, "I cannot accept this approach. . . . To do so would be to hand the decision as to what is cruel to the food industry completely, moved as it must be by economic . . . considerations."[41]

David J. Wolfson is an attorney in New York City, and the author of *Beyond the Law*, an in-depth discussion of how the laws enacted to protect farm animals from cruelty and abuse have been weakened. He writes,

> "The bizarre result of this trend is that farm animals have been placed in a legal time machine and transported to a time prior to the enactment of anticruelty statutes. . . . The delegation of power to the farming industry is breathtaking. It's difficult to imagine another non-governmental group possessing such influence over a criminal legal definition; for example, chemical corporations determining that they did not pollute (and, consequently, violate criminal law) so long as they released pollutants in amounts 'accepted,' or vested as 'customary,' by the chemical industry."[42]

What we are seeing are two simultaneous trends. On the one hand, ever more people are becoming increasingly appalled by factory farm methods and outraged that such methods should be allowed to continue. And on the other, the industries that profit from the exploitation of livestock are managing to obtain legislation exempting their practices from any laws that restrict cruelty to animals.

It is frightening to see the increasing divergence between the will of the people and the laws of an increasing number of states. Fortunately, there is another direction that we might follow, and we in the United States have a model for how we might begin, just across the Atlantic Ocean.

Hope in Europe

As 18 states in the United States were passing laws during the 1990s exempting farm animals from the statutes that prevent cruelty to animals, many European nations were doing just the opposite—passing legislation banning inhumane farming practices.[43]

It began in 1987, when Sweden passed an animal protection law granting all farm animals the right to a favorable environment where their natural behavior is safeguarded, virtually banning all factory farming.[44]

The European Parliament eventually followed suit, passing a recommendation to ban veal crates, phase out chicken cages, discontinue confinement of sows, and ban routine tail-docking and castration of pigs. By 1999, nations throughout the European community, including Sweden, Denmark, Austria, Ireland, Finland, Belgium, and the Netherlands, had enacted almost complete bans on veal crates.[45]

As well, in 1999, agriculture ministers from the European Union agreed to end all caged egg production in Europe by 2012, replacing it completely with free-range farming.[46] In 2000, scientists from the United Kingdom called for an end to *all* factory farming in Europe as the only sure way to halt Mad Cow disease.[47] And in 2001, the European Union proposed new animal welfare rules for pigs.[48]

Attorney David Wolfson commented, "The contrast is stark: the United States alters the law to allow cruel farming practices while Western European countries are banning cruel farming practices."[49]

Seeing such a dramatic contrast, I am reminded of the words of one of our world's great moral leaders, Mahatma Gandhi, who said, "The greatness of a nation can be judged by the way its animals are treated."

Fortunately, there are voices within the U.S. meat industry who understand the wisdom of the direction the Europeans are taking. Rather than resisting the public's growing awareness, they say, it would be good business to take animal protection issues seriously.

In 1999, the journal *Feedstuffs* carried a remarkably insightful piece titled, "Agribusiness Wise to Consider Animal Welfare," which stated,

> "The United States has lagged far behind other civilized countries in regard to farm animal welfare. Ironically, as other countries have passed laws to outlaw intensive confinement systems such as veal crates, battery cages, and sow gestation crates, many states in the United States have actually moved in the opposite direction, amending their anti-cruelty laws to exclude agricultural practices. When Americans learn about the disparity between farm animal protection laws in the United States compared with other countries, they are embarrassed and outraged. Public opinion polls have found more than 90 percent of U.S. citizens oppose intensive confinement systems commonly used in the United States, and this puts animal agriculture in a difficult position. It markets to a consuming public which is strongly opposed to practices it employs."[50]

Strongly opposed, yes, and getting stronger by the day.

Now What?

As I've learned what's done to farm animals in modern meat production, there have been times that I've not known how to live with the pain I felt. It can be overwhelming to think of each of these billions of creatures as individual beings with personalities and feelings, yet forced to endure such deprivation. I've wondered how I could stay in touch with the pain in a positive way, how I could avoid succumbing to abhorrence and outrage at what is being done to these creatures. I've sought to find a way to be around people in this society, and keep my heart open to all of us, without turning my back on the animals.

What I've learned is this: My complaint is not with the people who eat animal products. My problem is with the industry that treats the animals, each of them a sentient being, with no more respect than if they were garbage.

I don't want to demonize the farmers, many of whom went into the business out of a desire to work with nature and be close to the land, and don't like what's going on any more than you or me. But something has happened to the way animals are treated in modern meat production that is a disgrace to the human spirit, and a violation of the ancient human-animal bond.

My problem is not with people who are bombarded by misinformation and are doing what they have come to believe is best for themselves and their children. My complaint is not even with those who suspect what's being done to the animals and sometimes look away, unable to bear the pain. My criticism is with the industries that on the one hand tell the public that they treat farm animals like members of their own families, and on the other fight to get legislation passed exempting farm animals from any protection from cruel treatment.

The process of rearing farm animals in the United States has changed dramatically from the family farms of yesteryear. This reality, coupled with the exemption of farm animals from laws that forbid cruelty to animals, has produced a heartbreaking situation. More animals are being subjected to more torturous conditions in the United States today than has ever occurred anywhere in world history.

This is painful. It can be shattering to see that in our ignorance we have, perhaps for many years, unknowingly eaten the products of such a system. But this pain may serve a healing purpose. It may be the breaking of the shell that encloses our understanding. It may enable us to hear the call of our own humanity. It may be what we need to bring our lives and our society out of collusion and into compassion.

Seeing what we as a society do to animals so that we can mass produce their flesh has made me, at times, ashamed of my species. But when I see the results of polls that say more than 90 percent of Americans deplore such treatment of animals, I am filled again with hope. The more of us who know, the sooner we can put a stop to this crime against the animals, against nature, and against our own humanity.

It takes courage to lift the veil, and to see what animals in today's factory farms must endure. In the face of such tragedy, it's not easy to keep our eyes and our hearts open. In a culture where there is so much indifference and denial, we may fear that our pain at what is being done to animals is a failure on our part, evidence that we can't cope, a signal that we are the ones with the problem. But the feelings of grief and outrage and helplessness that arise when we see what is being done to today's animals are not signs of weakness. They are signs that our hearts are thawing from our previous collective apathy, and that feeling is returning where there has been numbness. Our distress at what is being done is real, and it is healthy. It speaks of our commitment to stopping this cruelty. It's a measure of our humanity.

The pain we feel at what is being done to our fellow creatures is not ours alone. It arises from our kinship with life. We hurt because we are not separate from the animals, nor from the people who are the perpetrators of such suffering. We hurt because these animals are our fellow mortals, part of the greater Earth community, and because the people administering such cruelty are our fellow human beings. We hurt because we are all connected, because we all are part of the great web of life.

In the heart of our grief we can find our connection to each other, and our ability to act. Our strength lies in our kinship with life. Our power lies in our deepest human responses. Our power does not lie in looking the other way.

Through history there have always been people who have chosen to be vegetarians because they did not feel it was right to kill animals for food when it was not necessary, when there was other nourishing food available. People like Mahatma Gandhi, Albert Einstein, and countless others have been ethical vegetarians for just such reasons. But today, because of the way animals are raised for market, the question of whether or not it's ethical to eat meat has a whole new meaning and a whole new urgency. Never before have animals been treated like this. Never before has such deep, unrelenting, and systematic cruelty been mass produced.

Never before have the choices of each individual been so important.

A Letter

The industries that are profiting from the misery of billions of pigs, cows, chickens, and other farm animals every year don't want PETA to campaign against McDonald's cruelty and force the giant corporation to change. They don't want the Humane Farming Association to expose the horrendous abuses in IBP's slaughterhouses, opening the world's largest meat packer to possible criminal and civil charges. They don't want people like the pig farmer to wake up to what they are doing.

But most of all, they don't want you to stop buying their products.

Among the many letters I have received since I wrote *Diet for a New America*, there is one that I would like to share with you. I received it in the mid-1990s, from a man in San Francisco, California. It represents, for me at least, a statement of hope for us all.

Dear Mr. Robbins,

Your book *Diet for a New America* has had quite an influence on my family. About two years ago, I would have liked to have killed you for it. Let me explain.

I am an extremely successful man. I am used to getting my way. When my daughter, Julie, was a teenager, she announced that she wanted to become a vegetarian. She had read your book. I thought this was ridiculous, and insisted that she stop this nonsense. When she did not obey, I became angry. "I am your father," I told her, "and I know better than you."

"I am your daughter," she replied, "and it's my life."

We had many fights over this. We weren't getting along very well, and there were tensions between us, but they seemed always to come to a head over the never-ending vegetarian debates. It drove me crazy. As far as I saw it, she was being disrespectful and willful, and just wanted to get her way. She said the same about me.

At first, my wife and I forced her to eat meat, but she made such a stink about it that meal times were completely ruined. So eventually, resenting it, we caved in and allowed her to eat her vegetarian meals. But I let her know how I felt about it. It's okay to be an idealist, I told her, but you've got to keep your feet on the ground. It's okay to be a lawyer, she told me, but you've got to keep your heart open. It was terribly aggravating.

For my birthday, one year, she made me breakfast in bed. But there was no bacon, no sausage, not even any eggs. It just turned into another bad situation.

I reminded her that it was my birthday, not hers. She set about telling me about how the pigs and chickens were treated, quoting chapter and verse from your book. This was not what I wanted to hear, first thing in the morning, on my birthday.

After she graduated from high school, Julie moved out. I was glad, actually, because I was sick and tired of it. Every meal it was an issue. I wanted her to eat meat, and she wouldn't. She wanted me to stop eating meat, and I wouldn't. There was no peace. But after she left, I missed her. Not the arguments, I didn't miss them, but I missed her a lot more than I thought I would.

Several years later, Julie found herself a husband, and a short while after that she became pregnant. When our grandchild was born, I was on top of the world. But of course it didn't last. Sure enough, Julie wanted to raise her son, our grandson, as a vegetarian. This time, I put my foot down. "You can ruin your own life if you want to," I told her, "but you cannot ruin the health of this innocent boy." As far as I was concerned, what she was doing was child abuse. I even considered calling the Department of Children's Services. I believed they would either force her to feed our grandson properly, or remove him from her clutches. It was only because my wife prevented me that I didn't take that step.

While I had found I could (barely) tolerate Julie being a vegetarian, I simply could not accept her doing this to our grandson. Eventually, it got so bad that she stopped seeing me entirely. Not only had this stupid vegetarian obsession of hers cost me my relationship with my daughter, it had also cost me my relationship with my grandson, because now she wouldn't bring him by, nor would she let me visit. I was completely cut off.

I thought I should at least try to keep the door open, though, so through my wife (Julie wouldn't even speak to me by then) I asked her what she wanted for her next birthday. She said what she most wanted was for me to read your book, *Diet for a New America*. I told her this would be impossible, because it would be too time consuming. She told me that if I would actually read it, for every hour it took me, she would let me see my grandson for an equal number of hours. She's a smart one. She knows where my soft spots are.

So, Mr. Robbins, I read your book. I read the whole thing, every word. What impacted me the most was your description of how animals are raised nowadays. I had no idea it was so severe. It's ghastly, and I totally agree with you that it must not be allowed to continue. I know cruelty when I see it, and this is extreme.

I'm sure you've heard this all before, but no book I have ever read has impacted me in this manner. I was overwhelmed.

I called her, when I was done reading. "I told you not to call me," she said as soon as she knew it was me. "Yes," I said, "but I've read the book, and I want you to come over for dinner and bring the boy."

Mr. Robbins, I am a proud man, and what I said next did not come easily to me. But I knew what I must do, and so I did it. "Dearest Julie," I said, "please forgive me. There won't be a fight if you come over. I have made a terrible mistake, and I understand that, now. If you come, there will be no meat served, to anyone."

There was silence on the other end of the phone. I learned later that she was crying, but I didn't know it at the time. I only knew there was something else I had to say. "And there won't be any meat served ever again in this house," I told her, "that comes from factory farms."

"Are you joking?" she asked in disbelief.

"I'm not joking," I said. "I mean it."

"We're coming," she said.

And I did mean it. There has been no meat served here since then. We simply don't buy it. Julie is teaching us how to eat vegetable burgers, tofu, and a variety of other things I used to mock. I don't mind a bit. I look upon it as a kind of adventure.

Since then, they have come over for many happy dinners, and many other happy times, too. Mr. Robbins, can you understand what this means to me? I've got my daughter back, and my grandson, too. My daughter is a wonderful human being. And our grandson has not yet had a single cold or ear infection or any of the other ailments children often have. She says it's because he eats so well. I say it's because he's got the best mother in the world.

What's being done to these animals is wrong, terribly and horribly wrong. You are right. Animals should never be treated like that. Never. Never. Never. Never. Never.

I pledge to you what I have pledged to Julie. I will never again let a bite of flesh cross my lips that comes from an animal that has been treated like that.

Now, when Julie says that animals are her friends, and she doesn't eat her friends, I don't argue, as I used to. I just smile, happy to know that I am no longer at odds with such a special person. And glad that I can look my grandson in the eye, and know I am helping to make the world a better place for him.

Yours with great respect,

(Name withheld by request)

The Journey

The lawyer who wrote the letter you have just read, and the pig farmer who opened up to his true feelings and changed his life, have something in common. They have each found a way to bring their lives into accord with their compassion.

We need people like that, people who have heard the call of their humanity and responded, people who stand for the integrity and kinship of life. They remind us that in both our suffering and our joy, we are connected to one another, and to all others who live.

Some say there's no need to extend our compassion to animals, because it says in the Bible that we are given dominion over them. But what does *dominion* really mean? Let's say you have two sons, and you go out for the evening, and as you do, you say to the elder one, "While I'm gone, you're in charge," and you say to the younger one, "While I'm gone, you've got to do what your older brother says." You are giving the older boy dominion over the younger one for the time you're gone, are you not?

But how would you feel if you came home later that night to find that the older boy had subjected the younger one to relentless cruelty?

Dominion means stewardship and respect. It means taking care of other beings, not abusing them.

In our time, there is an awakening sense of compassion toward animals. We can run from it. We can deny it. We can mock those who stand for it. But when we choose to eat with conscience, I truly believe that our world becomes a kinder and safer place for us all.

My biggest complaint, honestly, with the thousands of diet books that direct you toward animal products is not that they may increase your likelihood of heart disease, cancer, and other diseases, though we now know this to be true. My larger difficulty with them is that they never even mention the plight of the animals whose flesh they advise you to eat. They evidently consider it irrelevant that the meat they tout likely comes from an animal whose life has been one long sustained cry of agony.

I do not believe that anyone's true health can be sustained by eating products produced through systems that depend on the relentless and systematic suffering of billions of our fellow creatures.

We are bigger than that. We are not just physical beings with a need for so many grams of iron a day. I believe we are also spiritual beings, with a need for respect and compassion, with a need to make our caring visible, with a need to love and to honor life.

There are forces at work in our culture that tell us we are separate from life. But there are forces at work in our hearts that are helping us to awaken, and take our place on this Earth in harmony with the other beings who draw breath from the same source as we do.

We are not here to abuse and exploit other creatures. We are here to live and help live.

Every meal is part of the journey.

Our Food,
Our World

chapter 13 # Choices for a Healthy Environment

One of the major discoveries in history was that we live on a round planet. Up until only 350 years ago, most people believed that the Earth was flat.

Once we realized that the Earth is round, we began to see how the places on our planet are physically connected to each other. We saw that if we kept traveling in one direction, we would not fall off the edge of the Earth, but would instead go around in a circle and return to where we started. This was a crucial discovery for our ancestors. But we are learning something of even greater significance today.

Art Sussman has performed scientific research at Oxford University, Harvard Medical School, and the University of California at San Francisco. He describes the breakthrough in the simplest of terms:

"Now we are learning something much more important than how the places on our planet are physically connected. We are discovering how Earth works as a whole system. Earth is not flat. Earth is much more than round. Earth is whole. . . .

"All of the planet's physical features and living organisms are interconnected. They work together in important and meaningful ways. The clouds, oceans, mountains, volcanoes, plants, bacteria and animals all play important roles in determining how our planet works."

In urban settings, we are surrounded almost entirely by other people and by objects. Under such conditions, we can forget our dependence on the rest of life for our well-being and indeed for our very survival. We can think that it is the economy that delivers our food, air, water, and energy and deals with our sewage and waste.

But in reality, of course, it is the Earth itself that provides these services and makes our economy possible. Increasingly, today, people are remembering that we are biological beings, as dependent on the biosphere as any other life form. We undermine our own survival if we pollute our air and water, if we destroy the rainforests and deplete our natural resources, and if our activities release carbon dioxide and other greenhouse gases faster than the Earth can reabsorb them.

As the awareness has grown that we are part of our fragile planet and inextricably dependent upon it, people have begun to take notice of how their lives impact the environment. People are becoming more conscious, for example, about energy efficiency. They are insulating their hot water heaters with "blankets" to save energy. Stores that sell refrigerators, freezers, washing machines, dryers, water heaters, and other home appliances are prominently displaying the machines' energy efficiency ratings.

People are turning the heat down, or off, when rooms aren't occupied or in use. They are saving energy by caulking and weather-stripping, and insulating the heating ducts in forced-air heating systems. And they are reducing air conditioning costs by closing the blinds or curtains on hot days and opening the windows at night.

As well, increasing numbers of people are saving energy and money by using energy-efficient lighting, such as compact fluorescents. And by doing simple things like turning off the lights when they leave rooms.

As environmental awareness grows, it takes many forms. You see people realizing that they can't throw anything "away," because there is no such place, when you come down to it, as "away." It all ends up somewhere, be it a landfill, an incinerator, or the ocean. To save resources and reduce trash output, people are recycling their newspapers, glass, and aluminum cans. They're cutting down on disposable diapers. Some are composting yard and kitchen wastes.

Every day, more of our newspapers are printed on recycled paper. Our air conditioners and freezers no longer use CFCs (chlorofluorocarbon chemicals) that harm the ozone layer. Carpool lanes are springing up everywhere. Cities are instituting and expanding curbside recycling programs. Sales of Earth-friendly household products, like low-phosphate detergents, are booming. The nation's largest home builders and the nation's largest home improvement retailers (Home Depot, Lowe's) have vowed to stop using and to phase out sales of wood from old-growth trees.

Increasing numbers of people today are aware of the need to honor the Earth and live within its limits. Most of us are seeking to live more lightly on the Earth and to reduce, if we can, our "ecological footprint." Eighty percent of Americans, in polls, say they are environmentalists. Virtually everyone understands that the environment is deteriorating under the impact of human activities.

And yet, most of us have remained unaware of the one thing that we could be doing on an individual basis that would be most helpful in slowing the deterioration and shifting us toward a more ecologically sustainable way of life. Few of us realize there is something we all could do that would have a tremendous impact on reducing pollution, conserving resources, and protecting our precious planet and the life it holds.

There is indeed one action, within the grasp of each and every one of us, that could help to turn the tide. And yet most of us don't know what it is.

I am talking about what you eat.

Stewards of the Planet?

Traditionally, farm animals played a useful role in keeping agriculture on a sound ecological footing. They ate grass, crop wastes, and kitchen scraps that people could not eat, and turned them into food that people could eat. Their manure provided the soil with needed nutrients. And the animals pulled plows and provided other services that enhanced human life.

But all this has changed as traditional farming practices have increasingly given way to factory farms that process huge numbers of animals in gigantic industrial assembly lines. With the expansion and mechanization of animal farming, world meat production has quadrupled in the last 50 years.[1] There are now 20 billion livestock on Earth—more than triple the number of human beings.

Such a massive change could not have occurred without enormous implications for the environment. As the business of food production has increasingly been taken over by large-scale agribusiness, there have necessarily been profound ecological consequences.

Up until quite recently, most of the dairy farms in the United States were small operations, with the cows grazing on pastureland. In Wisconsin, which still calls itself "America's Dairyland," the rolling pastures were home to Holstein and Guernsey herds. But today, most of the small farms are gone, replaced by operations with thousands of cows each. One farmer said such operations are not agriculture, but are "60 acres of concrete and 10 acres of manure pits."[2]

Highly industrialized farming has carried the day because it seems more efficient. And it is, but only if you don't count some of the larger costs, such as the pollution caused by agrochemicals and the dislocation of rural cultures.

There is a trilogy of evil here. The very food production systems that are providing us with the foods that medical science is finding are harming our health—the very same factory farms and feedlots that are so painfully cruel to animals—are also, it turns out, undermining the life-support systems of our imperiled planet.

In recent years, impartial researchers and nonprofit environmental organizations like the Worldwatch Institute, EarthSave, the Union of Concerned Scientists, the Audubon Society, the Natural Resources Defense Council, the Environmental Defense Fund, and the Sierra Club have sought to alert the public and elected officials to the toll modern meat production is taking on the environment.

And it isn't only environmentalists. There are members of the animal industry, too, who see the price our fragile planet is paying for the growth of modern factory farms and feedlots. Peter R. Cheeke is a professor of animal agriculture at Oregon State University and serves on the editorial boards of the *Journal of Animal Science* and other industry journals. In 1999, he wrote,

> "Raising cattle in huge feedlots, consolidating dairy farms into confinement units with 1,000–10,000 cows, consolidating swine and poultry production into huge confinement units as the trend is now . . . [is] a frontal assault on the environment, with massive groundwater and air pollution problems."[3]

Where's Our Water Going?

Life on Earth began in water, and has always depended for its very existence on water. With water, life can flourish; deserts can be transformed into gardens, lush forests, or thriving metropolises like Tel Aviv or Los Angeles. Without water, we die.

Yet most of us are so used to having this precious resource at our fingertips that we have come to take it for granted. Sadly, we are fast approaching the time when we may be forced to learn the inestimable value of this natural treasure the hard way. Our supply of good water is disappearing at an alarming rate.

In 2000, the World Commission on Water predicted that the increase in water use in the future due to rising population will "impose intolerable stresses on the environment, leading not only to a loss of biodiversity, but also to a vicious circle in which the stresses on the ecosystem [will] no longer provide the services [necessary] for plants and people."[4]

Everywhere you look today, particularly in the western United States, people are seeking to conserve water. You see people washing their cars less often. People are installing low-flow showerheads and sink fixtures, and low-flow toilets. You see people using drought-resistant landscaping. The vigilant turn off the water at the sink when brushing their teeth, except to rinse the brush, and when shaving, except to rinse the blade.

These measures are prudent and helpful, but all of them combined don't save anywhere near the amount of water you would save by shifting toward a plant-based diet.

WHAT WE KNOW

Water required to produce 1 pound of U.S. beef, according to the National Cattlemen's Beef Association: 441 gallons[5]

Water required to produce 1 pound of U.S. beef, according to Dr. Georg Borgstrom, Chairman of the Food Science and Human Nutrition Department of the College of Agriculture and Natural Resources at Michigan State University: 2,500 gallons[6]

Water required to produce 1 pound of California beef, according to the Water Education Foundation: 2,464 gallons[7]

Water required to produce 1 pound of California foods, according to Soil and Water specialists, University of California Agricultural Extension, working with livestock farm advisors:[8]

1 pound of lettuce:	23 gallons
1 pound of tomatoes:	23 gallons
1 pound of potatoes:	24 gallons
1 pound of wheat:	25 gallons
1 pound of carrots:	33 gallons
1 pound of apples:	49 gallons
1 pound of chicken:	815 gallons
1 pound of pork:	1,630 gallons
1 pound of beef:	5,214 gallons

Here's one way to look at it. Let's say you take a shower every single day. And let's say your showers average seven minutes long. At that rate, you'd be in the shower 49 minutes each week (seven times seven). Let's round that off, for easier math, to 50 minutes per week.

Now, let's say the flow rate through your shower head is 2 gallons per minute. At the rate of 2 gallons per minute, and 50 minutes per week, you'd be using 100 gallons of water per week in order to shower each day.

You can multiply that figure of 100 gallons times 52 (since there are 52 weeks in a year) to discover that you would use, at that rate, 5,200 gallons of water to shower every day for a year.

When you compare that figure, 5,200 gallons of water, to the amount of water the Water Education Foundation calculates is used in the production of every pound of California beef (2,464 gallons), you realize something extraordinary. In California today, you may save more water by not eating a pound of beef than you would by not showering for six entire months. Using the figures of the Soil and Water specialists at the University of California Agricultural Extension is even more dramatic. By their analysis, you'd save more water by not eating a pound of California beef than you would by not showering for an entire year.

> "In California, the single biggest consumer of water is not Los Angeles. It's not the oil and chemicals or defense industries. Nor is it the fields of grapes and tomatoes. It's irrigated pasture: grass grown in a near-desert climate for cows. . . . The West's water crisis—and many of its environmental problems as well—can be summed up, implausible as this may seem, in a single word: livestock." (Marc Reisner, author, *Cadillac Desert*)

Meat produced in different parts of the country requires different amounts of water. Meat produced in the Southeast takes much less water than meat produced in other regions; you don't need to irrigate nearly as much thanks to more rain during the growing season in the Southeast. Arizona and Colorado meat, on the other hand, take even more water than California.

The reason that more water is used to produce a pound of beef than a pound of pork or chicken, by the way, is that the pork and poultry industries in the United States are generally concentrated in areas where grain fields need little or no irrigation, and because pigs and chickens are more efficient at converting feed to flesh than are cattle.

Of course, the cattlemen insist that meat production doesn't use that much water. But it's critically important that we not underestimate water use, in the same way that it's crucial not to underestimate how much gasoline it will take to get to a destination if there's no way to refuel en route.

In both cases, shortfalls don't show up until the very end. You can go on pumping water out of wells or aquifers unsustainably until the day you run out. It's like driving a car without a fuel gauge. You push down on the gas pedal and the car accelerates, leading you to conclude that you've got plenty of gas—until the moment when you suddenly run out.

But it's even more important that we don't underestimate water usage. There are alternatives to oil, such as hydrogen, solar, wind, and other resources, but there aren't alternatives to water. If we run out, we can't grow food or maintain other essential life functions.

> "Nearly half the water consumed in this country is used for livestock, mostly cattle." (*Audubon*, 1999)[9]

Running On Empty

It took nature millions of years to form the great Ogallala aquifer that stretches from South Dakota to Texas. This is the largest body of fresh water on Earth, and it lies underneath some of the richest farmland in the world—the great American grain belt. It is one of the reasons the United States is by far the world's largest producer of grain per capita, and has the world's largest food supply.

The famous "amber waves of grain" are so heavily irrigated from the Ogallala that nearly one-third of all the ground water used for irrigation in the United States comes from this one enormous aquifer. But things are changing. The Ogallala is a fossil aquifer, which means the water in it is left from the melted glaciers of the last Ice Age. It's not like a reservoir or river, which are replenished regularly from rainfall. When the water in the aquifer is gone, it's gone.

Fifty years ago, the great Ogallala aquifer remained virtually inviolate, hardly touched by the amount of water being pumped out of her enormous reservoirs. But with the advent of factory farming and feedlot beef, the amount of water drawn from the Ogallala has risen dramatically. At the present time, more than 13 trillion gallons of water are taken from this enormous aquifer every year, with the vast majority used to produce beef. More water is withdrawn from the Ogallala aquifer every year for beef production than is used to grow all the fruits and vegetables in the entire country. America's grain belt, often called "the bread basket of the world," actually produces far more grain for factory farm and feedlot animal feed than bread for humans.

Ominously, the Ogallala's water tables are dropping precipitously, and some wells are going dry. In northwest Texas, by the early 1990s, one-quarter of the Texas share of the aquifer had been depleted. By then, more than a third of the land in Texas that had been irrigated in the 1970s had lost its water, and had become parched and unable to grow food. Without water, these once fertile farmlands will be deserts forever.

If we continue pumping out the Ogallala at current rates, it's only a matter of time before most of the wells in Kansas, Nebraska, Oklahoma, Colorado, and New Mexico go dry, and portions of these states become scarcely habitable for human beings. This scenario may seem like bad science fiction, but it is being predicted by many leading environmentalists. And if it happens, says Ed Ayres, editor of *WorldWatch*, the consequences will be severe.

"The United States will lose much, if not all, of its grain surplus. In so doing, it will also lose much of its ability to . . . (provide) security for its own people. . . ."[10]

And it's not just the Ogallala. The same pattern is taking place all over the world. Aquifers, the vast storehouses of fresh water we have inherited from the ancient past and have come to depend on to feed ourselves, are being depleted at an alarming rate.

"Only within the last half-century have we acquired the ability to use powerful diesel and electric pumps to empty aquifers in a matter of decades. . . . Around the world, as more water is diverted to raising [cattle], pigs and chickens, instead of producing crops for direct consumption, millions of wells are going dry. India, China, North Africa, and the United States are all running freshwater deficits, pumping more from their aquifers than rain can replenish." (*Time* magazine, 1999)[11]

The National Cattlemen's Beef Association, however, has its own point of view. According to this organization,

"Water used in cattle production is not 'consumed' or 'used up.' It's quickly recycled as part of nature's hydrological cycle. . . . For example, water put on cropland mostly evaporates or runs off and appears as rain or in stream water in another location in the hydrological cycle. An acre of corn [for cattle feed] puts 4,000 gallons of water back into the hydrological cycle every 24 hours."[12]

It depends on what you mean by *put back.* The water used in cattle production remains in the greater planetary hydrological cycle, but most of it becomes unavailable to support human life. When water is taken from an aquifer (or from any other location where it's accessible to human use) and used to irrigate land, it eventually evaporates and comes to fall as rain—most of it in the ocean (71 percent of the Earth's surface is ocean) or somewhere else where it is no longer accessible for human use. Furthermore, irrigation water that runs off farmland and into waterways contributes to soil erosion and to the pollution of rivers and streams, making water downstream less usable. This is particularly likely if the land has been treated with synthetic fertilizers and pesticides—practices extremely common in feed grain production in the United States.

More than 97 percent of the water in the planet's hydrological cycle is salty. Saltwater is toxic for terrestrial organisms, which require unsalted water to sustain life. Of the water that is sufficiently free of salt to be able to drink, almost all is locked away in glaciers and ice sheets or is too deep underground to reach. Only about 0.0001 percent of fresh water is readily accessible.[13] It is incredibly important to conserve water.

> "The amount of water that goes into a 1,000 pound steer would float a (Naval) destroyer." (*Newsweek*)[14]

A cultural shift toward a plant-based diet would help plug the drain through which much of our water is being lost. It would enable us to conserve this most precious of natural resources. It would mean that our children would have more abundant sources of water—for drinking, cooking, cleaning, and for growing food.

If we are serious about wanting to leave our children, and their children, a habitable world, then we have to ask where our leverage lies, and where we can be most effective. There is no other single action that is as effective at saving water as eating a plant-based diet.

The Other End of the Cow, Pig, and Chicken

There are more chickens processed annually in the United States than there are people in the world—7.6 billion chickens versus 6 billion humans. There are more turkeys in the United States than there are Homo sapiens—300 million of the big birds versus 280 million of us. Plus there are now about 100 million hogs and 60 million beef cattle in the United States.[15] What do you think happens to the excrement from so many animals?

Properly handled, manure is not waste but a natural, biodegradable fertilizer. In years past, most of the manure from livestock returned to enrich the soil. But today, when huge numbers of animals are concentrated in feedlots and confinement buildings, there is no economically feasible way to return the animals' wastes to the land. As a result, our agriculture is experiencing an increasing dependence on chemical fertilizers and pesticides.

Deprived of manure and continually doused with chemicals, our nation's soils are losing their texture and ability to retain topsoil. Topsoil is the rich soil layer without which food production becomes seriously endangered. The amount of topsoil we are losing from Iowa alone would fill 165,000 Mississippi River barges a year. Losing topsoil, notes Worldwatch Institute's Ed Ayres, "has about the same effect on a terrestrial community as losing blood has on a person. Only so much can be lost."[16]

The production of every quarter-pound hamburger in the United States causes the loss of five times the burger's weight in topsoil.[17]

Unfortunately, instead of being returned to the soil and helping to rebuild topsoil, the wastes from today's livestock often end up in our water.

"Mass production of meat has become a staggering source of pollution. Maybe cow pies were once a pastoral joke, but in recent years livestock waste has been implicated in massive fish kills and outbreaks of such diseases as pfiesteria, which causes memory loss, confusion and acute skin burning in people exposed to contaminated water. In the United States, livestock now produces 130 times as much waste as people do. . . . These mega-farms are proliferating, and in populous areas their waste is tainting drinking water." (*Time* magazine, 1999)[18]

In 1997, the U.S. Senate Agricultural Committee issued a lengthy report on livestock waste in the country. In a synopsis of the report, the Scripps Howard news service wrote,

"Untreated and unsanitary, bubbling with chemicals and disease-bearing organisms . . . (livestock waste) goes onto the soil and into the water that many people will, ultimately, bathe in and wash their clothes with and drink. It's poisoning rivers and killing fish and sickening people. . . . Catastrophic cases of pollution, sickness, and death are occurring in areas where livestock operations are concentrated. . . . Every place where the animal factories have located, neighbors have complained of falling sick."[19]

Learning how profound these problems have become, I've at times felt horrified and disgusted. But when we know the cause, we can work to solve the problems and prevent more from occurring.

WHAT WE KNOW

Gallons of oil spilled by the Exxon-Valdez: 12 million

Gallons of putrefying hog urine and feces spilled into the New River in North Carolina on June 21, 1995, when a "lagoon" holding 8 acres of hog excrement burst: 25 million[20]

Fish killed as an immediate result: 10–14 million[21]

Fish whose breeding area was decimated by this disaster: Half of all mid-East Coast fish species[22]

Acres of coastal wetlands closed to shell fishing as a result: 364,000[23]

Amount of waste produced by North Carolina's 7 million factory-raised hogs (stored in open cesspools) compared to the amount produced by the state's 6.5 million people: 4 to 1[24]

Relative concentration of pathogens in hog waste compared to human sewage: 10 to 100 times greater[25]

As the pork industry has grown rapidly in North Carolina, so have problems with water pollution. The National Pork Producers' Council assures us we can trust them to handle things. Others have a different view. . . .

Is THAT SO?

> "Pork producers are dedicated to conserving the environment."
> —National Pork Producers' Council[26]
>
> "The contamination of the nations' waterways from [pork] manure run-off is extremely serious. Twenty tons of [pork and other] livestock manure are produced for every household in the country. We have strict laws governing the disposal of human waste, but the regulations are lax, or often nonexistent, for animal waste."
> —Union of Concerned Scientists[27]

The scientific name for a toxic microbe that has caused widespread human illnesses and massive fish kills in East Coast waterways in recent years is *pfiesteria piscicida*. More commonly, it's called "the cell from hell." If you're exposed, you may experience sores, severe headaches, blurred vision, nausea, vomiting, difficulty breathing, kidney and liver dysfunction, memory loss, and/or severe cognitive impairment.[28] These things can happen to you not just from drinking water in which these organisms live, but from mere skin contact with such water.

More than 1 billion fish have been killed by pfiesteria in North Carolina waters in the last few years.[29]

Pfiesteria has been around for centuries, but only recently has it turned into a devastating menace. What had made the difference? The pollution of waterways due to animal waste.[30] When hog waste gets into waterways, it creates conditions in which pfiesteria thrives.

> "North Carolina has been known for its natural beauty, mountains, and beaches. The hog industry is turning it into America's toilet bowl." (Don Webb, former hog producer)[31]

When large amounts of animal manure pollute waterways, the result is severe oxygen depletion in these aquatic ecosystems. Fish suffocate when there is prolonged oxygen depletion, or starve when their prey (smaller fish) are suffocated. As a result of animal waste pollution, there is now, in the Gulf of Mexico south of Louisiana, a "dead zone" of nearly 7,000 square miles that can no longer support most aquatic life.[32] And this kind of thing is happening everywhere. . .

"(When) 420,000 gallons of hog manure spilled into a creek only a small number of fish were killed—but only because an earlier spill had already wiped most of them out." (Sierra Club)[33]

All over the country, water pollution from factory farms and feedlots is causing enormous problems.

"Streams today in Missouri are little more than open sewers. People are getting sick with respiratory problems. Even the flies are sick." (Albert Midoux, former USDA food safety inspector)[34]

The industries responsible, however, would like you to believe that the problem has been greatly exaggerated, and actually, all is well. According to Dale Van Voorst, spokesman for one of the largest poultry producers in the United States, "The modern poultry producer manages manure so that none of it enters the waters of the area. There may be occasional accidents, as there are in any industry, but animal agriculture operates in strict accordance with the Clean Water Act. No one is out there trying to pollute. Everyone who is supposed to obtain a discharge permit is doing so."[35]

WHAT WE KNOW

Number of poultry operations (according to the General Accounting Office) that are of sufficient size to be required to obtain a discharge permit under the Clean Water Act: About 2,000[36]

Number (according to the General Accounting Office) that have actually done so: 39[37]

Number of the 22 largest animal factories in Missouri required to have valid operating discharge permits that actually have them: 2[38]

The volume of waste produced by factory farms is so enormous and so toxic that it is challenging to describe. The hog waste produced by a single Circle Four Farms hog plant in Milford, Utah, for example, is equal to the volume of human waste produced by the entire human population of the state of Utah. And ever since this Circle Four plant began to operate, health problems in the area have been increasing.

> "Milford residents have 20 times more diarrheal illness than Utahns as a whole . . . The rate of respiratory illness in Milford is seven times higher than the state average . . . according to the Utah Department of Health." (*Salt Lake Tribune*, 2000)[39]

Of course, Circle Four Farms insists it isn't their fault:

> "There isn't any data pointing the finger at Circle Four, or anyone else for that matter." (Circle Four Farms spokesman Brian Mauldwin)[40]

Americans know their water is not pure. Each year, Americans spend $2 billion for bottled water and home tap-water treatments. That's an amount more than half of Lebanon's gross national product.[41]

Meanwhile, the Union of Concerned Scientists tells us that the amount of water pollution generated in producing a pound of meat is a staggering 17 times greater than that generated in producing a pound of pasta.[42]

The Water You Drink

It is terribly sad to see our species polluting our water. It would be difficult to exaggerate the importance of clean water on Earth. Water blesses our planet and makes it appear beautifully blue from space. It is the presence of liquid water that clearly distinguishes Earth from all other known planets and moons. Water covers three-quarters of our planet's surface. And water makes up three-quarters of our own bodies. Art Sussman reminds us,

> "Think about one of our ancestors who lived in Africa a million years ago. Or think about a dinosaur that lived 70 million years ago. Or consider a buffalo that roamed the American Midwest millions of years before the arrival of humans. No matter which you choose to bring to mind, that organism drank water throughout its life. This water was present in every drink and in every grain, fish, or flesh that was consumed.

The water molecules became part of that organism's body, and then flowed back into the world as blood, sweat, urine, and exhaled water vapor."

Noting that every drop of water contains an enormous number of water molecules (about 3,000,000,000,000,000,000,000,000), he continues,

"Fill a glass with water. This glass that you hold in your hand today has more than ten million water molecules that passed through the body of the buffalo, more than ten million water molecules that passed through the dinosaur and more than ten million water molecules that passed through one of our African ancestors. The water that we drink connects us intimately with the living beings that inhabited the planet before us, that inhabit Earth today, and that will inhabit it in the future."

But today, increasingly, the water we drink connects us to the excrement of animals housed in factory farms and feedlots. California dairies are a disturbing example.

The excrement produced each year by the dairy cows in the 50-square-mile area of California's Chino Basin would make a pile with the dimensions of a football field and as tall as the Empire State Building. When it rains heavily, however, dairy manure in the Chino Basin is washed straight down into the Santa Ana River and into the aquifer that supplies half of Orange County's drinking water.[43]

WHAT WE KNOW

Number one milk-producing area in the United States: California's Central Valley

Amount of waste produced by the 1,600 dairies in California's Central Valley: More than the entire human population of Texas[44]

Total number of water quality inspectors in California's entire Central Valley: 4[45]

Cities that rely on California's Central Valley as an important source of drinking water: Los Angeles, San Diego, and most cities in between

Number of Californians whose drinking water is threatened by contamination from dairy manure: 20 million (65 percent of the state's population)[46]

Pathogen, stemming from dairy manure, that infected Milwaukee's drinking water in 1993, sickening 400,000 people and leading to the deaths of more than 100 people: Cryptosporidium[47]

Pathogen that Los Angeles metropolitan water district officials say is a constant threat to contaminate Los Angeles drinking water from Central Valley dairy waste: Cryptosporidium[48]

How is it, you may wonder, that the public is not more aware of the role played by animal agriculture in our water pollution problems? Part of the answer that the industry often denies responsibility. . .

Is that so?

"Essentially all livestock and poultry manure winds up as a natural fertilizer on the land . . . without polluting water supplies."
—National Cattlemen's Beef Association[49]

"Dairies are the single largest source of water pollution. . . . Our volunteers frequently encounter massive discharges of dairy waste that literally cauterize waterways and kill fish. . . . We're in the process of losing one of the most marvelous and diverse aquatic ecosystems in the world."
—Deltakeeper, an environmental group that monitors California's waterways[50]

A cultural shift toward a plant-based diet would mean far fewer animals in factory farms and feedlots, far less manure produced, and far cleaner water. It would mean that our water would be healthier and far less likely to harbor dangerous pathogens from animal waste. It would be a major step toward restoring the life-giving waters of our planet.

The choices we make, individually and collectively, have a profound effect on the water that flows through our veins, through our rivers and streams, and that will flow through the bodies of all those yet to be born. Every time you choose to eat plant foods rather than the products of today's factory farms and feedlots, you are helping to reduce water pollution. Each of us is ultimately responsible for the integrity and consequences of our actions.

A new direction for America's food choices would mean that the water in our children's lives might yet be clean and plentiful.

Wasting the West

Livestock today are raised in a variety of environments. In the United States and other industrialized countries, pigs and chickens are almost all housed and fed in factory farms. Cattle typically graze on rangeland for the first part of their lives, and then are moved to feedlots for their last three or four months, where they are fed grain and soybeans, supplemented, lest they get bored with the cuisine, with dried poultry waste, sewage sludge, and worse.

It is nearly impossible to overestimate the impact of cattle grazing on the western United States. Seventy percent of the land area of the American West is currently used for grazing livestock. More than two-thirds of the entire land area of Montana, Wyoming, Colorado, New Mexico, Arizona, Nevada, Utah, and Idaho is used for rangeland. Cattle, sheep, and other U.S. livestock graze roughly 525 million acres, nearly 2 acres for every person in the country. Just about the only land that isn't grazed is in places that for one reason or another can't be used by livestock—inaccessible areas, dense forests and brushlands, the driest deserts, sand dunes, extremely rocky areas, cliffs and mountaintops, cities and towns, roads and parking lots, airports, and golf courses. In the American West, virtually every place that can be grazed, is grazed.

What has been the environmental consequence?

Is that so?

"Cattle enrich our lives and enhance the planet. . . . [Cattle are] mother's nature's recycling machine. . . . Cows are . . . environmental protection machines."
—National Cattlemen's Beef Association[51]

"Although cattle grazing in the West has polluted more water, eroded more topsoil, killed more fish, displaced more wildlife, and destroyed more vegetation than any other land use, the American public pays ranchers to do it."
—Ted Williams, environmental author[52]

U.S. cowboys have traditionally been portrayed as the embodiment of rugged individualism and the epitome of self-reliance. And yet most of the land on which this grazing takes place is publicly owned. It belongs to the people, and to future generations.

Currently, 70 percent of the land in western National Forests and 90 percent of Bureau of Land Management land are grazed by livestock for private profit. Is the public getting a fair deal?

In 1994, the U.S. government paid $105 million to manage the publicly owned land used by cattle ranchers for grazing livestock. Yet, the U.S. government received only $29 million in revenue from ranchers for use of this land.[53]

The same pattern is repeated on state lands. Of the 9.3 million acres in Arizona's state public trust land, 94 percent are grazed by livestock. According to the Arizona Constitution, the Arizona Land Department is obligated to obtain the highest possible income from this land (while protecting it) for the benefit of the state's public schools. Yet the total gross revenue received by the Arizona Land Department from livestock grazing in 1998 was only $2.2 million.[54] That is exactly 26 cents an acre, a figure not even remotely comparable to the amount ranchers pay to graze cattle on private land.

It isn't any better in New Mexico. . .

WHAT WE KNOW

Amount paid by New Mexico Governor Bruce King in 1994 to graze his cattle on 17,372 acres of trust land: 65 cents/acre[55]

Amount paid by New Mexico's 1994 candidate for land commissioner Stirling Spencer to graze his cattle on 20,000 acres of trust land: 59 cents/acre[56]

New Mexico trust land that is open to livestock grazing: 99 percent

Amount New Mexico's livestock ranchers do not pay in property tax, sales tax, or other taxes due to special deductions and exemptions given to the cattle industry: Billions of dollars annually[57]

Number of states with higher taxes on the poor than New Mexico: 3[58]

Number of states with a greater percentage of women living in poverty: 0[59]

The cattlemen claim that grazing is the best possible use for the American West. According to the National Cattlemen's Beef Association, "When cattle are properly grazed, they benefit the land by 'aerating' the soil with their hooves, which means they loosen the soil when they walk on it. This allows more oxygen to enter the soil, helping grasses and plants grow better."[60]

In reality, however, when 1,000-pound animals walk on the earth, they trample plants and compact the soil. This makes it harder for grasses and plants to grow. And since compacted soil does not absorb water as freely, heavy rain then courses off the surface, carrying away topsoil, scouring deep gullies, and damaging streambeds.[61]

Undaunted, the cattlemen insist they are benefactors to the land. . .

Is THAT SO?

"Open space exists largely because of . . . America's cattle farmers and ranchers. . . . Cattlemen are the foundation for this country's open space and its abundant wildlife."

—National Cattlemen's Beef Association

"The impact of countless hooves and mouths over the years has done more to alter the type of vegetation and land forms of the West than all the water projects, strip mines, power plants, freeways, and subdivision development combined."

—Philip Fradkin, in Audubon[62]

The USDA's Animal Damage Control (ADC) program was established in 1931 for a single purpose—to eradicate, suppress, and control wildlife considered to be detrimental to the western livestock industry. The program has not been popular with its opponents. They have called the ADC by a variety of names, including, "All the Dead Critters" and "Aid to Dependent Cowboys."

In 1997, following the advice of public relations and image consultants, the federal government gave a new name to the ADC—"Wildlife Services." And they came up with a new motto—"Living with Wildlife."

This is an interesting choice of words. What "Wildlife Services" actually does is kill any creature that might compete with or threaten live-stock. Its methods include poisoning, trapping, snaring, denning, shooting, and aerial gunning. In "denning" wildlife, government agents pour kerosene into the den and then set it on fire, burning the young alive in their nests.

Among the animals Wildlife Services agents intentionally kill are badgers, black bears, bobcats, coyotes, gray fox, red fox, mountain lions, opossum, raccoons, striped skunks, beavers, nutrias, porcupines, prairie dogs, black birds, cattle egrets, and starlings.

Among the animals Wildlife Services agents unintentionally kill are domestic dogs and cats, and several threatened and endangered species.

All told, Wildlife Services, the federal agency whose motto is "Living with Wildlife," intentionally kills more than 1.5 million wild animals annually.

This is done, of course, at public expense, to protect the private financial interests of the cattlemen. This is their due, the cattlemen say, because they take such good care of the environment.

Is THAT SO?

"Ranchers are the ultimate environmentalists."
—National Cattlemen's Beef Association spokeswoman Julie Jo Quick, explaining why cattle should be encouraged throughout the American Southwest[63]

"Most of the public lands in the West, and especially the Southwest, are what you might call 'cow burnt.' Almost anywhere and everywhere you go in the American West you find hordes of cows. . . . They are a pest and a plague. They pollute our springs and streams and rivers. They infest our canyons, valleys, meadows and forests. They graze off the native bluestems and grama and bunch grasses, leaving behind jungles of prickly pear. They trample down the native forbs and shrubs and cacti. They spread the exotic cheatgrass, the Russian thistle, and the crested wheat grass. Even when the cattle are not physically present, you see the dung and the flies and the mud and the dust and the general destruction. If you don't see it, you'll smell it. The whole American West stinks of cattle."
—Edward Abbey, conservationist and author, in a speech before cattlemen at the University of Montana in 1985[64]

If we ate less meat, the vast majority of the public lands in the western United States could be put to more valuable—and environmentally sustainable—use. Much of the western United States is sunny and windy, and could be used for large-scale solar energy and wind-power facilities. With the cattle off the land, photovoltaic modules and windmills could generate enormous amounts of energy without polluting or causing environmental damage. Other areas could grow grasses that could be harvested as "biomass" fuels, providing a far less polluting source of energy than fossil fuels. And much of it could simply be left alone, providing habitat for wildlife and gracing our world with wilderness.

A shift toward a plant-based lifestyle would mean that the vast prairies of the West could gradually return to health. It would mean life instead of extinction for many of the species that federal programs currently target and kill.

It would mean that our children might yet live to see a way of life in harmony with the natural systems of the Earth.

chapter 14

Once Upon
a Planet

I was fortunate to be able to know and work with the late actor Raul Julia. A man who emanated enormous exuberance and joy, Raul was one of those special Hollywood celebrities who had an abiding concern for world issues, particularly hunger issues, and a deep sense of social responsibility. He and I once appeared together, along with River Phoenix and Lisa Bonet, on what was then the TV talk show with the largest viewing audience in the world. We had an hour to introduce the public to my work and to the enormous impact our food choices have on our health and the environment.

On many occasions, Raul and I pondered the fate of the tropical rainforests and their extraordinary biological diversity. For Raul, this was an extremely important and personal issue. He won both Golden Globe and Emmy awards for one of his last performances, his starring role in *The Burning Season*. He played Chico Mendes, the union leader who fought heroically to protect the homes and lands of the Brazilian peasants in the western Amazon rainforest. Mendes became world famous, and became the international symbol of the effort to save the rainforests, because of his work to prevent the building of a road that would have provided the cattle industry with easy access to the rainforest. Mendes was violently assassinated in 1990 by cattlemen who opposed his efforts. But his message and work live on.

Unfortunately, not everyone is as concerned about the rainforests and their fellow human beings as Raul Julia and Chico Mendes were. I remember a few years ago meeting a popular New Age guru. Some of his disciples had been telling him of my work and were urging him to support a vegetarian direction. He wasn't interested, and told me that he could eat veal and cheeseburgers and suffer no harm because he could "transform the vibrations." Telling me I needed to get over my hang-ups, he made a point of eating a hamburger in front of me.

If his intention was to make me uncomfortable, he succeeded. But I didn't take this as a lesson in letting go of attachment to preconceived ideas, as I believe he intended it. Instead, I spoke to him. "Maybe you have some special powers," I said, "so that you won't raise your likelihood of having a heart attack or cancer like the rest of us mortals would, but what good will that do for the veal calves, crammed into stalls hardly larger than their own bodies, standing knee-deep in their own excrement?"

He said that for an animal to be eaten by a holy person brought great karma to them.

My heart was by this point feeling quite heavy, and I wasn't at all sure there was any point in continuing the discussion. But I proceeded, nevertheless, to ask him one more question. What good, I asked, would his "transforming the vibrations" do for the rainforests, the jewels of nature that are being cut down so that he and others like him could have their burgers?

Rainforests and other earthly phenomena, he said, are just an illusion.

Well, they're a pretty convincing one, I responded, given that they produce a good portion of the world's oxygen.

"This is not a problem for me," he answered. "I create my own reality."

He certainly does create his own reality, I thought as I left. Unfortunately, it is one that does not engage with or even acknowledge the most pressing issues of our times. And it is a reality that, in its obliviousness, causes all-too-real real suffering to other creatures and to the world's endangered ecosystems.

Trading Tropical Rainforests for Cheeseburgers

The tropical rainforests are among the planet's most precious natural resources. They contain 80 percent of the world's species of land vegetation and account for much of the global oxygen supply. These forests are the oldest terrestrial ecosystems on Earth and have developed extraordinary ecological richness. Half of all species on Earth live in the moist tropical rainforests. And the rainforests are home to the world's most ancient indigenous peoples, tribes who have lived in harmony with their environment since before the time of the Pharoahs.

The biologist E. O. Wilson once found as many species of ants on one rainforest tree in Peru as exist in all of the British Isles. A naturalist counted 700 species of butterflies within a 3-mile radius in an Amazon rainforest. In constrast, all of Europe has only 321 known butterfly species. Twenty-five acres of Indonesian rainforest contain as many different tree species as are native to all of North America.[1]

We still know very little about the natural treasures of the tropical rainforests, yet it's clear that their preservation is essential to the planet's ecology. Currently, one-quarter of our medicines derive from raw materials found in these forests. A child suffering from leukemia now has an 80 percent chance of survival instead of only a 20 percent chance, thanks to the alkaloidal drugs vincristine and vinblastine, which are derived from a rainforest plant called the rosy periwinkle. Since less than 1 percent of the plant species of the tropical rainforests have been tested for medicinal benefits, researchers feel that here lie what could be the medicines of the future.

With all their beauty and importance, however, the tropical rainforests are being destroyed at a terrifying rate. Every second, an area the size of a football field is destroyed forever.[2]

What drives this devastation?

"The number one factor in elimination of Latin America's tropical rainforests is cattle-grazing. . . . [We are seeing] the 'hamburgerization' of the forests." (Norman Myers, author of *The Primary Source: Tropical Forests and Our Future*)[3]

In Central America, cattle typically graze on land that was rainforest before being cut down and burned to be used for rangeland. According to the Rainforest Action Network, 55 square feet of tropical rainforest, an area the size of a small kitchen, are destroyed for the production of every fast-food hamburger made from rainforest beef.[4]

> "Rainforest beef is typically found in fast food hamburgers or processed beef products. In both 1993 and 1994 the United States imported over 200,000,000 pounds of fresh and frozen beef from Central American countries. Two-thirds of these countries' rainforests have been cleared, primarily to raise cattle whose stringy, cheap meat is exported to profit the U.S. food industry. When it enters the United States, the beef is not labeled with its country of origin, so there is no way to trace it to its sources." (Rainforest Action Network)[5]

It has always struck me as the height of absurdity for Americans, whose cholesterol levels are already too high, to be eating hamburgers made from rainforest beef so they can save a little money. Particularly when the amount of money saved, according to the MacArthur Foundation, is small indeed.

> "Imports of beef by the United States from southern Mexico and Central America during the past 25 years has been the major factor in the loss of about half of the tropical forests there—all for the sake of keeping the price of hamburger in the United States about a nickel less than it would have been otherwise." (MacArthur Foundation Report)[6]

Rainforest beef imported into the United States is mixed with more fatty domestic cattle trimmings and sold mostly to fast food chains and food processing companies for use in hamburgers, hot dogs, luncheon meats, chilies, stews, frozen dinners, and pet foods. McDonald's and Burger King claim they no longer buy from tropical countries, but these claims are difficult to substantiate because, once the U.S. government inspects beef imports, the meat enters the domestic market with no origin lables. Though Central American beef exports to the United States have declined in recent years, they still approach 100,000,000 pounds annually.

WHAT WE KNOW

Number of species of birds in one square mile of Amazon rainforest: More than exist in all of North America[7]

Life forms destroyed in the production of each fast-food hamburger made from rainforest beef: Members of 20 to 30 different plant species, 100 different insect species, and dozens of bird, mammal, and reptile species[8]

Length of time before the Indonesian forests, all 280 million acres of them, would be completely gone if they were cleared to produce enough beef for Indonesians to eat as much beef, per person, as the people of the United States do: 3.5 years[9]

Length of time before the Costa Rican rainforest would be completely gone if it were cleared to produce enough beef for the people of Costa Rica to eat as much beef, per person, as the people of the United States eat: 1 year[10]

What a hamburger produced by clearing forest in India would cost if the real costs were included in the price rather than subsidized: $200[11]

The National Cattlemen's Association has downplayed the connection between U.S. beef and rainforest destruction. The organization's effort to refute *Diet for a New America* states, "Fast-food beef consumption by Americans contributes little or nothing to tropical rainforest destruction."[12]

Given how many fast-food hamburgers are eaten in the United States, I wish they were right. But many leading figures within the U.S. beef industry say otherwise. Dr. M. E. Ensminger is former Chairman of the Department of Animal Science at Washington State University and the author of ten books dealing with livestock raising. His classic 1,200-page textbook titled *Animal Science* is currently in its ninth edition. In this edition, he writes,

"Is a quarter pound of hamburger worth a half ton of Brazil's rainforest? Is 67 square feet of rainforest—an area about the size of one small kitchen— too much to pay for one hamburger? Should we form cattle pastures to produce hamburgers in the Amazon, or should we retain the rainforest and the natural environment? These and other similar questions are being asked too little and too late to preserve much of the great tropical rainforest of the Amazon and its environment. It took nature thousands of years to form the rainforest, but it took a mere 25 years for people to destroy much of it. And when a rainforest is gone, it's gone forever."[13]

We need our world's forests. They are vital sources of oxygen. They moderate our climates, prevent floods, and are our best defense against soil erosion. Forests recycle and purify our water. They are home to millions of plants and animals. They provide wood for our buildings and cooking fuel for much of humanity. In their biological integrity, they are a source of beauty, inspiration, and solace.

The world's forests are being depleted as a result of several developments in addition to beef cattle ranching: population resettlement, major power projects like dams, hydroelectric plants, and the roads that go with them, and logging. What can we do? We can reuse paper and wood products, reduce the amount of paper and wood we use, and use recycled paper whenever possible. We can stop all use of tropical hardwoods. (To stop importing tropical hardwoods, the United States would have to reduce its consumption of timber by only 2 percent.) We can support organizations involved in rainforest conservation. And, most important, we can eat less meat.

A cultural shift toward a plant-based diet would be a substantial step toward saving our remaining forests. It takes far less agricultural land to produce a plant-based diet than to produce meat, so with this shift we could feed our species without having to clear ever more forest land for food production. Since forests absorb carbon dioxide and produce oxygen, the movement toward a plant-based diet would provide our children with more plentiful oxygen to breathe, an atmosphere with fewer greenhouse gases, and a more stable climate.

There is still time to turn things around if we act now. Every time you choose to eat plant foods rather than meat, it's as if you were planting and tending a tree, helping to create a greener and healthier future for all generations to come.

The Heat Is On

If the Earth were the size of a basketball, the part of the atmosphere where weather occurs and all organisms live would be as thin as the film of water vapor from a single human breath. It's within this gossamer thin veil that all life on Earth exists. It's also here that the buildup of greenhouse gases is destabilizing our climate and throwing the viability of the biosphere into jeopardy.

The atmosphere is a complex mixture of gases that envelops the world. For countless centuries, the atmosphere has remained stunningly stable, as it must to maintain conditions conducive to life. If the concentration of oxygen, for example, were to increase by 20 percent, all vegetation on Earth would burst into flame and virtually all life on the planet would be destroyed, most of it within a few hours.[14]

The concentration of another of the atmosphere's gaseous constituents, carbon dioxide, has also remained remarkably stable over countless centuries—that is, until now. When we burn fossil fuels (coal, oil, and gas) and forests, we pump enormous amounts of carbon into the atmosphere. In what by any measure of Earth time is a mere microsecond, we have raised the level of carbon dioxide in the atmosphere by 25 percent. Most of that gain has occurred in only the last 40 years. As long as we keep on burning fossil fuels and forests, the amount of carbon dioxide in the atmosphere will continue to skyrocket out of control.

As the concentration of carbon dioxide continues to increase, which it inevitably will unless we make major changes, Earth's vegetation won't catch on fire. But many scientists expect the ice caps to break up, the seas to rise, storms to worsen, pests to spread, and entire ecosystems to die.

The Intergovernmental Panel on Climate Change was set up by the World Meteorological Organization and the United Nations Environment Program in the early 1990s to ascertain what is certain, and what is speculative, about climate change. The panel, made up of leading climate scientists from 98 countries, studied the problem exhaustively and issued a 1995 report warning the world that global warming is an indisputable reality. The report did not have one or two lead authors, as is usual for scientific papers, but 78 lead authors and 400 contributing authors from 26 countries, whose work had been reviewed by 500 additional scientists from 40 countries, and then re-reviewed by 177 delegates representing every national academy of science on Earth.[15]

The findings of the Intergovernmental Panel on Climate Change were unequivocal. There is simply no question any longer. Our burning of fossil fuels is destabilizing the world's climate and is likely to unleash devastating weather disturbances and disasters. It is absolutely imperative that we cut carbon emissions all over the world, but particularly in the industrial nations where these emissions are the heaviest.

In 2001, the Intergovernmental Panel on Climate Change published a new report, revising its estimates. Global warming, they said, was nearly twice as serious and dangerous as their own previous calculations, done five years earlier, had indicated.

Of course, human beings have always altered the world. We've always been busy as beavers, building houses, damming rivers, plowing fields, cutting trees, and changing things in countless other ways to suit ourselves. But huge increases in population and even greater increases in technological capability have exponentially amplified our ability to create change.

Living indoors in heated and air-conditioned buildings, as many of us do today, we can forget how vulnerable we are to atmospheric conditions. Stephen Schneider is a climatologist who spent twenty years at the National Center for Atmospheric Research in Boulder, Colorado. He is currently a professor at Stanford University and an advisor to the Intergovernmental Panel on Climate Change. He recently described what even a four-degree warming over the next century—now a very conservative estimate of what we may encounter—would mean.

> "By and large, most of us can adapt to one degree. But four degrees is virtually the difference between an ice age and a warm epoch like we're in now. It takes nature ten thousand years to make those kinds of changes, and we're talking about changes like that on the order of a century. There isn't an ecologist anywhere who thinks that we can adapt to that without dramatic dislocation to the species in the world, and to agriculture and other patterns of living that depend on climate."[16]

If a four-degree increase would cause that much disruption, imagine the impact of a much larger increase, which the 2001 Intergovernmental Panel on Climate Change report indicates is likely. According to this report, the next century is expected to bring an increase of anywhere from 2.7 to 11 degrees. If they are correct, global food security will be dealt brutal blows by the loss of biodiversity and by massive flooding of coastal areas. Such flooding would devastate coastal croplands.

This can sound like bad science fiction and seem unbelievable at first. But it is unfortunately all too real. The changes we are causing go far beyond a simple rise in temperature. If we continue to radically alter the envelope of gases that surround the planet and sustain life, there will be all kinds of other effects, from bizarre weather to localized crop failures to ecosystem collapses. Schneider says we can only speculate about some of them. The Gulf Stream could change direction or stop, and if it did, while the world was warming, Europe would freeze. The destruction of the West Antarctic ice sheet could raise sea levels by tens of feet, flooding coastlines and inundating island nations.[17]

There have been many extreme weather events in the past. Yet as Bill McKibben, author of the environmental bestseller about global warming, *The End of Nature*, points out,

> "Climate changes all the time, but it changes slowly. We're doing it at an enormous rate of speed. . . . That has real consequences. . . . Natural systems can't adapt to that sort of speed of change. . . . With the ability to change climate, you change everything. You change the flora and the fauna that live at a particular place. You change the rate at which the rain falls and at which the rain evaporates. You change the speed of the wind. You change the very ocean currents. . . . Nothing that we've ever done as a species is as large in its effect as this. . . . An all-out nuclear war would have been a consequence of the same magnitude. But happily, we stepped back from that brink. Unhappily, we're not stepping back from this one."[18]

What would it take to step back? We'd have to dramatically reduce our burning of fossil fuels, and convert to sustainable energy sources such as solar, wind, and hydrogen. To avoid devastating consequences, it is imperative that we dramatically reduce the amount of carbon dioxide, methane, and other greenhouse gases that we are emitting into the atmosphere.

Unfortunately, much as the meat industry has sought to confuse the public about the harm it causes, the coal and oil industries have hampered efforts to bring about needed changes. Even as weather extremes were wreaking staggering damage in 2000, Exxon/Mobil declared in an ad on the op-ed page of the *New York Times,* "Some . . . claim that humans are causing global warming, and they point to storms or floods to say that dangerous impacts are already under way. Yet scientists remain unable to confirm either contention."[19]

Actually, scientists were nearly unanimous in confirming both contentions. Scientific groups ringing the alarm bell included the Geophysical Fluid Dynamics Laboratory of the National Oceanic and Atmospheric Administration at Princeton; the Goddard Institute of Space Studies of NASA in New York; the National Center for Atmospheric Research in Boulder, Colorado; the Department of Energy's Lawrence Livermore National Laboratory in California; the Hadley Center for Climate Prediction and Research in the United Kingdom; and the Max Planck Institute for Meteorology in Hamburg.[20]

Meanwhile, the Greening Earth Society, a creation of the Western Fuels Coal Association, was citing the opinion of a few "greenhouse skeptics," without mentioning that most of them are on Western Fuels' payroll, and then proclaiming that more warming and more carbon dioxide is good for us because it will promote plant growth and create a greener, healthier natural world.

Ross Gelbspan is a veteran reporter for the *Philadelphia Bulletin,* the *Washington Post,* and the *Boston Globe.* He is also the author of *The Heat Is On: Climate Crisis and Coverup,* an award-winning book that documents the fossil fuel industry's efforts to spread confusion and prevent public officials from taking needed actions. He responds, "They forget to mention that peer-reviewed science indicates the opposite. While enhanced carbon dioxide creates an initial growth spurt in many trees and plants, their growth subsequently flattens and their food and nutrition value plummets. As enhanced carbon dioxide stresses plant metabolisms, they become more prone to disease, insect attacks, and fires."[21]

In fact, rising levels of carbon dioxide and methane, along with corresponding changes to the gaseous composition of the atmosphere, have already raised global temperatures and caused enormous damage. The frightening thing is that we may be only beginning to witness what will unfold.

In the last 35 years of the twentieth century, the Arctic Ocean ice thinned by 40 percent. In 2000, the polar ice at the top of the world melted for the first time in human memory. If any explorers had been trekking to the North Pole that summer, they would have had to swim the last few miles. Many scientists believed there had not been so much open water in the polar region in 50 million years. Other scientists predicted that summer ice in the Arctic Ocean could disappear entirely by 2035.[22]

It was no secret why this was happening. Rising carbon dioxide levels in the atmosphere had increased the Earth's temperature. In 2000, it was announced that of the 25 hottest years that had occurred since Earth temperature record keeping began in 1866, 23 of them had occurred after 1975.[23]

That same year, *E* magazine, for only the second time in its history, dedicated an entire feature section to a single topic—global warming. The magazine's editor, Jim Motavalli, explained that crazy and extreme weather episodes had been increasing, but that was only part of the story. Scientists had confirmed:

> "Dramatic and permanent environmental changes. Sea level is rising in the Pacific, inundating small islands and threatening larger ones. Reefs around the world are dying from coral bleaching. Coastal resorts from New Jersey to Antigua are losing their beaches, and making a desperate attempt to hold back restless seas. The populations of California's tidal pools and Washington State's glacial slopes are changing dramatically. In the Antarctic, huge ice floes the size of American states are breaking off, and insect pests are killing the great coniferous forests of Alaska. Coastal cities like New York are battening down the hatches, and giant ozone clouds hide the Indian Ocean in gloom.
>
> "Worldwide climate change on this scale cannot be explained as part of a natural cycle. . . . The crisis is manmade, but the responsibility is not spread evenly over the Earth. Some 73 percent of carbon dioxide emissions come from industrialized nations, according to the White House Office of Science and Technology Policy. The largest single source is the United States, which alone accounts for 22 percent of total world emissions, or five tons of carbon dioxide per U.S. citizen, per year."[24]

November 1996 brought a once-in-200-years flood to the Potomac River in Washington, D.C. The assumption, when the flood subsided, was there would not be another one for two centuries. The next once-in-200-years flood occurred, however, three weeks later.[25]

Even taking into account the growth in urban populations, the increase in damage from severe climate events has been staggering. In 1992, Hurricane Andrew hit Florida, wreaking greater damage than any storm to hit the region in 300 years. In 1996, China was hit by a flood that killed more than 3,000 people and caused $26 billion in damages, breaking the record set by Andrew for the costliest natural disaster in world history. In 1998, China was struck by an even more devastating flood, this one causing $36 billion in damages, exceeding by itself *the entire world's* damages from all natural disasters in any year prior to 1995. In one watershed, 56 million people were flooded from their homes. During the same summer, Bangladesh was struck by a flood that put two-thirds of the densely populated country under water and left 21 million homeless. A couple months later, Hurricane Mitch killed 18,000 people in Central America.[26]

As the intensity of extreme weather events has increased, international aid agencies have struggled valiantly to respond. In 2000, the International Federation of Red Cross and Red Crescent societies said that climate change was manifesting "in a catalogue of disasters such as storms, droughts, and flooding unparalleled in modern times."[27]

WHAT WE KNOW

Economic losses from weather-related disasters, worldwide, 1980: $2.8 billion[28]

Average annual economic losses from weather-related disasters, worldwide, 1980–1984: $6.5 billion[29]

Economic losses from weather-related disasters, worldwide, 1985: $7.2 billion[30]

Average annual economic losses from weather-related disasters, worldwide, 1985–1989: $9.2 billion[31]

Economic losses from weather-related disasters, worldwide, 1990: $18.0 billion[32]

Average annual economic losses from weather-related disasters, worldwide, 1990–1994: $27.6 billion[33]

Economic losses from weather-related disasters, worldwide, 1995: $40.3 billion[34]

Average annual economic losses from weather-related disasters, worldwide, 1995–1999: $58.5 billion[35]

Economic losses from weather-related disasters, worldwide, 1999: $67.1 billion[36]

(All figures in 1998 dollars)

Gas Pains

For almost all of the past 10,000 years, the level of carbon dioxide in the atmosphere has remained constant, at about 280 parts per million. Then, about 100 years ago, it began, slowly at first, to rise. Now we're at 360 parts per million, a concentration of carbon dioxide that has not existed on Earth for at least 400,000 years.

While there are many human activities that are driving this alarming trend, agriculture turns out to be surprisingly significant. But not all forms of agriculture are equally to blame. Different food choices and different forms of food production have vastly different impacts on global warming.

The use of large amounts of nitrogen fertilizers in the United States is a driving force behind climate change, because ammonium nitrate, the most common form of nitrogen fertilizer (and also an ingredient in explosives), is essentially congealed natural gas, a fossil fuel.[37]

The impact on the atmosphere is extreme. Alan Durning and John Ryan of the Northwest Environment Watch say the U.S. economy consumes nearly a pound of ammonia per person per day, mostly as nitrogen fertilizer. They add that one-quarter of the nitrogen fertilizer used in the United States is applied to corn eaten by livestock.[38]

The production of any kind of food uses energy, and as long as that energy is derived from coal, oil, and gas, carbon dioxide will be released into the atmosphere. But when it comes to carbon dioxide emissions, not all foods are the same. Not nearly. . .

WHAT WE KNOW

Calories of fossil fuel expended to produce 1 calorie of protein from soybeans: 2[39]

Calories of fossil fuel expended to produce 1 calorie of protein from corn or wheat: 3[40]

Calories of fossil fuel expended to produce 1 calorie of protein from beef: 54[41]

Amount of greenhouse-warming carbon gas released by driving a typical American car, in one day: 3 kilograms[42]

Amount released by clearing and burning enough Costa Rican rainforest to produce beef for one hamburger: 75 kilograms[43]

Since beef requires the burning of 54 fossil fuel calories for the production of a calorie of protein, and soybeans require only two, people deriving their protein from soybeans are, in effect, consuming only 4 percent as much energy—and producing only 4 percent as much carbon dioxide—as people deriving their protein from beef.

By the same token, since corn or wheat require the burning of only 3 fossil fuel calories to produce a calorie of protein, people deriving their protein from beef are, in effect, burning 18 times as much energy—and producing 18 times as much carbon dioxide—as people deriving their protein from corn or wheat.

This is not just the opinion of anti-meat activists. In 1996, the *Journal of Animal Science* agreed, in an article titled "Ecosystems, Sustainability, and Animal Agriculture." The article's authors stated that "results [of extensive research at the Fort Keogh Livestock and Range Reserve Laboratory at Miles City, Montana] pointedly reveal the high level of dependency of the U.S. beef cattle industry on fossil fuels."[44]

Scientists, even those writing in animal industry journals, agree that modern meat production is responsible for a vastly disproportionate amount of carbon dioxide and other greenhouse gases. This doesn't prevent the cattlemen, however, from denying there is a problem. . .

Is THAT SO?

> "The overall energy efficiency of beef often is comparable, or even superior, to the energy efficiency of plant-source foods."
> —National Cattlemen's Beef Association[45]
>
> "American feed (for livestock) takes so much energy to grow that it might as well be a petroleum byproduct."
> —Worldwatch Institute[46]

Next to carbon dioxide, the most destabilizing gas to the planet's climate is methane. Methane is actually 24 times more potent a greenhouse gas than carbon dioxide, and its concentration in the atmosphere is rising even faster.[47] Concentrations of atmospheric methane are now nearly triple what they were when they began rising a century ago. The primary reason is beef production.

According to the EPA, the world's livestock are responsible for 25 percent of the world's anthropogenic methane emissions (those that are based in human activity).[48] Once again, however, when challenged, the U.S. meat industry manages to maintain its unique perspective.

Is THAT SO?

> "[It's a] myth that U.S. cattle produce large amounts of methane, a 'greenhouse' gas, thereby contributing significantly to possible global warming problems."
> —National Cattlemen's Beef Association[49]
>
> "Livestock account for 15 percent to 20 percent of (overall) global methane emissions."
> —Worldwatch Institute[50]

In 1999, the Union of Concerned Scientists published a book analyzing American society and explaining how things we do in our daily lives affect the environment. Focusing on global warming, the report concluded that the two most damaging things residents of this country do to our climate are drive vehicles that get poor gas mileage and eat beef.[51]

Deeply implicated, the U.S. meat industry has joined with the coal and oil industries in seeking to deny the existence of what may well be the most momentous development in human history.

Is THAT SO?

"The evidence of global warming has been inconclusive at best . . . whether [there exists] a warming trend is unclear."
—National Cattlemen's Beef Association[52]

"Global warming has emerged as the most serious environmental threat of the 21st century. . . . Only by taking action now can we insure that future generations will not be put at risk."
—Letter to the president from 49 Nobel Prize-winning scientists[53]

Stabilizing our climate would help resolve what many scientists consider to be the gravest environmental danger humankind has ever faced. Each of us has a part to play in shifting our culture toward a way of life that respects the natural world. The choices we make and the way we live can play roles in turning the tide. By eating in a way that is congruent both with our own health and the health of the biosphere, we can help our society to face and to turn around the enormous environmental challenges of our times. The more people move toward plant-based food choices, the greater the possibility that our species will not only survive, but will thrive.

A cultural shift toward a plant-based diet would be a step toward environmental sanity. It would be an act of love for all generations yet to come.

Saving Species, One Bite at a Time

Living immersed in human-made environments, surrounded by and interacting constantly with artifacts produced by people, many of us are unaware of our absolute dependence on the greater environment. Not only is every single thing we ever touch, see, feel, smell, or taste composed ultimately of materials from the natural world, but the diversity of species within the greater Earth community together create the conditions that enable human life to exist.

During the past 500 million years, there have been five major disruptions that the scientific community calls "mass extinctions." The most famous of these occurred about 65 million years ago, probably caused by a large meteorite colliding with the Earth. It marked the end of the dinosaurs.

Mass extinctions occur naturally, but they do so only every 100 million years or so, and life on the planet takes a long time afterward to recover. And when it recovers, it does so because new life forms have evolved, not because the old ones have returned. Extinction truly is forever.

Biologists surveyed by the American Museum of Natural History in New York say that we are now in the midst of the sixth of Earth's great mass extinctions, only this one is the fastest in Earth's history, even faster than when the dinosaurs died.[54] And this one is caused not by a giant meteorite from outer space, but by a two-legged creature that fancies itself the pinnacle of Creation.

Extinctions occur even in normal times, but we have precipitated a flood of extinctions that go way beyond anything resembling normalcy. Biologists estimate the "normal" level of extinctions at about 10 to 25 species per year. We are, however, now losing at least several thousand species per year, and possibly tens of thousands.

We need to save not only whales, cheetahs, pandas, and other impressive and/or cuddly creatures. We also need the plants (including plankton, microscopic organisms that are the basis for ocean food chains) and the fungi, bacteria, and insects. You won't see these creatures on refrigerator magnets, at the zoo, or featured in TV specials. But they are instrumental to life on Earth—probably far more necessary, in fact, than we are.

Harvard biologist Edward O. Wilson, who first coined the term "biodiversity," says that even the lowly ant may be far more important to the survival of life on Earth than human beings. "If all humanity disappeared," he points out, "the rest of life, except for domestic animals and plants, which represent only a minute fraction of the plants and animals of the world, would benefit enormously."[55] The forests would return, and atmospheric gases would stabilize. The fish in the oceans would recover, and most endangered species would slowly come back. There would be no humans left, and that would certainly be a great loss, but as far as the survival of other species goes, given how we've been behaving, the planet might actually be better off without us.

In contrast, says Wilson, if all ants were to disappear, the results would be disastrous. Ants turn and aerate a very large part of the Earth's soils. They're major predators of other insects, and they remove and break up more than 90 percent of many small, dead creatures as part of the soil-nutrient cycle. They even pollinate many plants. "If they were to disappear, there would be major extinctions of other species and probably partial collapse of some ecosystems."[56]

There are countless species of bacteria, fungi, and other micro-organisms that, like ants, are critical to the survival of entire ecosystems. How many species can disappear before the web of life unravels? No one knows.

But we know enough to be certain that the loss of a species to extinction is a tragedy not only for that species. The more species of plants, animals, and other life forms there are in any given bio-region, the more resistant that area will be to destruction, and the better it can perform its environmental roles of cleansing water, enriching the soil, maintaining stable climates, and generating the oxygen we breathe.

WHAT WE KNOW

World's mammalian species currently threatened with extinction: 25 percent[57]

Leading cause of species in the tropical rainforests being threatened or eliminated: Livestock grazing[58]

Leading cause of species in the United States being threatened or eliminated (according to the U.S. Congress General Accounting Office): Livestock grazing[59]

Today, cattle and other ruminant animals (such as sheep and goats) graze an astounding half of the planet's total land area. And they, along with pigs and poultry, eat feed raised on much of the world's cropland. These agricultural realities have had enormous consequences to wildlife habitat and biodiversity.

As vast reaches of the American West have been given over to cattle grazing, wildlife has paid a terrible price. Pronghorn sheep have decreased from 15 million a century ago to less than 271,000 today. Bighorn sheep, once numbering over 2 million, are now less than 20,000.[60] The elk population has likewise plummeted. Tens of thousands of wild horses and burros have been rounded up because they competed with cattle, many ending up in slaughterhouses. Meanwhile, cattle ranchers have sought to block the reintroduction of wolves into the wild, despite the fact that it's required by the Endangered Species Act.

In 1999, University of Wyoming law professor Debra Donahue, who also holds a master's degree in wildlife biology, wrote a book in which she said the most important thing that could be done to protect species from extinction and preserve biodiversity is to remove livestock from nearly all public lands. In response, Wyoming Senate president and cattleman Jim Twiford proposed a bill that would dismantle the university law school.[61]

Is THAT SO?

"Cattlemen graze livestock on more than half the land area of the United States. . . . These lands provide habitat for many of the species listed as threatened or endangered. The cattle business is often affected adversely by the Endangered Species Act because regulations to protect species habitat restrict land uses and limit ranchers' management options."

—National Cattlemen's Beef Association, explaining its opposition to the Endangered Species Act[62]

"Loss of species and climate change [exemplify how] current methods of rearing animals around the world take a large toll on nature. Overgrown and resource-intensive, animal agriculture is out of alignment with the Earth's ecosystems."

—Worldwatch Institute[63]

Some cattlemen I have spoken to echo the words of Ruben Ayala, the former California state senator. The senator, explaining why he opposed legislation to protect endangered species, said, "The dinosaurs went extinct and I don't miss them." These people take the position that species extinction is part of life. It has been going on since prehistoric times, and is how nature evolves. We need not worry about species extinction, they say, because the species that are dying out today are simply the ones that aren't adaptable enough to survive.

There might be some semblance of reality in this, except for the minor fact that today's unprecedented extinction rate is estimated by some biologists to be 1,000 to 10,000 times higher than existed in prehistoric times.

But I understand why the cattlemen would want to minimize the problem of species extinction. A major 1997 study of endangered species in the American Southwest by the U.S. Fish and Wildlife Service found that nearly half of the endangered species that were studied were threatened by cattle ranching.[64]

The driving force behind the escalating rate of extinction in the United States, the tropical rainforests, and elsewhere, is the destruction of wildlife habitat. When the Union of Concerned Scientists analyzed the environmental impact of human activities, they concluded that the damage to wildlife habitat from producing 1 pound of beef is 20 times greater than that from producing 1 pound of pasta.[65]

A cultural shift toward a plant-based diet would save many of the species that are currently endangered and threatened. It would be a statement that we no longer hold ourselves above the rest of Creation, with the right to do to other life forms anything we might want, including extinguish their very existence. It would be a statement that we are ready to accept with humility and honor our role in preserving and protecting other species, rather than playing the conqueror and ending up ourselves destroyed.

Extinction is irreversible: we cannot re-create what no longer exists. Yet, Nature has extraordinary powers of restoration and replenishment. When we decrease our assault on a given environment, Nature can restore itself. As more people move toward a plant-based lifestyle, the demands we place upon the planet grow lighter, and we are able to satisfy our needs and to grow in health and prosperity without sacrificing other members of our greater Earth family.

Once Upon a Planet

The production of modern meat in factory farms and feedlots has enormous health, humanitarian, and environmental costs. I want all of us to become aware of these costs, but I cannot criticize people who are not aware of them and whose actions follow from what they've heard and learned. Thanks to the misinformation campaigns of the meat industry and its efforts to silence its critics, most people have no clue as to the greater impact of their food choices.

My complaint is not with people who act in accord with what they've been told. My criticism is with the industries that are damaging our planet and our future, while telling us how wonderful they are. And also with the media, which has a responsibility to tell us what's really going on, but too often doesn't.

In 1992, 1,600 senior scientists from 71 countries, including over half of all living Nobel Prize winners, signed and released a document titled "World Scientists' Warning to Humanity." It began with the words, "Human beings and the natural world are on a collision course," and then continued,

> "Human activities inflict harsh and often irreversible damage on the environment and on critical resources. If not checked, many of our current practices put at serious risk the future that we wish for human society and the plant and animal kingdoms, and may so alter the living world that it will be unable to sustain life in the manner that we know. Fundamental changes are urgent if we are to avoid the collision our present course will bring about. . . .
>
> "No more than one or a few decades remain before the chance to avert the threats we now confront will be lost and the prospects for humanity immeasurably diminished. We the undersigned, senior members of the world's scientific community, hereby warn all humanity of what lies ahead. A great change in our stewardship for the Earth and life on it is

required, if vast human misery is to be avoided and our global home is not to be irretrievably mutilated."

You or I might think the release of such a powerful and historic statement would have been front-page news. But when the "World Scientists' Warning to Humanity" was released to the press, virtually every major newspaper in the United States and Canada deemed it "not newsworthy." That day, the *New York Times* did, however, find space on the front page for a story about the origin of rock and roll, while the front page of one of Canada's major newspapers, the *Globe and Mail*, included a large photograph of cars forming an image of Mickey Mouse.[66]

This is the kind of thing that gets me quite upset.

Similarly, just before the turn of the millennium, Worldwatch Institute released a report on ocean fisheries. It had just been discovered that overfishing was decimating not only the adult fish populations, but the juveniles as well, thus accelerating the destruction of the oceanic food web. The *Toronto Star* was all set to run a feature on the report but, due to a late-breaking story deemed to be of far more significance, had to cancel it. The story that was considered more newsworthy concerned a member of the Spice Girls, a pop singing group, who had announced she was leaving the group.[67]

It's enough to make you despair. Yet every so often something happens to balance all this. Once in a while, the media steps up and does something you never would have expected in a million years, restoring your faith in humanity and suggesting there is hope for us humans, after all.

Waking Up in the Most Unlikely of All Places

A few years ago, I got a phone call from a media person that I found utterly surprising. As a result, I was totally unprepared for how things developed.

I was sitting at home one day, more or less minding my own business, when the phone rang. There was an upbeat female voice on the line, though not one I recognized. She said she was with a television show, and they wanted to do a program on me and my work.

When *Diet for a New America* first came out, I had been eager to spread the message wherever I could, and had agreed to almost every request for an interview, no matter how large or small the publication, radio station, or TV show. After trudging out to tiny cable stations at 2:00 in the morning, and appearing on obscure local shows that reached viewers of the Home Shopping Channel at 3:00 A.M., however, I had become more selective.

"What's the name of your show?" I asked.

"*Lifestyles.*"

"Never heard of it."

"We're in every major market in the country."

Well, well, well, a national show, that's interesting. Could be good. But then again could be very bad. The name *Lifestyles* sounded innocent enough, but you never know with these big networks. I needed more information.

"What time are you on in my area?"

After she told me the particulars, I put the phone down and fetched a newspaper to check if the show was in my local listings. This seemed like a straightforward thing to do, and not one likely to cause problems, but when I found the spot, I was shocked. For what it said, right there in front of me, in my own local newspaper, was *Lifestyles of the Rich and Famous.*

Hardly believing what was happening, I returned to the phone, and told her what it said in my paper.

"Well, yes, that's the full name of our show."

I probably should have been diplomatic and tactful. My efforts in that direction, however, were not very effective. "I hate your show," I told her. "You glorify the shallowest parts of people. You exalt conspicuous consumption. Your motto should be 'Shop 'til the planet drops.'"

"I'm sorry you feel that way," she replied, seemingly unfazed, "but on our behalf, let me say that we are a positive show. We don't put people down, the way other shows like *Current Affair* and *Hard Copy* do. We try to be positive."

I wasn't impressed, and took the occasion to tell her so. When every religion and spiritual lineage known to humankind has taught that happiness cannot be attained through material acquisition, what kind of television show is it that preaches just the opposite? With the world ecology teetering on the edge, what kind of show glorifies an orgy of unsustainable consumption?

"I can't believe you're calling me," I said, finally. "I'm the total opposite of everything you're about. Are you sure you aren't looking for the author Harold Robbins?"

"No, John Robbins, author of *Diet for a New America*."

"Well that's me, but I can't understand why in the world you would be calling me."

"Let me explain," she said. "Once a year we're allowed to do a different kind of show. Once a year we do a show on philanthropists who donate to humanitarian causes. On people who use their wealth for the good of their fellow human beings."

"That's very nice," I replied. "I wish you did that show every week, and once a year you did your stupid show."

She laughed, which confused me all the more. I was totally serious. Twenty-five years earlier, I had walked away from the kind of lifestyle her show made such a fuss about, to live a far more simple and Earth-friendly life. As far as I was concerned, her show had no place in a world that is groaning under the weight of our out-of-control consumption.

Then it occurred to me what must be happening. She must be assuming I was still connected to Baskin-Robbins, and that I was rich. That's it, I thought, that explains why she's calling me.

I tried to be patient as I told her that I had walked away from all that years before, had been totally on my own ever since, and had no connection to any of the Baskin-Robbins money.

Telling her this, I thought, would take care of the matter. But I was wrong. To the contrary, she now seemed if anything to intensify her efforts to talk me into being on the show.

"Well, you *could have been* rich," she said.

Right, I thought, "Lifestyles of the *Could Have Been* Rich and Famous."

I decided to make one more stab at straightening things out. "Could you just tell me one thing? Why in the world would you want to do a show on me? I'm not rich, and quite frankly, I find your show disgusting."

She sighed, but she persisted. "Well, yes, I understand, but you see, some of us on the staff here have read your books, and we think they are the most important books we've ever read, and we want to use the program to get your message out to a large audience of people who otherwise might never be exposed to it."

So this was why she had called! Now it made sense, and I must admit I was flattered. But, still, even though she meant well, it seemed hopeless. I tried to explain to her how we lived. Our home was small, so tiny in fact that the room my wife and I slept in was also our living room and kitchen. Our only car was a fifteen-year-old Datsun station wagon that had been driven more than 200,000 miles, and looked it. It ran, and we were happy, but our lifestyle was quite a far cry from anything I thought they would ever be interested in filming.

"That doesn't matter," she assured me. "We'll find a way to make it work. We'll think of something."

I'm not sure what came over me, but I said okay, and we made a date for them to come.

When the time arrived, we cleaned up. Not that it took that long. You could vacuum the whole place in about ten minutes.

And then it happened. Outside, on the street, a gigantic van pulled up. On its side, in the gaudiest possible script, were the words, "Lifestyles of the Rich and Famous." I knew because I was peeking through the blinds. My first thought was, "What will the neighbors think?"

The van door opened, and out piled an entire crew, who I later learned included people to work the lights, the cameras, and the sound equipment, plus a producer and a director and someone they called a "gopher," whose job it was to go get hamburgers for them at lunch time. Plus what seemed like mountains of equipment. I looked around our living room/kitchen (we had put the bedding away) and concluded there was no way, no way at all, that all those people and their stuff could fit.

One rather heavyset fellow, who I later learned was one of the cameramen, approached the door first. He knocked, and I answered. "Excuse me," he said. "Sorry to bother you. But we're looking for the home of a John Robbins, and we seem to have gotten lost. Your house number is the same as his."

Oh God, I thought. I knew this was going to happen. But at this point I figured I had better make the best of it.

"That's me," I said cheerfully. "Come in and make yourself at home."
His face dropped. "This," he said doubtfully, "is where you live?"

"Yes," I said. "Please come in."

He turned toward the van and the others. "This is the right place," he shouted. Then he laughed. "Doesn't look like the places we go to, usually."

As they entered, I attempted to be a good host. "Have a seat," I said to the cameraman, gesturing toward our only chairs. We had four vinyl-covered chairs that had been purchased several decades before as a Sears dinette set. Over the years, one of our cats, a brown Siamese named Brownfellow, had decided that these chairs were his personal scratching posts, and had lacerated the vinyl. At first I had tried to stop him, but it was to no avail, and I had eventually given up the effort. He had enjoyed himself shredding the chairs, so that by this time there was more stuffing showing than vinyl. I had come, over the years, to look upon the chairs as a kind of art form, the artist in this case being a cat.

That did not seem, however, to be the way the cameraman saw things. "No thank you," he said stiffly. "I'd rather stand."

Perhaps his reluctance was because Brownfellow chose that particular moment to add something of his own creation to one of the chairs, something that indicated rather clearly that he had not been enjoying his food as much as I might have hoped.

Before long, they were all inside. It wasn't easy, but they and their equipment somehow managed to fit. Then I met the woman who had made the original call, a delightful woman, actually, and before long we were underway.

They interviewed me quite a few different times over the next few days, and also filmed an EarthSave fund-raiser where I spoke, plus got footage of the EarthSave office. Whenever I introduced them to colleagues or friends of mine, I always got a look that said, in no uncertain terms, "You don't really expect us to believe that these people are from *that* show, do you?"

After the first morning of shooting, it was time for the gopher to go for lunch, but they decided, and I think it was quite respectful of them, to all go "veggie" for the days they would be with us. My wife, Deo, made us all a fabulous lunch each day, with fresh organic vegetables from our garden and from the local farmer's market. A cameraman told me that he'd been with the show for years, filming all kinds of palatial estates, private islands, and mansions, and he'd never before been invited to have lunch with the people they were filming. Not once. I told him I thought that was sad, but I was glad, at least, that he was having a different experience now.

As time went along, I talked a good deal on camera about the environmental situation, and how our ethic of consumption was damaging the world and the future of all life. I spoke about the urgent need for all of us to create lifestyles and public policies that helped us to walk more lightly on the Earth, that did not create so much waste or use so much energy. I pointed with dismay to the ever-widening gap between the rich and the poor. And of course, I talked about a plant-based diet, and its many wonderful benefits.

When the time came to say good-bye, I realized how much fun it had been. The entire crew had indeed remained veggie for our time together, and had been much more than respectful toward me. The cameraman and other crewmembers told me they had enjoyed themselves very much, learned a great deal, and were going to eat far less meat in the future. The woman who had made the original call was ecstatic, and told me I had no idea how much this had all meant to her. She hugged me, and while she was at it, she told me that doing this show was one of the highlights of her life. "I'm so happy and proud," she said.

I was moved, and the feeling lingered for a while after they all left, until it dawned on me that I had no idea what in the end would appear on television. They had, after all, taken hours of footage and would create a show out of it all by cutting and splicing in the editing room. I had no idea what to expect.

It was therefore with some trepidation that I turned on the television the day they first aired the show. But actually, they did a marvelous job, and the program, which turned out to be one of their most popular ever, has since been aired thousands of times on stations all over the world. Robin Leach called me "the prophet of nonprofit." I rather liked that, especially considering some of the other things I've been called. There was one thing that I was sure they would cut, but they left it in—me saying that I admire Thoreau, and quoting him, saying, "I make myself rich by making my wants few."

At one point, the camera is sweeping across the room (they used a special lens to make the room look larger) and there, before you, are the chairs. Robin Leach announces, and to this day I have no idea where he got this, that "every stick of furniture in their house is recycled."

And then, at the end, they bring up on the screen for everyone to see the beautiful picture of the Earth from space. I'm sure you know the photo. Our precious blue-green planet, suspended among the stars like an exquisite jewel. Our beautiful Earth, more perfectly spherical than a billiard ball, a geometric marvel. Our world, with no political borders, just oceans and continents, so achingly fragile and beautiful. They leave this photo up there for a long time, instead of jumping from one image to the next every microsecond, as is so often done on TV today, and they have beautiful music behind the image of our gorgeous planet. And then Robin Leach, of all people, says something I can hardly believe I am hearing on *this* of all shows: "This man's life goes to prove that whoever believes, 'He who dies with the most toys wins,' doesn't see the whole picture." And here's the picture of the whole Earth from space.

I don't want to make too much of this, because I know it was just a television show. But I was moved by what transpired, because there's something in this that speaks to me of the paramount issues of our times. If a show like *Lifestyles of the Rich and Famous* could, even for a few minutes, broadcast these words of sanity, words that Americans so deeply need to hear, then maybe we have reason to hope.

Maybe we won't have to wait until the last river has been poisoned, the last acre of fertile ground has been paved over, and the last forest has been converted into a shopping mall, to learn that we can't eat money.

Maybe the day is not that far off when we will honor those who excel at giving, not those who excel at getting. Perhaps it won't be long before we recognize and appreciate the many courageous people who work day in and day out, not just to make the biggest buck, but to make the world a better place.

Maybe soon we will be giving our esteem and attention not just to those who make the most money, but to those who grow food that is healthy for our bodies and the Earth, and to those who repair damaged ecosystems and preserve endangered species.

Maybe the work so many people are doing to create a thriving and sustainable way of life for all might actually be taking root—even in some of the most unlikely places.

Like blades of grass bursting through a crack in a thick slab of concrete, something is seeking to break through the walls we have put between us and our kinship with the Earth. It is the awesome power of Creation itself. It is the same force that turns the tides, brings rain to parched earth, entices the bee to the flower, and ignites new life in countless species.

Maybe we aren't on a one-way road to oblivion. Maybe we're standing at a crossroad, facing what may be the most important choice human beings have ever faced, a choice between two directions. In one direction is what we will have if we do nothing to alter our present course. By doing nothing, we are choosing a world of pollution and extinctions, of widening chasms and deepening despair, a world where humanity moves ever farther from achieving its highest aspirations and ever nearer to living its darkest fears.[68]

Our other choice is to actively engage with the living world. On this path we work responsibly and joyfully to make our lives, and our societies, into expressions of our love for ourselves, for each other, and for the living Earth. In this direction we honor our longing to give our children, and all children, a world with clean air and water, with blue skies and abundant wildlife, with a stable climate and a healthy environment.

If you live with fear for our future, you are not alone.

If you live with dreams of a better world, you are not alone.

We all live, now, with both the pain and the possibility we carry in our hearts, both the despair and the hope that we may yet learn to live in harmony with our precious and endangered Earth. There is not a person alive today who does not, at some level, know we are facing these two directions, and understand how much is at stake.

At such a crossroad, the steps that we take toward an Earth-friendly lifestyle are important, both for the ground they cover and for the direction they lead. Each step makes possible the next step, and the next. We will not, of course, turn things around merely because we do a few convenient things to save the Earth. But as more of us do the things that matter, as more of us lead by example, others will find themselves pulled along. One step always leads to the next. As more of us find ways of expressing our love for the Earth, others will be swept up in the power of our caring and the integrity of our example.

I am aware how strong are the forces of ignorance, greed, and denial in our society. I know it is possible that we won't make it.

But I am also aware of how strong is the longing and the love of life in the human heart. And so I know it is possible that we will make it, that we will create a sustainable economy that protects the living systems of the Earth, that we will come to be part of the world's repair. The power of darkness in our world is great, but it is not as great as the power of the human spirit. We can learn to provide for our needs and limit our numbers while cherishing this beautiful planet and its creatures. It is in our nature to honor the sacredness of life.

What is at stake today is enormous; it is the destiny of life on Earth. At such a time, walking a path of honoring ourselves and the living planet is our responsibility as citizens of the planet, but it is something more, as well.

It is also a joy, and a privilege.

chapter 15 # Reversing the Spread of Hunger

At the first world food conference, held in Rome in 1974, U.S. Secretary of State Henry Kissinger promised that by 1984, no man, woman, or child on Earth would go to bed hungry.[1]

Many things have changed since then. At that time, there were barely 4 billion people on the planet. Today there are more than 6 billion.

During the 1970s, the world grain harvest per capita was growing. However, it peaked in 1984, the very year by which Kissinger hoped world hunger would end, and has been falling ever since.[2] And there is every indication this decline will accelerate in coming years as aquifers are depleted and water for irrigation becomes increasingly scarce.

At the same time, the state of the world's farmland has degraded. In 2000, using satellite photos, maps, and other data, the International Food Policy Research Institute completed the most comprehensive study ever made of agricultural land around the world. The findings were unmistakable. Due to problems like erosion and nutrient depletion, nearly 40 percent of the world's agricultural land had become seriously degraded, raising doubts about its ability to produce food in the future. Ismail Seragldin, World Bank vice president and chairman of a consortium of international agricultural research centers, commented,

"The results raise all kinds of red flags about the world's ability to feed itself in the future."[3]

Today, more than a billion people on this planet do not have enough to eat. Nearly one-third of the children in the developing world are chronically hungry, making them vulnerable to infectious disease and diarrhea, which often lead to permanent mental and physical impairment or death.[4] Meanwhile, McDonald's is opening five new restaurants a day—four of them outside the United States.

Is McDonald's in Ethiopia the answer to world hunger?

Is THAT SO?

"[It's a] myth [that] beef cattle production uses grain that could be used to feed the world's hungry."

—National Cattlemen's Association[5]

"In a world where an estimated one in every six people goes hungry every day, the politics of meat consumption are increasingly heated, since meat production is an inefficient use of grain—the grain is used more efficiently when consumed directly by humans. Continued growth in meat output is dependent on feeding grains to animals, creating competition for grain between affluent meat eaters and the world's poor."

—Worldwatch Institute[6]

In traditional livestock production systems, domestic animals turned grass and other things people could not eat into things people could. And still, in many parts of the world (including most of Africa), people depend on animals to convert vegetation that does not compete with human food crops into edible protein. To raise meat output, however, livestock producers in the industrialized world have adopted intensive rearing techniques that rely heavily on grains and legumes to feed their animals.

Virtually all of the pigs and poultry in industrial countries now reside in gigantic indoor facilities where their diets include grain and soybean meal. Most cattle spend their last months in feedlots where they gorge on grain and soybeans. Overall, nearly 40 percent of the world's grain is fed to livestock. And the nations that eat the most meat dedicate the largest share of their grain to fattening livestock. In the United States, livestock now eat twice as much grain as is consumed by the country's entire human population.

The more grain that is fed to livestock, the less is left to feed people. Dr. M. E. Ensminger, former Chairman of the Department of Animal Science at Washington State University, is one of the leading figures in the U.S. beef industry. In *Animal Science*, he writes,

> "There can be no question that more hunger can be alleviated with a given quantity of grain by completely eliminating animals. . . . It's not efficient to feed grain to animals and then to consume the livestock products."[7]

Who Eats? And Who Doesn't?

In nation after nation today, the world's wealthy are following in the meat-eating footsteps of the United States. Does this trend have consequences for the food security of the world's poor? As countries increase their consumption of animal products, ever more of their grain goes to animals and ever less to people, and they must import ever-increasing amounts of grain. In a world where per-capita grain production stopped rising in 1984, and has been falling ever since, how can this be sustained?

In the most populous nation in the world, China, the share of grain fed to livestock increased between 1978 and 1997 from 8 percent to 26 percent.[8] In the early 1990s, China was a net exporter of grain, but today, thanks to an increasing appetite for meat, China is the world's second largest grain importer, trailing only Japan.[9]

> "As Chinese eat more grain-fed meat, the country's need for grain will continue to grow. This . . . could quickly make China the world's leading grain importer, overtaking even Japan . . . potentially disrupting world grain markets . . . meaning rising food prices for the entire world. . . . China cannot import the grain it needs without driving world grain prices up, leaving the 1.3 billion people in the world who subsist on $1 a day at risk." (Worldwatch Institute)[10]

If food prices rise throughout the world, the wealthy will still eat, but the poor will increasingly be left with nowhere to turn. In recent years, grain prices have been kept reasonably stable only through massive over-pumping of aquifers worldwide for irrigation. But as a result, water tables are now falling rapidly throughout the world's agriculturally productive areas—including China, India, and the United States, which together produce half the world's food. The International Water Management Institute, the world's premier water research group, estimates that India's grain harvest may before long be reduced by one-fourth as a result of aquifer depletion.[11]

Thirty years ago, the U.S.S.R. was self-sufficient in grain; but in the 1990s, the former Soviet Union became the world's third largest grain importer. Russian livestock now eat three times as much grain as Russian people.[12] Hardly existent in Russia 20 years ago, hunger and human starvation are now widespread and severe.

Throughout the world, increases in grain-fed livestock have forced countries to import more feed. Twenty years ago, only 1 percent of Thailand's grain was fed to animals. Today the figure has risen to 30 percent.[13] At the same time, a growing number of people in Thailand and throughout Asia live on the perilous edge of food deprivation. Millions are dying from lack of adequate food. Many watch their children starve.

Vandana Shiva is the director of the Research Foundation for Science, Technology, and Natural Resource Policy, and one of the world's foremost experts on global food issues. She says we are seeing "the McDonaldization of the world. . . . As more grain is traded globally, more people go hungry in the Third World."[14]

Middle Eastern countries similarly maintain high levels of meat consumption only by depending heavily on imported grain. Twenty years ago, Egypt was self-sufficient in grain. Then, livestock ate only 10 percent of the nation's grain. Today, livestock consume 36 percent of Egypt's grain, and the country must import 8 million tons every year.[15] Jordan now imports 91 percent of its grain, Israel 87 percent, Libya 85 percent, and Saudi Arabia 50 percent.[16]

As livestock industries pour grain into producing animal products for the wealthy, almost all Third World nations must now import grain. That more and more countries are looking to the world market for food can only translate into food scarcity for the world's poor.

Remarkably, the world's nations depend massively on one nation for grain. The United States is responsible for half of the world's grain exports, shipping grain to more than 100 countries. Yet the U.S. grain harvest is notoriously sensitive to climate conditions, including droughts. In a time of global warming and climate destabilization, the possibility of a weather-induced drop in U.S. grain harvest is all too real.[17] And with the depletion of the Ogallala aquifer, experts are predicting that before long the United States will lose much, if not all, of its grain surplus.[18] With the world's agricultural economy devouring rapidly increasing quantities of grain for livestock production, the consequences to the world's less fortunate people could be tragic.

> "Higher meat consumption among the affluent frequently creates problems for the poor, as the share of farmland devoted to feed cultivation expands, reducing production of food staples. In the economic competition for grain fields, the upper classes usually win." (Worldwatch Institute)[19]

Since 1960, the number of landless in Central America has multiplied fourfold. International lending agencies such as the World Bank and the Inter-American Development Bank have responded with billions of dollars in loans. But these loans have not challenged the tightly concentrated distribution of economic power, nor the use of resources to benefit the wealthy at the expense of the poor. Often, the money has been lent to support livestock operations.

The hope has been that the resulting heightened beef production would be of use to the impoverished masses of these poor countries. But over half of Latin America's beef production is exported to the world's wealthier countries, and what remains is too expensive for any but the wealthy to purchase.[20] From 1960 to 1980, beef exports from El Salvador increased more than sixfold.[21] During that same time, increasing numbers of small farmers lost their livelihood and were pushed off their land. Today, 72 percent of all Salvadoran infants are underfed.[22]

Where does the income from the sale of beef go? Not to the poor, but to the very few who own the land. A handful of wealthy families own more than half the agricultural land in Costa Rica, grazing 2 million cattle.[23] In Guatemala, as is typical for Latin American countries, 3 percent of the population owns 70 percent of the agricultural land. Most of

Mexico's wealth is in the hands of about 30 families, while half of the people live on less than $1 a day.[24]

Only 35 years ago, sorghum was almost unknown in Mexico. But now it literally covers twice the acreage of wheat. What caused sorghum's incredible takeover of Mexican agricultural land? Sorghum is fed to livestock. Twenty-five years ago, livestock consumed only 6 percent of Mexico's grain. Today, the figure is over 50 percent.[25]

In Guatemala, much of the land and other resources for food production are given over to meat, while 75 percent of the children under five years of age are undernourished. The meat produced goes to those who can afford it. Guatemala is a nation where babies have only a 50–50 chance of reaching the age of four because of widespread malnutrition. Meanwhile, every year Guatemala exports 40 million pounds of meat to the United States.[26]

We see the same trend throughout the Third World. Copying, and providing for, the United States' meat-oriented diet, ever-larger percentages of the resources of poor nations go into meat production. In country after country the demand for meat among the rich is squeezing out staple production for the poor.[27]

In Costa Rica, beef production quadrupled between 1960 and 1980. Today, even with much of its original tropical rainforest land sacrificed to beef production, the average family in Costa Rica eats less meat than the average American house cat. Most Costa Rican beef is exported to the United States. As more and more Costa Rican land is being turned over to meat production, the population has less and less to eat.

With the help of the World Bank and other international lending institutions, Brazil has mounted an enormous effort to increase agricultural production, but this has been primarily meat-oriented and for export. Twenty-five years ago, there were virtually no soybeans planted in Brazil. Today, this crop is the nation's number one export, with almost all of it going to feed Japanese and European livestock. Twenty-five years ago, one-third of the Brazilian population suffered from malnutrition. Today, the number has risen to two-thirds. Now, half of the basic grains produced in Brazil are used for livestock feed. The country has the largest commercial cattle herd in the world, while the majority of the rural poor suffer from malnutrition.[28]

Is THAT SO?

"To get more grain to the poor and hungry, taxpayers or organizations must buy it and distribute it."

—National Cattlemen's Association[29]

"Two thirds of the agriculturally productive land in Central America is devoted to livestock production, yet the poor majority cannot afford the meat, which is eaten by the well-to-do or exported."

—Frances Moore Lappé, author, *Diet for a Small Planet*; co-founder, Institute for Food and Development Policy

Throughout the Third World, the production of meat is monopolizing the best local land, undermining the local food supply, and undercutting the efforts of the people to become food self-reliant. There are today millions of human beings in less-developed countries who are going hungry while their land, labor, and resources are being used to feed livestock so wealthy people can eat meat.

It's painful that as a species we can put a man on the moon, but haven't come close to ending the scourge of hunger. In a world where a child dies of hunger-caused disease every two seconds, only our own ignorance allows us to continue to view meat as a status symbol.

Feeding Cows, Not People

Dr. Walden Bello is Executive Director of the Institute for Food and Development Policy, and a leading expert on global food realities. He notes,

"Every time you eat a hamburger you are having a relationship with thousands of people you never met. Not just people at the supermarket or fast food restaurant but possibly World Bank officials in Washington, D.C., and peasants from Central and South America. And many of these people are hungry. The fact is that there is enough food in the world for everyone. But tragically, much of the world's food and land resources are tied up in producing beef and other livestock—food for the well-off—while millions of children and adults suffer from malnutrition and starvation. . . .

In Central America, staple crop production has been replaced by cattle ranching, which now occupies two-thirds of the arable land. The World Bank encouraged this switch-over with an eye toward expanding U.S. fast-food and frozen-dinner markets. The resulting expansion of cattle ranching has deprived peasants of access to the land they depend on for growing food. And because of ranching's limited ability to create jobs (cattle ranching creates 13 times fewer jobs per acre than coffee production), rural hunger has soared. . . . What does all this have to do with our hamburgers? The American fast-food diet and the meat-eating habits of the wealthy around the world support a world food system that diverts food resources from the hungry."

WHAT WE KNOW

Number of *underfed* and malnourished people in the world: 1.2 billion[30]

Number of *overfed* and malnourished people in the world: 1.2 billion[31]

Experiences shared by both the hungry and the overweight: High levels of sickness and disability, shortened life expectancies, lower levels of productivity[32]

Children in Bangladesh who are so *underfed* and *underweight* that their health is diminished: 56 percent[33]

Adults in United States who are so *overfed* and *overweight* that their health is diminished: 55 percent[34]

In the past, as the number of people on Earth grew, it was always possible to clear more land and grow more grain. But sadly, this is no longer the case. After 10,000 years of continuous expansion, the amount of land planted worldwide in grains—the primary crop on every continent—reached a peak in 1981. It has declined by 5 percent since then.

Ed Ayres is the editorial director of the Worldwatch Institute. In 1999, he described how the rapid expansion of cities all over the world has contributed to a decline in the world's agricultural acreage:

"The locations of most centers of population were originally chosen because the land was good for farming, so as cities have exploded in size they have spread over fertile land at a disproportionately rapid rate. The rivers that provided good soil and water also provided means of transport that became important to trade, so the tendency of people to settle near water—and therefore on good farmland—was reinforced. In the past quarter century, millions of acres of the world's richest farmland have been covered with housing developments, industrial parks, and pavement."[35]

In 2000, the United Nations Commission on Nutrition Challenges of the 21st Century said that unless we make major changes, 1 billion children will be permanently handicapped over the next 20 years due to inadequate caloric intake.[36] The first step to averting this tragedy, according to the commission, is to encourage human consumption of traditional grains, fruits, and vegetables.

What we know

Cattle alive today on Earth: More than 1 billion

Weight of world's cattle compared to weight of world's people: Nearly double

Area of Earth's total land mass used as pasture for cattle and other livestock: One-half[37]

Grassland needed to support one cow under optimal conditions: 2.5 acres[38]

Grassland needed to support cow under far more common marginal conditions: 50 acres[39]

In the United States, the National Cattlemen's Beef Association has not taken kindly to charges that U.S. beef production contributes to human hunger, and has mounted a campaign to convince the public, and public officials, of its point of view.

"Most of the grain fed to cattle," say the cattlemen, "is feed grain, not food grain."[40] This is true, but there is absolutely no reason why the land, water, energy, and labor that are currently used to grow feed grains could not easily be used to grow food grains.

The cattlemen also tell us, "If grain were not fed to livestock, more grain would not necessarily be available to feed the hungry."[41] In reality, however, if grain were not fed to livestock, it—and/or the resources needed for its production—would be available for a variety of uses, including feeding the hungry.

The National Cattlemen's Beef Association points to grazing as a wise use of the land: "Were it not for grazing animals like cattle, hundreds of millions of acres of U.S. grazing land would have no productive value. No more than 15 percent of the grazing land could be used to produce crops."[42] Actually, however, the food value to humans of growing grain and other crops for human consumption on the 15 percent of land currently used for grazing that would be suitable for such crops would be comparable to the food value now produced by grazing cattle on the entire amount. Further, if the remaining 85 percent wasn't grazed, it would return to wilderness, where it would provide habitat for countless species, many of them currently endangered as a direct result of cattle grazing. Trees would return to this land, reducing carbon dioxide in the atmosphere, beautifying the environment, providing oxygen, and helping stabilize our precarious climate.

WHAT WE KNOW

U.S. corn eaten by people: 2 percent[43]

U.S. corn eaten by livestock: 77 percent[44]

U.S. farmland producing vegetables: 4 million acres[45]

U.S. farmland producing hay for livestock: 56 million acres[46]

U.S. grain and cereals fed to livestock: 70 percent[47]

Human beings who could be fed by the grain and soybeans eaten by U.S. livestock: 1,400,000,000

World's population living in the United States: 4 percent

World's beef eaten in the United States: 23 percent[48]

The amount of grain needed to produce 1 pound of U.S. beef, according to the National Cattlemen's Beef Association is 4.5 pounds.[49] In a world where people starve, this would be wasteful enough. However, according to figures from the USDA Economic Research Service and Agricultural Research Service, the amount of grain needed to produce 1 pound of U.S. feedlot beef is far more—16 pounds.[50]

The cattlemen take issue with this. According to them, "The statement that it takes 12–16 pounds of grain to produce a pound of beef is absolutely false. This estimate is based on the false assumption that beef animals are fed grain diets from birth to market weight."[51]

In reality, however, the statement that it takes 12–16 pounds of grain is *not* based on the assumption that beef animals are fed grain diets from birth to market weight. It's based on USDA figures, according to which the animals are kept in feedlots for approximately 100 days and fed about 20 pounds of grain a day. In this time, the animals gain approximately 300 pounds, of which (at most) only 120 pounds, or 40 percent, is beef for human consumption (the other 60 percent are those parts of the animal that are inedible). Thus feeding the animal 2,000 pounds of grain yields 120 pounds of beef. By these figures, it takes nearly 17 pounds of grain for each pound of beef returned.

In 2000, the founder of Worldwatch Institute, Lester Brown, estimated that cattle require 7 pounds of grain to add 1 pound of live weight.[52] Since 40 percent of live weight is edible for humans, this figure indicates it actually takes slightly more than 17 pounds of grain to produce a pound of beef.

While the National Cattlemen's Beef Association regularly seeks to downplay the costs of U.S. beef production, others in the industry are more sober. Peter R. Cheeke, Professor of Animal Agriculture at Oregon State University, takes note of reality:

> "Beef has become a symbol of the extravagant, resource-consuming American who is destroying the global environment to live a life of luxury, while most of the rest of the world suffer pestilence and famine. . . . Strictly on a scientific basis, there can be no dispute that corn and soybean meal are used with more efficiency, and can provide food for more people when they are eaten directly by people rather than being fed to

swine or poultry to be converted to pork, chicken meat, or eggs for human consumption."[53]

What we know

Number of people whose food energy needs can be met by the food produced on 2.5 acres of land:[54]

If the land is producing cabbage:	23 people
If the land is producing potatoes:	22 people
If the land is producing rice:	19 people
If the land is producing corn:	17 people
If the land is producing wheat:	15 people
If the land is producing chicken:	2 people
If the land is producing milk:	2 people
If the land is producing eggs:	1 person
If the land is producing beef:	1 person

Grain needed to adequately feed every one of the people on the entire planet who die of hunger and hunger-caused disease annually: 12 million tons

Amount Americans would have to reduce their beef consumption to save 12 millions tons of grain: 10 percent

Fishful Thinking

As the number of people on Earth has mounted and the amount of farmland has shrunk, the world has looked increasingly to the oceans for food. From 1950 to 1990, the world's oceanic fish catch climbed from 19 million tons to 89 million tons. But since 1990, there has been no growth in the catch.[55] For the first time in history, the world can no longer rely on the oceans for an expanding food supply. In fact, most of the world's fisheries are now depleted or in steep decline—developments that have serious implications for world hunger.

In 1997, the United Nations Food and Agriculture Organization reported that 11 of the world's 15 major oceanic fishing grounds had gone into serious decline as a result of overfishing. Thirty-four percent of all fish species were vulnerable to, or in immediate danger of, extinction.

A year later, the journal *Science* concluded that the destruction of life in the oceans had progressed farther than anyone had suspected.[56]

As fish stocks have decreased and fish factories have had more difficulty filling their quotas, fishing ships have been dropping their nets ever deeper, hauling in and discarding ever-higher percentages of unusable fish.[57] Further, they have been willing to take ever-smaller fish. Worldwatch Institute's Ed Ayres describes the chain of events:

> "The small species are normally the food for larger ones, so as the nets reach down the food chain to the smaller varieties, the larger ones lose their sustenance and begin to die off. At the same time, in their efforts to take more of the smaller fish, the floating factories also haul in more of the juveniles of the larger species—thus undermining future fish populations as well as exhausting the existing ones. That, in turn, not only steals food from future human generations to feed the present, but pushes more oceanic species to the brink, or over the brink of extinction."[58]

Restaurant patrons in the eastern United States may have noticed a recent campaign to remove swordfish from menus until the species, stressed now to the point of collapse, has a chance to recover. At present, nearly two-thirds of swordfish caught in the North Atlantic today are too young to breed.[59]

Most of us think of fish as a renewable harvest resource, like wheat, rather than species that are endangered, like panda or tiger.[60] But as the technology used to vacuum every last fish from the ocean has become increasingly sophisticated, species after species has been pushed toward extinction. As *Rachel's Environment and Health Weekly* notes,

> "Trawlers are now using technology developed by the military to fish waters as deep as a mile, catching species that few would have considered edible or useful a decade ago. Now that the shallow fisheries are in serious decline, trawl nets fitted with wheels and rollers are dragging across the bottom of the deep oceans, removing everything of any size. . . .

Radar allows ships to operate in the fog and the dark; sonar locates the fish precisely; and GPS (geographical positioning system) satellites pinpoint locations so that ships can return to productive spots. Formerly-secret military maps reveal hidden deep-sea currents of nutrient-rich water, where fish thrive. Combined with larger nets made from new, stronger materials, modern fishing vessels guided electronically can sweep the oceans clean—and that is precisely what is happening. As a result, the ocean's fish are disappearing."[61]

WHAT WE KNOW

Amount of fish caught per person, worldwide, sold for human consumption in 1996: 16 kilograms[62]

Amount of marine life that was hauled up with the fish and discarded, per person, in 1996: 200 kilograms[63]

Amount of world's fish catch fed to livestock: Half[64]

In 1992, Don Tyson, the Arkansas chicken tycoon, purchased the Arctic-Alaska Fisheries Company and three other fishing companies. These companies operate a fleet of industrial super-trawlers that each cost $40 million to build and are each the length of a football field. They pull nylon nets thousands of feet long through the water, capturing everything in their path, typically taking in 800,000 pounds of fish in a single netting.[65]

WHAT WE KNOW

Nation's leading *surimi* producer (*surimi* is deboned fish tissue that can be used to make fish sticks, synthetic "crab meat," and other products): Tyson Foods[66]

Reason President Clinton's first Secretary of Agriculture, Mike Espy, was fired: Inappropriately accepted "gifts" from Tyson Foods[67]

Fines paid by Tyson Foods upon pleading guilty to federal gratuities statutes on December 29, 1997: $4 million, plus $2 million investigation costs[68]

Federal subsidies received by Tyson's factory-trawler fleet: $200 million[69]

Likely result if current overfishing trends continue: Wholesale collapse of marine ecosystems[70]

Salmon have long captured the imaginations of human beings. Spending part of their lives in streams and part in the sea, these fish, by using a sense of smell thought to be 1,000 times more acute than that of dogs, return to their birthplace to spawn. But in recent years, their numbers have plummeted.

In 1994, hundreds of millions of dollars were spent to help salmon in the Snake River in Washington State, but the effort was a failure. That fall, only 800 Chinook returned, and only a single Sockeye made it.[71]

To my eyes, this is a tragedy, and not just for the fish. Healthy and plentiful wild salmon play a crucial and irreplaceable role in the functioning of a vast array of ecosystems, including rivers, lakes, and forests. David Suzuki explains the mechanism:

> "Salmon spend their adult lives at sea, thousands of kilometers from their birthplace in forested and mountain streams. Marine carbon and nitrogen isotopes leave a unique 'signature' that scientists can detect, and of course, after years in the ocean, salmon carcasses are full of these two important atomic nutrients. After the adult salmon make the arduous journey from the ocean back to their natal streams, they spawn and die. Various predators—bears, eagles, wolves—catch them and leave their remains on land. . . . They nourish fish, mammals and birds throughout the forest. In the water, the dead salmon are digested by fungus, which in turn nourishes bacteria that sustain insects, copepods and other invertebrates in the stream. And like fallen logs in the forest, their decaying flesh provides nourishment for their own offspring. When the fry emerge from the gravel, a banquet awaits: 25 to 40 percent of the carbon and nitrogen in juvenile salmon comes from the remains of their parents. Isotope studies show that 30 percent of the vital nitrogen and carbon in aquatic algae and insects, and 18 percent in vegetation along the river, comes directly from salmon."[72]

In order to thrive, forests need the salmon. Biologists tell us that in a single season, a bear will carry about 700 partially consumed salmon carcasses into the forest. After consuming salmon, bears (and also eagles, wolves, and ravens) defecate, spreading the salmon remnants throughout the forest, providing the trees with their primary source of nitrogen fertilizer. There is in fact a direct correlation between the width of tree rings (a measure of tree growth) and the amount of marine carbon and nitrogen, reflecting the size of that year's salmon run.

Although grizzly bears went extinct in Oregon in 1931, hides of these animals have been preserved and studied, so we know that up to 90 percent of the nitrogen and carbon in the bears' bodies was of marine origin.

If we continue to think of fish, and indeed the whole of the natural world, as existing primarily to fulfill our immediate needs, we will pay a stupendous price for our ignorance.

Is Fish Farming the Answer?

In an effort to compensate for falling wild fish stocks, and to help feed ever-growing populations, more and more fish are being farmed. Aquaculture output is today the fastest growing sector of both the United States and the world food economy.[73]

In 1985, barely 5 percent of the world's fish for food was produced by aquaculture. But by 2000, the share produced by fish farms accounted for nearly a third of the world's total fish consumption.[74] By then, virtually all the catfish and rainbow trout, half the shrimp, and one-third the salmon eaten in the United States were the product of fish farms.

Unfortunately, the promise of aquaculture to alleviate pressure on marine ecosystems has thus far proven disappointing. The farming of shrimp, salmon, trout, bass, yellowtail, and other carnivorous species has actually increased demands on marine production in order to provide feed for the farmed fish. It takes 5 pounds of wild ocean fish to produce a single pound of farmed saltwater fish or shrimp.[75]

In 2000, Rosamond Naylor, a senior research scholar at Stanford's Institute for International Studies, wrote in a cover story in the journal *Nature* that "aquaculture is . . . a contributing factor to the collapse of fisheries stocks around the world."[76]

She and the articles' other authors, representing institutes of aquaculture from all over the world, added that as a result of fish farming, some populations of herring, mackerel, sardines, and other fish low in the marine food chain are in danger of disappearing from the world's oceans.[77]

Aquaculture contributes to the decline of oceanic fish in another way as well. Diseases and parasites thrive in the densely populated conditions of fish farms, and can easily spread to wild populations. There were 800,000 wild Atlantic salmon in 1975, but by 2000 their numbers had been reduced to a mere 80,000. When the World Wide Fund for Nature and the North Atlantic Salmon Conservation Organization cited the three reasons for this loss, one of them was disease and parasites stemming from salmon farms.[78]

As is the case with cattle, poultry, and pigs, raising large numbers of fish in confined environments puts abnormal stress on the fish, which increases vulnerability to outbreaks of disease both on the farm and in surrounding waters. The result, as with the factory farming of livestock, is greater use of antibiotics and other chemicals. Fish farmers are using chemicals to kill bacteria, herbicides to prevent the growth of vegetation in ponds, and other drugs to treat diseases and parasites.

Fish farming is one of the most intensive forms of animal agriculture. As many as 40,000 fish may be crammed into a cage, with each fish given the equivalent of half a bathtub of water in which to spend its life.[79] The wild salmon migrates thousands of miles, but the caged fish goes nowhere. The wild fish develops its pinky-orange color partially from eating krill, but the caged fish is often fed artificial pigments to create this desired color, as well as vaccines and hormones.

Consumers, presented with salmon wrappers that portray leaping salmon, mountains, and glistening streams, typically do not know their fish comes increasingly from fish farms. In 1990, only 6 percent of the salmon consumed in the world were the product of fish farms. But by 1998, the number had risen to 40 percent.[80]

The value of salmon as a healthy food is primarily due to their extremely high concentration of Omega-3 fatty acids. No salmon, or any other fish or animal, manufactures Omega-3s, but wild salmon get them by eating particular algae that make these important nutrients, and then storing them in their body fat. Wild salmon are a plentiful source of Omega-3s. Farmed salmon, however, have far less of these essential nutrients.

The situation is similar in cattle and other livestock kept in confinement. Meats from grain-fed feedlot cattle have far less Omega-3s than meats from pastured animals. Milk, butter, and cheese from grain-fed cows are markedly deficient in Omega-3s. And supermarket eggs have only 5 percent as much Omega-3s as do eggs laid by free-range chickens.[81]

There are some substances, however, that farmed fish, like factory farmed livestock, provide in abundance. Unfortunately, they are not substances you want to eat. As with factory cattle, pigs, and chickens, the food given to farmed fish frequently contains potentially dangerous levels of toxic chemicals. In 2001, independent studies conducted in Canada, Scotland, and the United States found that farmed fish contained much higher levels of pollutants, including ten times more polychlorinated biphenyls (PCBs), than wild fish. "The results were very, very clear," noted Dr. Michael Easton, a Vancouver-based geneticist and expert in ecotoxicology. "Farmed fish and the feed they were fed appeared to have a much higher level of contamination with respect to PCBs, organochlorine pesticides, and polybrominated diphenyl ethers than did wild fish. In short, it was extremely noticeable." These pollutants affect the central nervous system, the immune system, and can cause cancers.[82]

Many people think that farmed fish is environmentally more benign. But there is yet one more parallel between aquaculture and factory farms—enormous waste problems. The caged salmon grown in Scotland, for example, contaminate Scottish coastal waters with an amount of untreated waste equivalent to that produced by 8 million people.[83] Yet the entire human population of Scotland is itself barely more than 5 million.

And it's not just salmon. In the last few decades, the growth of high-intensity manmade shrimp farms has been staggering. In Ecuador, for example, 500,000 acres have been given over to shrimp farms, with 80 percent of the shrimp exported, more than half going to the United States. The costs of this growth, however, have been equally staggering, including coastal pollution, the displacement of local people from their land, and the clearing of large tracts of coastal mangrove forests.

Mangrove forests are the breeding grounds for countless species of fish, and when they are replaced by shrimp farms, offshore fish catches plummet. There were originally 1,250,000 acres of mangrove forests in the Philippines. Today, only 90,000 acres remain, the rest having been converted into shrimp farms producing for foreign markets.

So great is the ecological destruction caused by fish farming, particularly of shrimp, that a 2000 report published in the *New Internationalist* compared the environmental damage caused by fish farming to that caused by replacing tropical rainforests with cattle ranches.[84]

The point, of course, is to produce more food for people to eat. But intensive shrimp and prawn industries typically locate in areas that have traditionally grown rice—the primary staple for most of the world's people. With every new shrimp pond, rice paddies are lost, and with them, food for local people.[85]

So far, the fish farming industry is following directly in the footsteps of the livestock industries, feeding primarily the rich at the expense of the planet, the animals, and the poor. As Jean-Michel Cousteau writes, "(Aquaculture) means that we are taking vast amounts of small fish that form the basis of the poor person's diet in the oceanic world and using them to produce one large fish that is enjoyed primarily by the upper echelons in industrial nations."[86]

Meanwhile, 22 million tons of wild fish were used by the livestock industry for pig and cow feed in 1997.[87] That is a figure greater than the combined weight of the entire human population of the United States.

May All Be Fed

"The law, in its majestic equality, forbids the rich as well as the poor to sleep under bridges, to beg in the streets, and to steal bread." (Anatole France)

Reversing the spread of hunger is one of humanity's paramount challenges. It will mean overcoming the fatalistic belief that chronic, persistent hunger is inevitable. It will mean reversing the trend toward ever greater concentration of wealth in ever-fewer hands. It will mean building our lives upon the certainty that all humanity is connected.

When humanity finally sheds the onerous and degrading specter of starvation, it will be because we have decided not to treat food, and the resources needed to produce it, just like any other commodity, but have come to see food as a basic and universal human right. It will be because we have found ways to stabilize our numbers and to heal the planet's deeply injured life-support systems. It will be because we have realized that only when none of us fears hunger can any of us truly find peace.

And it will be because we have returned to the efficiency of a plant-based diet, making it possible for more people to eat. It is increasingly obvious that environmentally sustainable solutions to world hunger can only emerge as people eat more plant foods and fewer animal products. To me it is deeply moving that the same food choices that give us the best chance to eliminate world hunger are also those that take the least toll on the environment, contribute the most to our long-term health, are the safest, and are also far and away the most compassionate toward our fellow creatures.

Reversing the spread of hunger will mean learning to create a world based on cooperation and on the affirmation of the human spirit. It will mean organizing our societies in ways that assure every person the chance to live a healthy and productive life in harmony with Nature. It will mean examining all of our public policies and personal lifestyles in the light of our desire to touch as many people as possible with a message of hope for a better world.

> "The day that hunger is eradicated from the Earth there will be the greatest spiritual explosion the world has ever known. Humanity cannot imagine the joy that will burst into the world on the day of that great revolution." (Frederico Garcia Lorca)

PART IV

Genetic Engineering

chapter 16

Pandora's Pantry

C an answers to world hunger, human health, and environmental problems be found in the genetic engineering of our food supply? Gentetic engineering involves the permanent alteration of the genetic blueprint of a seed. By modifying a seed's hereditary makeup, scientists hope that a plant grown from the seed, and its descendants forever, will have certain characteristics.

For example, the first genetically engineered food sold in the United States was the "FlavrSavr" tomato. The Calgene Corporation (now a subsidiary of Monsanto) isolated the tomato gene that codes for a ripening enzyme, then found a way to alter the gene to block the expression of that enzyme. The company hoped thereby to produce a tomato that would have an extended shelf life; after it was picked, it would not continue to ripen but would instead remain firm.

The FlavrSavr tomato was announced with great fanfare in 1995, and the company planned to bring the variety to market as a high-end gourmet product. But things didn't work out as the people who created it had wanted. The tomato turned out to have reduced yields and disease resistance. And contrary to Calgene's expectations, the tomatoes were so soft and bruised so easily that they had no appeal at all as fresh produce.

At first, Calgene put labels on the tomatoes saying they were genetically engineered, hoping that the scientific aura of such a label would heighten demand for the tomatoes and allow them to be sold for a higher price. But when consumers responded warily to the labels, not only Calgene but the entire genetic engineering industry learned a lesson it would not forget.[1] Since that time, the industry has not labeled any genetically engineered foods. And it has gone further than that. With its political allies, the industry has fought unceasingly against labeling requirements for genetically engineered foods.

Having been burned when it informed consumers that the FlavrSavr tomato was genetically engineered, Calgene next tried marketing the very same genetically altered tomatoes under the friendly sounding "MacGregor" brand name. The new name was deliberately chosen to obscure the reality that the tomato had an altered genome. The company had learned well the value of nondisclosure.[2]

Genetically engineered foods go by different names. They are sometimes called "genetically modified," "genetically altered," "transgenic," and "biotech" foods—all of which mean the same thing. Of course, though the terms are synonymous, they carry different emotional associations. The corporations behind genetic engineering greatly prefer the term "biotech," and have spent tens of millions of dollars on marketing campaigns with the goal of getting Americans to refer to the industry as "biotechnology" instead of one of the "emotionally charged labels" such as "genetically modified organisms" or GMOs.

As it turned out, the MacGregor tomato also flopped, even though consumers didn't know that it was genetically altered. Calgene's genetic "miracle" was a bust because the altered gene turned out to have many other effects besides the one they had planned. The engineered tomato looked like the real thing, but serious questions arose about its nutritional value. Furthermore, there was evidence that pathogenic bacteria in the intestines of people who ate the tomato could become resistant to antibiotics.[3]

The FlavrSavr (or MacGregor) tomato was pulled from the market in 1996, only a year after its introduction—the same year that Calgene was purchased by Monsanto.

Grand Hopes

For countless centuries, plant breeders have sought to alter the characteristics of plants in order to create desired effects. But they have been limited to working with characteristics that were already present in the species. An orange could be crossed with a different kind of orange, but it could not be crossed with a gorilla. You had no choice but to deal with "apples and apples."

In genetic engineering, on the other hand, genes are usually taken from one species and then inserted into another species in an attempt to transfer a desired trait. After the FlavrSavr, for example, the next engineered food in line to be grown commercially was a strawberry that had a gene from an arctic fish (the flounder) inserted into it to make the strawberry more frost-resistant. It, however, also failed.

Though the technology is still in its relative infancy (the first large-scale commercial plantings of genetically engineered crops took place in 1996), many people have dreamed that genetically engineered foods could be an answer to humanity's prayers. We have hoped that they might bring solutions to world hunger, that they might allow us to do away with pesticides, that they might provide healthier foods, and that they might help the Third World to leapfrog over the environmental dangers of the Industrial Revolution into a brighter, healthier, and more sustainable future.

In 2000, *Time* magazine ran a cover story titled "Grains of Hope."[4] The article excitedly described the development of a genetically engineered "golden rice," so named because it incorporated genes from viruses and daffodils and produced beta-carotene, something no variety of rice had ever done before. Golden rice, said *Time*, could be a godsend for the half of humanity that depends on rice for its major staple. Nearly a million children die every year because they are weakened by vitamin A deficiencies, and an additional 350,000 go blind. The human body converts beta-carotene into vitamin A.

It was, it seemed, compelling and inspiring evidence that genetically engineered crops could help reduce malnutrition. *Time* quoted Jimmy Carter, reminding everyone what was at stake. "Responsible biotechnology," said the former president, "is not the enemy, starvation is."

But in all the excitement about golden rice, several facts seemed to escape attention. One was that we have no assurance, yet, that the genetically engineered strain will grow in the kinds of soil that it must to be of value to the world's hungry. Researchers said it would take millions more dollars and another decade of development at the International Rice Research Institute to produce golden rice varieties that could actually be grown in farmer's fields. And even then, they would require large amounts of water, water that might not be available in precisely those areas where vitamin A deficiency is most a problem.[5]

Also overlooked in the hoopla was that there are alternative ways to alleviate vitamin A deficiency that are far less costly and do not carry the dangers of genetically engineered foods. In Bangladesh, for example, the Food and Agriculture Organization of the United Nations (FAO) began such a project in 1993. Working with Helen Keller International and other nongovernmental organizations, they introduced a program to help develop small home gardens with improved cultivation methods. Families without land were shown how to grow vitamin A-rich plants (pumpkins, squashes, and beans) up the walls of their homes. The project swiftly snowballed as the health benefits became apparent. By 1998, the program was helping at least 3 million people grow foods at home that are high in vitamin A. Independent analyses found that very small areas of land were required to generate sufficient vitamin A, and that the greater variety of vegetables and fruits people ate, the better their intake of vitamin A and other vitamins.[6] Health benefits to the poor from programs like this are enormous.

Advocates of genetic engineering imply that if we don't get over our queasiness about eating genetically modified food, kids in the Third World will go blind. But on March 4, 2001, both the *New York Times Magazine* and the *St. Louis Post Dispatch* revealed that an eleven-year-old would have to eat 27 to 54 bowls of golden rice to satisfy the minimum daily requirement for vitamin A.

And a larger issue in all of this is that the golden rice effort, although held up as a shining example of genetically engineered foods benefiting humanity, is not even remotely representative of the genetic engineering industry as a whole. The research that is being done on "wonder crops" such as golden rice is conducted almost solely by a small number of institutions dependent on philanthropy or public funds. But such projects are far from the norm. The vast majority of genetic engineering is undertaken for private profit, funded by corporations such as Monsanto.

In a tactic that has led to enormous public confusion, these biotech corporations have not hesitated to refer to crops like golden rice repeatedly in PR campaigns designed to increase public acceptance for genetic engineering, omitting the fact that the vast majority of their efforts focus in a very different direction.

The Biotech Industry

The Monsanto Corporation, founded in 1901 by a chemist to manufacture saccharin, the first artificial sweetener, is by far the largest player in the world of genetic engineering today. "I want to emphasize," Monsanto's CEO, Bob Shapiro, said in 1999, "that we will remain fully committed to the promise of biotechnology, because we believe that it can be a safe and sustainable and useful tool in agriculture and nutrition, in human health, and in meeting in particular the world's needs for food and fiber."[7]

It sounds as if his goal is to help the world. But Monsanto, like Astra-Zeneca, DuPont, Novartis, and Aventis, is governed by the profit motive. These five top biotech companies together account for nearly 100 percent of the market in genetically engineered seeds. They also account for 60 percent of the global pesticide market. And, thanks to a flurry of recent acquisitions, they now own 23 percent of the commercial seed market.[8]

Whatever their PR might say, their efforts are filtered through, and focused on, the pursuit of corporate profit. Unlike the developers of golden rice, their intention is not to make the world a better place. It is to make money.

Phil Bereano is a professor of technical communications at the University of Washington, and helped found the Council for Responsible Genetics. He asks, "Who in the corporations determines the design criteria for what form of genetic engineering they're going to have? It's the money boys. . . . It's the guys who are dealing with the bottom line. The projects that are likely to make the most money are the projects that are going to be developed, not the projects that correspond to some authentic ordering of human needs."[9]

Most of the public, at least in the United States (the home of the genetic engineering industry), believes that the technology is being employed to make food healthier, or to increase yields, or to make the food taste better, or to reduce pesticide use, or to enhance some other characteristic that would benefit humanity or the environment. Unfortunately, up until now at least, that is not the way the industry has functioned.

How does it function? What kinds of crops are being grown? In 1999, the great majority (nearly 80 percent) of the total global transgenic acreage was planted in varieties of soy, corn, cotton, and canola that had been genetically altered by agrochemical companies to withstand massive dousings of their own commercial brands of herbicides.[10] Herbicides, a type of pesticide, are chemicals that kill plants or disrupt their photosynthesis, and are also known as "weedkillers."

Up until now, farmers could spray herbicides before planting, but not after, because any herbicide that would kill weeds would also kill the intended crop. They had to use other means to combat weeds. But now, with genetically modified varieties, farmers can spray all they want throughout the growing season and their crops won't die, as long as they use the weedkiller that their crop has been engineered to withstand.

In their eagerness to make their products appear beneficial to the public, the biotech companies repeatedly say that genetically engineered crops require less pesticide. This sounds wonderful, but the reality is decidedly different.

With so called herbicide-tolerant crops, otherwise impossible amounts of a given herbicide can be oversprayed on the crop to kill surrounding weeds while leaving the commodity virtually unscathed.[11] Thus, almost 80 percent of the world's genetically modified acreage is planted in crops whose only advantage is their ability to tolerate virtually unlimited applications of particular herbicides.

And the other 20-plus percent of the planet's genetically modified acreage? This land is planted in crops that have been engineered to produce pesticides in every cell of the plants throughout their entire life cycle.[12] One of these, a potato Monsanto has given the welcoming name

"New Leaf" potato, is typical. The name "New Leaf" makes it seem as though the variety was the kind of organic food you'd find in a health food store. But in reality, Monsanto's New Leaf potato technology, which kills any potato beetle that dares take a bite, is itself required to be registered as a pesticide with the EPA.[13]

Rounding Up Profits

By the year 2000, 80 million acres worldwide, an area far larger than the entire land mass of the United Kingdom, were planted with genetically engineered herbicide-resistant varieties of soy, corn, and canola.[14] In every case, the agrochemical companies that created and sold these varieties also manufactured and sold the corresponding herbicide.

It is no coincidence that the five largest biotech companies in the world also include the world's five largest herbicide companies, and, indeed, are the world's leaders in all kinds of pesticides. The genetically altered varieties they have developed ensure a continuous and ever-expanding market for their agrochemicals.

The bestselling herbicide in the world is Monsanto's Roundup. In 2000, this one brand of weedkiller brought in almost $3 billion to Monsanto, and the corporation was planning for sales to grow prodigiously in the future. The reason? Monsanto's "Roundup Ready" varieties of soy, corn, and canola had come to account, by themselves, for more than half of all the transgenic plantings in the world.

Roundup Ready crops are genetically engineered to withstand repeated doses of Roundup, enabling farmers to spray their fields and kill weeds without killing the Roundup Ready crop. This is the crops' only benefit, and no farmer ever grows a Roundup Ready variety without applying the herbicide.

In 1998, Monsanto was on track to spend nearly a billion dollars building new factories worldwide to manufacture more Roundup.[15] And it was doing this unfazed by the fact that the U.S. patent on Roundup ran out in the year 2000. This was not a problem, because Monsanto had come up with a clever plan to extend its monopoly rights on the herbicide indefinitely. It's actually quite simple. Farmers who grow

Monsanto's Roundup Ready crops are required to sign a contract that requires them to buy only Monsanto's brand of the herbicide.[16] Despite high-minded talk of golden rice and ending hunger, Monsanto seems to have a few other motives.

Is Roundup safe? By pesticide standards, it's relatively benign, and certainly does not belong in the same toxicity class as DDT, Alachlor, or Butachlor, which Monsanto also makes. But that doesn't mean it's harmless. In fact, the U.S. Fish and Wildlife Service has identified 74 plant species that are potentially endangered by excessive use of glyphosate, the primary active ingredient in Roundup.[17] Glyphosate kills fish in concentrations as low as 10 parts per million, impedes the growth of earthworms and increases their mortality, and is toxic to the soil microbes that help plants to take up nutrients from the soil.[18] In the early 1990s, it was also the third most commonly reported cause of all forms of pesticide-related illness in California (the only state that keeps track of such statistics).[19] Symptoms include eye and skin irritation, cardiac depression, and vomiting.[20]

In 1997, Monsanto was forced to remove advertisements that billed Roundup as "totally safe" and "environmentally friendly" after the New York attorney general's office complained about the toxicity of Roundup's supposedly inert ingredients, one of which had been cited as the cause of toxicity in nine deaths.[21] As well, studies have linked exposure to glyphosate to an increased risk for non-Hodgkin's lymphoma, a serious cancer that affects young people, and the third fastest-growing cancer in the United States.[22]

Monsanto's key selling point for Roundup Ready seeds has been to tell farmers that one or two good dousings with Roundup will solve all their weed problems. The corporation placed print ads telling farmers that Roundup was "the only weed control you'll ever need," even while, in the words of University of California Professor of Biochemistry and Molecular Biology J. B. Neilands, "the quantities of Roundup Monsanto is planning to apply to their proprietary Roundup Ready cultivars [varieties] humbles the imagination."[23]

Because so much Roundup is used on Roundup Ready crops, the residue levels in the harvested crops greatly exceed what until very recently was the allowable legal limit. For the technology to be commercially viable, the FDA had to triple the residues of Roundup's active in-gredients that can remain on the crop.[24] Many scientists have protested that permitting increased residues to enable a company's success reflects an attitude in which corporate interests are given higher priority than public safety, but the increased levels have remained in force.

Advertisements and glossy brochures, seeking to convince farmers to plant Roundup Ready seeds, speak proudly of "clean fields"—*clean* in this usage meaning enormous fields with nothing growing in them but soybeans or cotton or canola. This is intended as a selling point, and many farmers go for it, but it is an odd use of the word. The fields are ac-tually so chemicalized that they bear little resemblance to a healthy, flourishing, and biodiverse ecosystem. The soil, deprived of decaying plant matter (other than the crop itself), and often impoverished of worms, insects, and bacteria becomes increasingly dependent on chemi-cal fertilizers.

Ironically, we're spraying our fields and food with a toxic substance to make use of a sophisticated technology that is largely unnecessary. There are simpler mechanical ways to deal with weeds, including no-till farming, mulching, and companion cropping. But of course, none of these Earth-friendly methods can be patented and sold for profit, and none fit with massive mono-cultures and reliance on chemicals, so they hold no interest for Monsanto and the other agricultural chemical com-panies that dominate the business of genetic engineering.[25]

The clean fields, devoid of all weeds, that Monsanto likes to tell us will help end malnutrition, may be doing something very different. Dr. Vandana Shiva, director of India's Research Foundation for Science, Technology, and Resource Policy, points out that killing every single weed in a field can deprive the poor of needed sources of key nutritional elements. "In India," she says, "at least 80 to 90 percent of the nutrition comes from what the agricultural industry terms 'weeds.' (Agribusiness) has this attitude that the weeds are stealing from them, so they spray (Roundup or other herbicides) on a field which has sometimes 200 species that the women of the area would normally use in various ways as food, medicinal plants, or fodder."[26]

Shiva goes on to say that in many cases, people are suffering from vi-tamin A deficiency not because they don't have access to golden rice, but because their fields have been doused with too many chemicals. "At the moment," she says, "about 40,000 children in India are going blind for lack of vitamin A, only because industrial farming has destroyed so many wild field plants, the sources of vitamin A that were available to the poorest people in the rural areas. With biotechnology they will increase this lunacy."[27]

Meanwhile, conservation organizations are telling us that increased use of Roundup means trouble for wildlife. Many of the plants the herbicide eradicates are food for other species. In the United Kingdom, the Royal Society for the Protection of Birds has warned that increased use of Roundup and other herbicides will kill the plants that support the insects and produce the seeds that birds consume. This, they say, could mean extinction for many bird species—including the skylark—that are already in decline due to industrialized farming practices. Graham Wynne, chief executive of the conservation group, says, "The ability to clear fields of all weeds using powerful herbicides which can be sprayed onto genetically engineered herbicide-resistant crops will result in farmlands devoid of wildlife and spell disaster for millions of already declining birds and plants."[28]

It's not just Monsanto. Other agrochemical manufacturers are busy genetically engineering crops to tolerate their herbicide brands. AgrEvo, for example, manufactures the herbicide glufosinate. The company expects sales for the weedkiller to increase by more than half a billion dollars in the next few years, because it is developing genetically modified crops that will be resistant to glufosinate.

The company says glufosinate is "environmentally friendly." The EPA, on the other hand, says it is toxic to many aquatic and marine invertebrates, even at very low concentrations.[29] Glufosinate is water soluble and readily leaches into groundwater.[30]

Similarly, Calgene/Monsanto has developed a strain of cotton plants (called BXN Cotton) that can withstand direct spraying with the toxic herbicide bromoxynil (sold under the brand name Buctril). Bromoxynil is recognized by the EPA as a possible carcinogen and as a teratrogen (a substance that causes birth defects).[31]

When the EPA licensed bromoxynil for use on Monsanto's genetically modified BXN Cotton, the agency assumed that bromoxynil had no way to enter the human food chain. But at certain times of the year in the southern United States, cattle in feedlots are fed silage containing up to 50 percent cotton slash and cotton debris. Thus, bromoxynil is today making its way into the human food chain through meat.[32]

What about World Hunger?

The global area planted in genetically engineered foods grew nearly 25-fold in the three years after 1996, the first year of large-scale commercialization. Yet this enormous growth took place almost entirely in only three countries. In 1999, the United States by itself accounted for 72 percent of the global area. Argentina was responsible for another 17 percent, and Canada weighed in with another 10 percent. These three countries together accounted for 99 percent of the entire planet's genetically engineered plantings.[33]

WHAT WE KNOW

Total global area planted in genetically engineered crops, 1995: Negligible[34]

Total global area planted in genetically engineered crops, 1996: 4 million acres[35]

Total global area planted in genetically engineered crops, 1997: 27 million acres[36]

Total global area planted in genetically engineered crops, 1998: 69 million acres[37]

Total global area planted in genetically engineered crops, 1999: 99 million acres[38]

Monsanto and other proponents of biotechnology continually tell the public that genetic engineering is necessary if the world's food supply is to keep up with population growth. But even with nearly 100 million acres planted in 2000, and with genetically engineered crops covering one-quarter of all cropland in the United States, their products had yet to do a thing to reverse the spread of hunger. No commercial acreage had been planted in crops which had been engineered to produce greater yields or that had any kind of enhanced nutritional value. There was no more food available for the world's less fortunate. In fact, the vast majority of the fields were growing transgenic soybeans and corn that were destined for livestock feed.[39]

One of the clearest independent voices in the sometimes raucous debate about genetically modified foods is *Rachel's Environment and Health Weekly*, published by the Environmental Research Foundation in Annapolis, Maryland. In 1999, the journal noted,

> "Neither Monsanto nor any of the other genetic engineering companies appears to be developing genetically engineered crops that might solve global food shortages. Quite the opposite. If genetically engineered crops were aimed at feeding the hungry, then Monsanto and the others would be developing seeds with certain predictable characteristics: a) ability to grow on substandard or marginal soils; b) plants able to produce more high-quality protein with increased per-acre yield, without the need for expensive machinery, chemicals, fertilizers, or water; c) they would aim to favor small farms over larger farms; d) the seeds would be cheap and freely available without restrictive licensing; and e) they would be for crops that feed people, not meat animals. None of the genetically engineered crops now available, or in development (to the extent that these have been announced) has any of these desirable characteristics. Quite the opposite. The new genetically engineered seeds . . . produce crops largely intended as feed for meat animals, not to provide protein for people. The genetic engineering revolution has nothing to do with feeding the world's hungry."[40]

If genetically engineered plants were designed to reverse world hunger, you would expect them to bring higher yields. But there is no evidence that they do, and in fact increasing evidence that they do just the opposite. Ed Oplinger, a professor of agronomy at the University of Wisconsin, has been conducting performance trials for soybean varieties for the past 25 years. In 1999, he compared the soybean yields in the 12 states that grew 80 percent of U.S. soybeans, and found that the yields from genetically modified soybeans were 4 percent lower than conventional varieties.[41]

When other researchers compared the performance of Monsanto's transgenic soybeans (the number one genetically engineered crop in the world in terms of acreage planted) with those of conventional varieties grown under the same conditions, they found nearly a 10 percent yield reduction for the genetically engineered soybeans.[42] And research done by the University of Nebraska in 2000 found the yields of genetically engineered soybean plants to be 6 to 11 percent lower than conventional plants.[43]

Of course, just because today's genetically engineered crops have lower yields doesn't mean that the technology will never produce greater harvests. Stephen Dofing, an expert in plant breeding and genetics, points out that developing and incorporating herbicide resistance in plants is far easier than increasing yields. The reason is that herbacide resistance can often be conferred by altering a single enzyme or pathway, whereas yield involves hundreds or thousands of genes, interacting among themselves and the environment.[44] It is possible that, given enough time, genetic engineering could be successfully used to increase nature's bounty.

Thus far, though, this hasn't happened. And Dr. Vandana Shiva, one of the world's foremost experts on world hunger and transgenic crops, is not convinced that it ever will. She rejects the claims that biotechnology will help feed the world. The argument, she says, "is on every level a deception. First of all, the kinds of things they're producing don't feed the Third World. . . . Soybeans go to feed the pigs and the cattle of the North. . . . All the investments in agriculture are about increasing chemical sales and increasing monopoly control. . . . All this is taking place in the private domain, by corporations that are not in the business of charity. They are in the business of selling. The food they will produce will be even more costly."[45]

Similarly, delegates from 18 African countries at a meeting of the UN Food and Agriculture Organization responded to Monsanto's advertisements with a clear statement: "We . . . strongly object that the image of the poor and hungry from our countries is being used by giant multinational corporations to push a technology that is neither safe, environmentally friendly, nor economically beneficial to us. We do not believe that such companies or gene technologies will help our farmers to produce the food that is needed. . . . On the contrary . . . it will undermine our capacity to feed ourselves." The representative from Ethiopia added, "We strongly resent the abuse of our poverty to sway the interests of the European public."[46]

Not that any of this has sobered Monsanto, which continues to promote genetic engineering as the answer to world hunger.

Is THAT SO?

"Biotechnology is one of tomorrow's tools in our hands today. Slowing its acceptance is a luxury our hungry world cannot afford."
—Monsanto advertisement[47]

"Genetically engineered crops were created not because they're productive but because they're patentable. Their economic value is oriented not toward helping subsistence farmers to feed themselves but toward feeding more livestock for the already overfed rich."
—Amory and Hunter Lovins, Founders of Rocky Mountain Institute, a resource policy center[48]

One thing is certain. Monsanto and the other biotechnology companies will not soon stop telling us that genetically engineered foods can alleviate world hunger. In 2000, a coalition of biotech companies began a $50 million marketing campaign to keep fears about genetically altered foods from spreading through the United States. Bankrolling the campaign, which included $32 million in TV and print advertising, were Monsanto, Dow Chemical, DuPont, Swiss-based Novartis, the British Zeneca, Germany's BASF, and Aventis of France. The ads, complete with soft-focus fields and smiling children, pitched "solutions that could improve our world tomorrow" and aimed to convince the public that biotech foods could help end world hunger.[49]

Suicide Seeds

There is something absolutely miraculous about seeds, tiny units of life that have the capacity to grow into whole plants that will in turn produce thousands of new seeds. Seeds are one of life's fundamental mysteries, and one of Nature's most elegant means of continuance. Seeds that have been found in Egyptian tombs have been viable after having lain dormant for thousands of years.

For countless centuries farmers have fed humanity by saving the seed from one years crop to plant the following year. But Monsanto, the company that claims its motives are to help feed the hungry, has developed what it calls a "Technology Protection System" that renders seeds sterile. Commonly known as "terminator technology," and developed with taxpayer funding by the USDA and Delta & Pine Land Company (an affiliate of Monsanto), the process genetically alters seeds so that their offspring will be sterile for all time. If employed, this technology would ensure that farmers cannot save their own seeds, but would have to come back to Monsanto year after year to purchase new ones.

At least Melvin J. Oliver, the molecular biologist who is the primary inventor of the terminator technology, doesn't try to convince us that the point of the technology is to halt the spread of world hunger. "Our mission," he says, "is to make us competitive in the face of foreign competition."[50]

Critics call the genetically engineered seeds "suicide seeds." "By peddling suicide seeds, the biotechnology multinationals will lock the world's poorest farmers into a new form of genetic serfdom," says Emma Must of the World Development Movement. "Currently 80 percent of crops in developing countries are grown using farm-saved seed. Being unable to save seeds from sterile crops could mean the difference between surviving and going under."[51]

In October 1999, after facing intense and sustained public opposition to its terminator technology, Monsanto reluctantly declared that it had no immediate plans to commercialize terminator seeds. This was viewed as a victory for those opposed to the technology. But Monsanto also stated, at the same time, that it would continue closely related research designed to enable it to switch off other genetic traits critical to seed reproduction.[52]

When I first learned about Monsanto's plans to render seeds sterile, I found the prospect chilling. But I have been dismayed to learn that it's not just Monsanto that's doing this. Alarmingly, there are others in the biotechnology industry who see the profit potential and have similar aspirations.

AstraZeneca, for example, has patented a genetic process that makes plant growth and germination dependent upon repeated application of the company's chemicals. Similarly, Novartis has patented a technique that turns off the genes upon which plants depend to fight infections from many viruses and bacteria. Lo and behold, the only way to turn the genes back on is the application of chemicals sold by Novartis.[53]

As of 1999, twelve different companies had obtained more than two dozen patents on genetically sterilized or chemically dependent seeds.[54] It is unlikely these companies went to the expense of obtaining these patents or developing these systems if they didn't have plans to use them. These agribusiness corporations recognize the astounding profit potential inherent in gaining a substantial measure of control over the food supply of any nation that widely adopts their company's genetic technologies.

To these companies, the terminator and other seed sterilizing technologies are simply business ventures that have been designed to produce profit. In this case, there is not even the implication of agronomic benefit to farmers or nutritional benefit to consumers. "Monsanto's goal," says *Rachel's Environment and Health Weekly*, "is effective control of many of the staple crops that presently feed the world."[55]

Robert T. Fraley, co-president of Monsanto's agricultural sector, seems to agree. After the company bought up yet another competing seed company, he said, "This is not just a consolidation of seed companies. It's really a consolidation of the entire food chain."[56]

This shines an interesting light on Monsanto's corporate slogan—"Doing well by doing good."

Are the Risks Overblown?

There is a great deal of controversy about the safety of genetically engineered foods. Advocates of biotechnology often say that the risks are overblown. "There have been 25,000 trials of genetically modified crops in the world, now, and not a single incident, or anything dangerous in these releases," said a spokesman for Adventa Holdings, a U.K. biotech firm. "You would have thought that if it was a dangerous technology, there would have been a slip up by now." Similarly, during the 2000 presidential campaign, then-candidate George W. Bush said that "study after study has shown no evidence of danger." And the secretary of agriculture during the Clinton administration, Dan Glickman, said that "test after rigorous scientific test" had proven the safety of genetically engineered products.[57]

Is this the case? Unfortunately not, according to a senior researcher from the Union of Concerned Scientists, Dr. Jane Rissler. With a Ph.D. in plant pathology, four years of shaping biotechnology regulations at the EPA, and a dozen more in biotech science and policy, she is one of the nation's leading authorities on the environmental risks of genetically engineered foods. Dr. Rissler has been closely monitoring the trials and studies. "The observations that 'nothing happened' in these . . . tests do not say much," she and her colleague Dr. Margaret Mellon (a member of the USDA Advisory Committee on Agricultural Biotechnology) write. "In many cases, adverse impacts are subtle and would almost never be registered by scanning a field. . . . The field tests do not provide a track record of safety, but a case of 'don't look, don't find.'"[58]

When scientists actually look, what they see can be terrifying. A few years ago, a German biotech company engineered a common soil bacterium, *Klebsiella planticula*, to help break down wood chips, corn stalks, wastes from lumber businesses and agriculture, and to produce ethanol in the process. It seemed like a great achievement. The genetically engineered Klebsiella bacterium could help break down rotting organic material and in the process produce a fuel that could be used instead of gasoline, thus lessening the production of greenhouse gases. And, it was assumed, the post-process waste could afterward be added to soil as an amendment, like compost. Everybody would win. With the approval of the EPA, the company field-tested the bacterium at Oregon State University.

As far as the intended goals were concerned—eliminating rotting organic waste and producing ethanol—the genetically engineered bacterium was a success. But when a doctoral student named Michael Holmes decided to add the post-processed waste to actual living soil, something happened that no one expected. The seeds that were planted in soil mixed with the engineered Klebsiella sprouted, but then every single one of them died.[59]

What killed them? The genetically engineered Klebsiella turned out to be highly competitive with native soil micro-organisms, and to suppress activities that are crucial to soil fertility. Plants are only able to take nitrogen and other nourishment from the soil with the help of fungi called "mycorrhysal." These fungi live in the soil and help make nutrients available to plant roots. But when the genetically engineered Klebsiella was introduced into living soils, it greatly reduced the population of mycorrhysal fungi in the soil. And without healthy mycorrhysal fungi in soils, no plants can survive.[60]

To me, it is testimony to the amazing powers of science that researchers were able to track the mechanism by which the genetically engineered Klebsiella prevented plants from growing. There are thousands of different species of micro-organisms in every teaspoon of fertile soil, and they interact in trillions of ways.

But the scientists discovered something else in these experiments, something that sent chills down their spines. They found that the genetically modified bacteria were able to persist in the soil, raising the possibility that, had it been released, the genetically engineered Klebsiella could have become established—and virtually impossible to eradicate.[61]

"When the data first started coming in," says Elaine Ingham, the soil pathologist at Oregon State University who directed Michael Holmes' research on Klebsiella, "the EPA charged that we couldn't have performed the research correctly. They went through everything with a fine tooth comb, and they couldn't find anything wrong with the experimental design—but they tried as hard as they could. . . . If we hadn't done this research, the Klebsiella would have passed the approval process for commercial release."[62]

Geneticist David Suzuki understands that what took place was truly ominous. "The genetically engineered Klebsiella," he says, "could have ended all plant life on this continent. The implications of this single case are nothing short of terrifying."[63]

Meanwhile Monsanto and the other biotech companies are eagerly developing all kinds of genetically modified organisms, hoping to bring them to market. How do we know if they're safe? David Suzuki says, "We don't, and won't for years after they are being widely used."[64]

It's not a prospect that helps calm the nerves and restore confidence in our collective future. And in fact it can seem incredible that these things actually are happening. Surely, I've wanted to believe, when the chips are down, they would never do anything that would jeopardize life on Earth. Surely, the people who run these companies or the government officials who oversee them would never allow something that dangerous to occur. Surely, I've wanted to believe, the dangers of genetic engineering can't be that great.

But then again, this wouldn't be the first time that I've wanted to believe something that turned out to be only wishful thinking. And it wouldn't be the first time that corporations like Monsanto have brought us new products they promised would make life better for everybody and that turned out to do something very different. This is the same company, after all, that brought us PCBs and Agent Orange. Even the product the company was originally formed to produce, the artificial sweetener saccharin, was later found to be carcinogenic.

Of course, Monsanto tells us that this time we don't have to worry. . . .

> "These [genetically engineered] products are absolutely safe. For the most part you wouldn't know [if you were eating them] but the point being that you wouldn't need to know." (Bryan Hurley, Monsanto spokesman)[65]

The Industry No One Will Insure

You and I are repeatedly told by the biotech industry that genetically engineered crops are completely safe. The Biotechnology Industry Organization, for example, tells us, "Crops and foods improved through biotechnology have been modified with incredible precision. They have also been examined in advance in more depth and detail than any other crops and foods in human history. . . . Each and every food allowed on the market has been found to be at least as safe as the foods already available to consumers."[66]

The insurance industry, however, does not seem to agree. To date, no insurance company has been willing to insure the biotech industry.

"How do commercial interests usually protect themselves from liability claims?" asks geneticist Dr. David Suzuki. "Through insurance. In fact, in our society, the litmus test for safety is insurance. You can be insured for almost anything if you pay enough for the premium, but if the insurance industry isn't willing to bet its money on the safety of a product or technology, it means the risks are simply too high or too uncertain for them to take the gamble."[67]

There is today no insurance whatsoever against the kinds of catastrophic losses and tragedies that could ensue from introducing transgenic organisms into the environment and into the human food chain. The insurance industry has consistently not been willing to place insurance premiums on the potential for loss that is involved.[68]

The European Community has expressed a few concerns as well. In 1999, London's newspaper, the *Independent*, announced that "European governments are drawing up contingency plans for a nuclear fallout-style emergency involving genetically modified organisms (GMOs). A five-point Emergency Response Plan has been formulated by the European Commission, designed to cope if genetically modified plants result in widespread illness or the death of wildlife. . . . The plan is designed to prevent a human health disaster and stop genetically modified plants from breeding wildly with native species."[69]

chapter 17 **Farmageddon**

I don't particularly enjoy contemplating the difficulties and dangers that could develop as a result of genetic engineering. It's far more exciting to think that the technology might open the door to a brighter future. It can feel wonderful to imagine the possibilities for good and the expansion of human power and potential the technology might bring. The industry tells us we're going to put vaccines into common foods like bananas, thereby saving millions of lives. We're going to have fish that grow faster, pigs whose excrement is less toxic, and cows that produce less methane. Foods like golden rice will be designed to contain higher levels of the things we want, like vitamins, and fewer of the things we don't, like cholesterol and saturated fat. Pigs will be bred to grow human organs for transplants. Scientists are even isolating DNA from species long extinct, such as mastodons and Neanderthal people, in the hope of restoring them to life.

It sounds as if the sky is no longer the limit. Genetic engineering and the biotech companies can seem to hold the key to the promised land.

Dr. David Suzuki's genetics research lab was once the largest in Canada, and he co-wrote the most widely used introductory genetics textbooks in the world. He introduces a note of balance into the discussion:

"Genetics has enormous implications; it is full of promise to benefit and improve human lives, but equally heavy with potential to destroy and cause untold suffering. . . . The word 'engineering' conjures up images of roads and bridges and buildings, all designed and constructed to precise specifications. But as a geneticist, I can assure you that genetic engineering is based on trial and error, rather than on precision. For instance, if I want to insert a gene from a fruit fly into a daffodil, I can't pluck out just that gene and set it down exactly where I want it to go in its new home. The technique just doesn't work like that. Some geneticists even use a kind of molecular shotgun to blast the genes into the cells. And they never know exactly where they'll end up."[1]

Most of us think that a characteristic can be transferred from one species to another simply by moving the gene responsible for the given characteristic into the new species. But it's far from being that simple. For example, you might have a gene that in a mouse produces a hormone that regulates growth. But that gene will not necessarily produce the same hormone with the same effect in another species. It could produce a totally different effect, and there's no way of knowing. As genes are moved from one species to another, the effects are almost totally unpredictable. The science of genetics allows us to predict how genes will be expressed within a given species. But once we cross species boundaries, as the techniques of genetic engineering allow us to do, we have, according to David Suzuki, "absolutely no idea what might happen."[2]

To make things even more uncertain, conditions in the environment affect the way a gene is expressed in a plant. The same gene can produce different effects, depending on soil conditions, climate, chemical exposures, and a host of other environmental variables. This is why a plant that appears predictable and safe after a few years of observation on a small test plot may turn out to have entirely different consequences when grown in the variety of conditions that occur in the real world.

Suzuki is concerned that we are rushing ahead with a staggeringly powerful technology without adequate understanding of what we are doing. "The biotechnology industry makes anybody who brings up such matters look hysterical," he says. "Unfortunately, history shows us that all kinds of things—petrochemicals, CFCs, toxic dumps and nuclear power—that we thought, even insisted, were benign, turned out to be extremely dangerous. History informs us that caution is well warranted when it comes to buying into a powerful new technology."[3]

When genetic engineers shot "eye genes" from mice into fruit fly DNA, they produced fruit flies with extra eyes, all right, but the eyes were all over the flies' bodies. The scientists were not able to predict or control how many extra eyes would exist or where they would appear. In fact, they created flies with eyes on their wings and legs.[4]

Those extra eyes were visible and obvious. We don't know what other changes took place in the flies. Similarly, it is entirely possible that the transgenic plants we are releasing into the global ecosystem, and growing by the tens of millions of acres, could carry tragic flaws that are not apparent at first observation.

Of course, the lack of precision and certainty that we note in genetic engineering is normal with any new technology. The difference is that, in this case, with staggering potential consequences, we are growing hundreds of thousands of square miles of genetically modified crops without having conducted any long-term testing whatsoever.

Proponents of genetic engineering say it is simply the latest in a seamless continuum of biotechnologies practiced by human beings since the dawn of civilization, from bread and winemaking to selective breeding.[5] They do not pretend that there are no risks associated with genetic engineering. But they say these risks are no different from those for similar plants bred using traditional methods.

This can seem persuasive. But in traditional forms of breeding, traits are developed and accentuated that already exist within a species. In genetic engineering, on the other hand, we're taking genes from one species, or from several species, and inserting them into a completely different species.

We're taking flounder genes and putting them into tomatoes. We're taking human genes and putting them into salmon. We're taking genes from bacteria and from rats and putting them into broccoli. The Roundup Ready varieties that in 1999 made up more than half of the entire U.S. soybean crop and a third of the entire U.S. corn crop contain genes from viruses and petunias.

It is this crossing of, and violation of, Nature's species barriers that makes the process unprecedented and uniquely powerful. It is also, however, what makes it uniquely dangerous.

Nature has not made it easy to cross species boundaries. Dogs cannot breed with cats, much less fish with tomatoes. But genetic engineering overcomes the formidable barriers that Nature has erected, and that have almost never before in billions of years of life on Earth been transgressed, by creating "vectors." Derived from viruses and bacteria, these vectors are specifically designed to break down species barriers and to shuttle genes between a wide variety of species.

In genetic engineering, these vectors are attached to the genes that are to be transported, and then together they are shot into the genetic material of the recipient species. This is what makes the technology possible. But it is also what raises the likelihood that the genetic traits being transferred can jump from their new home into yet other organisms. The genetically modified crop isn't necessarily the end of the line. The same vector that enabled the trait to get into the transgenic organism can enable it to spread from there.

Contemplating some of the nightmarish scenarios that could occur can be frightening. There's a part of me that doesn't want to do it, that just wants to believe that things will be fine. No doubt we'll make a few messes and screw up plenty, I want to think, but we'll find a way to muddle through.

Perhaps. But if we are going to tamper with the code that generates all life, shouldn't we first know what we are doing? If we are going to plant 100 million acres in transgenic crops after only four years of commercial deployment, shouldn't we consider every danger?

The biotech industry frequently implies that those who question it are reacting from emotion rather than reason, and that concerns about safety or health are irrational and exaggerated. But the more I've learned, the more I've seen that there are bona fide issues here of scientific uncertainty, health risks, and environmental dangers. And the more it seems to me that it's not the people who challenge genetic engineering who are blinded by emotion, but rather those who want to rush headlong into it, reckless with the excitement of overcoming Nature's most ancient and inviolate boundaries.

Is that so?

"The biggest mistake that anyone can make is moving slowly, because the game is going to be over before you start."
—Hendrik Verfaillie, Monsanto's Senior Vice President and Chief Financial Officer[6]

"I have a feeling that science has transgressed a barrier that should have remained inviolate.... You cannot recall a new form of life.... It will survive you and your children and your children's children. An irreversible attack on the biosphere is something so unheard of, so unthinkable in previous generations, that I only wish that mine had not been guilty of it."
—Erwin Chargaff, Professor Emeritus of Biochemistry, Columbia University, and discoverer of "Chargaff's Rules," the scientific foundation for the discovery of the DNA double helix[7]

John Fagan is a molecular biologist who for more than twenty years was funded by the National Institutes of Health to conduct genetic engineering research. But in 1994, he returned more than $600,000 to the NIH and withdrew his proposals for another $1.25 million. Then he launched a global campaign to alert the public about the hazards of genetic engineering. According to Dr. Fagan,

"Genetic engineers can cut and splice genes very precisely in a test tube, but the process of putting those genes into a living organism is extremely imprecise, inaccurate, and uncontrolled. Such manipulations can cause mutations that damage the functioning of the organism. Once a gene is inserted into an organism, it can cause unanticipated side effects. Mutations and side effects can cause genetically engineered foods to contain toxins and allergens and to be reduced in nutritional value."[8]

Dr. Richard Strohman is a renowned molecular biologist. Past chair of the prestigious department of molecular biology at the University of California at Berkeley, he agrees with Dr. Fagan that the stakes are high.

The trouble with genetically engineering, he says, "is that it often doesn't work. And when you put a biological entity out into the environment, or into a human being, and you're not completely certain—and you can never be certain in this business, in my opinion—your ability to do damage is very, very high."[9]

Strohman and others point to the dangers inherent in gene-splicing techniques. When scientists snip a bit of DNA from one organism and insert it into another, it doesn't travel alone. It can include genetic parasites, such as viruses. Genetic parasites are naturally specific to certain species. They are contained by genetic species barriers, and indeed this is one of the reasons why Nature has kept species barriers so intact and inviolate. But with genetic engineering, we are transgressing the gene-transfer barriers that normally exist. In the eyes of many scientists, this is deeply troubling, because in the past few years, there have been an increasing number of reports of new pathogens arising from the kind of horizontal (across species barriers) gene transfer that is the basis for genetic engineering.

Within the past twenty-five years, we have seen a rash of new diseases arising, including Ebola, AIDS, hepatitis C, Lyme disease, and hantavirus, and no doubt we will see more emerge in coming years. There is much we don't know about these emerging diseases, but we know they take a terrifying toll on humanity. And we know that many of these new pathogens seem to stem from horizontal gene transfer. This means they have come from other species and have jumped to us.

This happens rarely in Nature, which is fortunate, because when it does, the results can be disastrous. The flu pandemic of 1918, which killed more than 22 million people worldwide, is thought to have been caused by horizontal gene transfer. AIDS is now thought to stem from a virus that originated in chimpanzees and somehow jumped to humans who ate the chimps or exchanged blood with them. Mad Cow disease is now understood to be the result of horizontal transfer of an infectious protein that kills sheep.

With so much at stake, you might think that those involved would be moved to humility. Sometimes, they are. Then again, sometimes they aren't. . .

Is THAT SO?

"Those of us in industry can take comfort. . . . After all, we're the technical experts. We know we're right. The 'antis' obviously don't understand the science, and are just as obviously pushing a hidden agenda—probably to destroy capitalism."

—Bob Shapiro, Monsanto's CEO[10]

"(Genetic engineering) faces our society with problems unprecedented, not only in the history of science, but of life on the Earth. It places in human hands the capacity to redesign living organisms, the products of some three billion years of evolution. . . . Up to now, living organisms have evolved very slowly, and new forms have had plenty of time to settle in. Now whole proteins will be transposed overnight into wholly new associations, with consequences no one can foretell. . . . Going ahead in this direction may be not only unwise, but dangerous. Potentially, it could breed new animal and plant diseases, new sources of cancer, and novel epidemics."

—George Wald, M.D., Nobel Laureate in Medicine,
Professor of Biology, Harvard University

It's quite an experiment to be undertaking without any long-term testing and without the consent or knowledge of the people involved.

Genetic Roulette

Medical authorities estimate that one-quarter of the population experiences allergic reactions to one or more foods—most commonly dairy products, eggs, wheat, and nuts. We don't know why some people react adversely and others don't. But the consequences can be serious, and can result in many problems, including life-threatening anaphylactic shock.

In 1996, researchers at Pioneer Hi-Bred inserted a protein from Brazil nuts into soybeans. Because the genetically engineered soybeans were regarded as "substantially equivalent" to non–genetically engineered soybeans, Pioneer Hi-Bred was not required to test for allergic responses in human beings. But when researchers at the University of Nebraska tested the genetically engineered soybeans on samples of blood serum drawn from people who were allergic to Brazil nuts, they found that if these people had eaten the soybeans, they would have suffered serious, even fatal, allergic reactions.[11] Pioneer Hi-Bred withdrew the product.

In discussing the situation in the *New England Journal of Medicine*, the researchers emphasized that tests on laboratory animals are not sufficient to discover allergic reactions to genetically modified organisms.[12] Only tests on humans can do that.

In this case, we were lucky. Knowing that Brazil nuts can be allergenic, Pioneer Hi-Bred undertook the tests of its own accord. But with genetic material from bacteria and viruses continually being inserted across species boundaries into genetically engineered foods, it is seemingly only a matter of time until a genetically engineered food causes adverse reactions in the unsuspecting public. It may in fact already be happening, though impossible to trace to its source.

Today, the FDA requires allergy testing when the organism from which the gene is taken is a known and common allergen. But such tests have never been required of Monsanto's Roundup Ready soybeans, even though the genetic engineering process has incorporated genes from petunias and viruses into the soybeans, because petunias and viruses are not known allergens. Of course they aren't; no one's ever eaten them before. How would anyone know if they were allergic to petunias? Since soy products are widely dispersed in the American diet, it is entirely conceivable that members of the public are already experiencing harm from transgenic foods.

At present, we can only speculate what adverse reactions might already be occurring. The lack of labeling effectively prevents any attempt to monitor the human health impact of consuming these foods.

Laura and Robin Ticciati are the authors of the 1998 book *Genetically Engineered Foods: Are They Safe? You Decide.* They ask questions like:

> "What if we find out in twenty years that genetically engineered foods aren't safe after all? What if we discover some bizarre disease in the next generation that ends up linked to the (soy or canola) oil we pour on our salads today? What if the French fries our kids devoured last week cause birth defects in our grandchildren? What if we learn that manipulating

the DNA of our foods has an effect on a growing fetus after all? Or that genetically engineered foods contain some unknown allergen that produces a reaction that just can't be cured?"[13]

When a spokesperson for one of the largest producers of genetically engineered seeds called the Ticciatis to task, comparing them to someone who was afraid to cross the street because "what if" a car came just at that moment and hit them, they had an answer. "We look both ways before stepping off the curb," they said. "Don't you?"

The L-Tryptophan Story

The food supplement L-tryptophan was safely used by tens of millions of people for decades as an aid to relaxation and sleep. The process by which the supplement was produced involved a particular bacteria. In fact, it's not too much of an oversimplification to say that the bacteria actually produced the L-tryptophan.

But then, in 1989, Showa Denko, a Japanese company that manufactured L-tryptophan, genetically engineered the bacteria *(Bacillus amyloliquefaciens)* to greatly increase the amounts of L-tryptophan the bacteria was able to produce. Shortly thereafter, thousands of people who were taking L-tryptophan began to suffer from an extremely serious disease, Eosinophilia Myalgia Syndrome (EMS), that left at least 37 people dead and thousands with permanent disabilities, including paralysis.[14]

Because the batch of L-tryptophan that had been made by genetically engineered bacteria had not been labeled any differently than other L-tryptophan, it was not immediately apparent that it was the cause of the outbreak. And Showa Denko didn't help matters any by destroying all batches of the genetically engineered bacteria once investigators came knocking. But extremely toxic compounds (Peak E, Peak 97, and EBT) were subsequently found in the L-tryptophan that had been made using the genetically engineered bacteria, and have never been found in brands produced with non–genetically engineered bacteria.[15] And no one has ever been known to contract EMS from non–genetically engineered L-tryptophan.

The batch of L-tryptophan that was made by Showa Denko using the genetically engineered bacteria, like all genetically engineered products, was considered "substantially equivalent" to the L-tryptophan produced normally and had not been subjected to any kind of testing by authorities.

L-tryptophan was subsequently banned for sale in the United States, but sadly, the L-tryptophan tragedy could potentially be a harbinger of things to come. Bacteria are also used to produce many vitamins. In 1996, the United Kingdom approved a new process to manufacture riboflavin (vitamin B-2) using genetically engineered bacteria. They did so based on data that identified only those contaminants found at levels greater than 0.1 percent. But this would not have been a fine enough screen in the case of the L-tryptophan made by genetically engineered bacteria, because the toxic compounds in that L-tryptophan constituted only 0.01 percent of the marketed product by weight. "Under current international safety regulations," notes genetic engineering expert and author Luke Anderson, "a product which contained contaminants as dangerous as those found in the (genetically engineered) L-tryptophan could still be passed as safe for human consumption."[16]

Unfortunately, because of the lack of labeling, there is no way for consumers to tell today whether or not their vitamins and other supplements have been made with the aid of genetically engineered bacteria. One company, NOW Foods of Bloomingdale, Illinois, has begun to augment its vitamin line with non-GMO supplements. "The challenge," said James Roza, the company's director of quality assurance, "is enormous. Not only do we have to worry about the contamination of raw materials like corn and soy, but . . . all of the genetically engineered processing aids used to make vitamins as well."[17]

I wish I could tell you the name of a particular brand of vitamins that you could purchase knowing they were guaranteed to be free from GMOs. But I can't. It's ironic, because you can buy a safer car, or one that gets better gas mileage. You can choose an energy-efficient freezer. But the lack of labeling makes it very difficult to choose foods and supplements that don't contain genetically altered substances.

Milk from Drugged Cows

For some time, bovine growth hormone (BGH) has been used to stimulate milk production in cows. The hormone was too expensive for widespread use, however, until Monsanto came up with a genetically altered hormone, called rBGH (recombinant bovine growth hormone), sold under the brand name Posilac. This genetically engineered hormone is now injected into about a quarter of the cows in U.S. dairies.[18]

There is no controversy about whether rBGH increases milk production. It does. But there are other points of contention. For one thing, the need for the technology has been questioned, because since 1950 U.S. dairy farmers have been producing vastly more milk than Americans can consume. In fact, in 1986–1987, the federal government paid farmers to kill their cows and stop dairy farming for five years, in an effort to reduce the amount of milk produced. More than 1.5 million U.S. milk cows were slaughtered. Even this drastic program, however, did not solve the problem of milk overproduction in the United States.

Another issue is that milk from cows that have been injected with Monsanto's genetically engineered rBGH contains 2 to 10 times as much IGF-1 (insulin-like growth factor) as normal cow's milk.[19] This is significant, because studies have found that the risk of prostate cancer for men over 60 years of age with high levels of IGF-1 to be 8 times greater than for men with low levels,[20] and the risk of breast cancer for premenopausal women with increased IGF-1 to be up to 7 times greater.[21]

Consultants paid by Monsanto say that milk from injected cows is absolutely safe for human consumption because IGF-1 is destroyed by pasteurization. FDA researchers, on the other hand, report that IGF-1 is not destroyed by pasteurization.[22]

Monsanto also says the hormone is safe because IGF-1 is completely broken down by digestive enzymes and does not enter the human intestinal tract.[23] But researchers not paid by Monsanto say that IGF-1 may not be totally digested, and that some does make its way into the colon and cross the intestinal wall into the bloodstream.[24]

It makes you wonder.

Meanwhile, cows treated with the genetically engineered hormone have a 25 percent increase in udder infections (mastitis) and a 50 percent increase in lameness. To counter the health problems among cows injected with rBGH, Monsanto suggests a greater use of antibiotics. As it just so happens, the company also sells the very antibiotics it recommends.

Health Problems from Eating Genetically Engineered Foods?

Does eating genetically engineered foods pose potential health risks to people? In 2001, the *Los Angeles Times* published an exposé revealing that Monsanto's own research had raised many questions about the safety of their Roundup Ready soybeans.[25] Remarkably, the FDA did not call for more testing before allowing these soybeans to flood the marketplace. Since half the soybeans grown in the United States are now Monsanto's Roundup Ready variety, and because soy is contained in such a wide array of processed foods, tens of millions of people are unknowingly eating these experimental foods daily.

According to Monsanto's own tests, Roundup Ready soybeans contain 29 percent less of the brain nutrient choline, and 27 percent more trypsin inhibitor, a potential allergen that interferes with protein digestion, than normal soybeans. Soy products are often prescribed and consumed for their phytoestrogen content, but according to the company's tests, the genetically altered soybeans have lower levels of phenylalanine, an essential amino acid that affects levels of phytoestrogens. And levels of lectins, which not infrequently are allergens, are nearly double in the transgenic variety.[26]

What might be expected from consuming soybeans containing higher levels of trypsin inhibitor and lectins? At the very least, slower growth in children. And possibly, unexpected and even dangerous allergic reactions.

Dr. Arpad Pusztai, senior scientist at the Rowett Research Institute in Aberdeen, Scotland, has published 270 scientific papers, and is widely known as the world's leading expert on lectins.[27] When he began conducting experiments in which he fed genetically engineered potatoes to rats, he considered himself a "very enthusiastic supporter" of gene splicing biotechnology. However, the rats fed on genetically modified potatoes showed a variety of unexpected and disturbing changes, including smaller livers, hearts, and brains—and weakened immune systems. "Feeding transgenic potatoes to rats induced major and in most instances highly significant changes in the weights of some or most of their vital organs," he concluded. "Particularly worrying was the partial liver atrophy. . . . Immune organs, such as the spleen and thymus were also frequently affected."[28] Sadly, the rats' growth was impaired, and some developed tumors and showed significant shrinkage of the brain after only ten days of eating genetically modified potatoes.[29]

I'm not a big fan of animal studies, because I've found that a great number of them are cruel and unjustified and their relevance to humans is often questionable. Still, the results of Pusztai's tests were shocking. "I was totally taken back. No doubt about it," Pusztai said. "The longer I spent on the experiment, the more uneasy I became."[30] When he appeared on the major British TV program *World In Action*, Pusztai was asked, point blank, whether he personally would eat genetically modified potatoes. "No," he answered, adding that "it is very, very unfair to use our fellow citizens as guinea pigs."

For this, Dr. Pusztai was suddenly and inexplicably fired. Only later was it discovered that the Rowett Institute is partially funded by Monsanto.

A subsequent panel of twenty independent scientists from thirteen countries, however, confirmed both Dr. Pusztai's data and his findings, and the Institute eventually was forced to reinstate Dr. Pusztai. Meanwhile, a ban was imposed on growing genetically engineered crops of any kind in the United Kingdom for three years.

There are now laws in the United Kingdom requiring the labeling of genetically modified foods, and almost every major food chain in the country has pledged to be "gene-free." Yet amazingly, the industry has continued to forge ahead unabated in the United States, where the federal government, rather than testing and regulating the industry, has been its cheerleader.

The *Lancet*, widely recognized to be one of the most prestigious medical journals in the world, describes the situation candidly:

"It is astounding that FDA has not changed their stance on genetically modified food. . . . Governments should never have allowed these products into the food chain without insisting on rigorous testing for effects on health.[31]

Regulatory Agencies Out to Lunch

There are three federal agencies that in different ways regulate genetically engineered crops and foods in the United States: the Food and Drug Administration (FDA), the U.S. Department of Agriculture (USDA), and the Environmental Protection Agency (EPA). You'd like to think that these agencies are protecting the public and looking out for the common good. But on this issue, according to *Rachel's Environment and Health Weekly*,

"The heads of all three agencies are on record with speeches that make them sound remarkably like cheerleaders for genetic engineering, rather than impartial judges of a novel and powerful new technology. All three agencies have set policies that:

- No public records need be kept of which farms are using genetically engineered seeds.

- Companies that buy from farmers and sell to food manufacturers and grocery chains do not need to keep genetically engineered crops separate from traditional crops, so purchasers have no way to avoid purchasing genetically engineered foods.

- No one needs to label any seeds, crops, or any food products, with information about their genetically engineered origins, so consumers have no way to exercise informed choices in the grocery store."[32]

These policies have two principal effects. They keep the public unaware of the rapid arrival of transgenic foods onto the family dinner table. And they prevent epidemiologists from tracing health effects, if any appear, because no one will know who has been exposed to novel gene products and who has not.

It is astounding how casually the federal agencies have taken the transition to genetically modified foods. Before the first altered foods came onto the market, the FDA determined that these foods were "substantially equivalent" to traditional foods, and therefore should be regarded and regulated as if they were no different. At present, except in cases where there are demonstrably major changes in nutrient composition, or in cases where specific proteins known to cause allergic reactions have been incorporated, transgenic foods in the United States are not subject to any pre-market approval process, public notification, or labeling.

The government essentially leaves it up to the biotech industry to decide when and whether to consult with the FDA. Any safety testing is done by the industry of their own products, and they are asked to notify the FDA only if they suspect a problem. Thus we have a situation where the very companies that stand to profit are the ones that decide whether or not their products are hazardous.

If the goal of public policy regarding genetic engineering is to reduce regulatory costs for the biotech corporations, it is certainly being achieved. But whatever happened to the goal of protecting the public from harm?

The FDA simply allows Monsanto and the other biotech companies to decide for themselves whether their products are "generally recognized as safe." If the companies decide that they are, no safety testing is required before these new products are introduced into the food supply.

Can we trust these companies to do the job? When independent researchers looked at Monsanto's tests on Roundup Ready soybeans, they found that the soybeans Monsanto tested were not an accurate representation of the Monsanto soybeans that appear in the store as food. They had not been treated with herbicide, although no one grows any Roundup Ready variety without using Roundup on the fields. When an independent testing firm reconducted the study, genetically altered soybeans grown under real world conditions and sprayed with the herbicide were found to have a 12 to 14 percent reduction in phytoestrogens—nutrients that help protect against heart disease, osteoporosis, and breast cancer.[33]

Suzanne Wuerthele is a toxicologist who has worked for the EPA for 13 years. She says,

"This technology is being promoted, in the face of concerns by respectable scientists and in the face of data to the contrary, by the very agencies which are supposed to be protecting human health and the environment. The bottom line in my view is that we are confronted with the most powerful technology the world has ever known, and it is being rapidly deployed with almost no thought whatsoever to its consequences."[34]

What is the reasoning behind these policies? The FDA and the biotech industry say that labels and testing would "mislead" people by implying that there is a "tangible difference" between genetically engineered foods and their natural counterparts. They continue to tell us that transgenic foods are "substantially equivalent" to their natural predecessors. The FDA has steadfastly maintained this position, even when many of the agency's own scientists expressed grave doubts about the safety of transgenic crops, and even in the case of Monsanto's New Leaf potato, which has been genetically modified to incorporate a pesticide into every cell (to kill potato beetles), and is itself registered with the EPA as a pesticide.[35]

It's hard to avoid the conclusion that the FDA and the biotech industry are talking out of both sides of their mouths. When it comes to labeling, transgenic foods are "substantially equivalent" and do not need to be labeled or tracked in any way. But when it comes to patenting, they are whole new organisms, and can be patented, owned, and sold for a profit.

In late 1999, a consortium of large organizations supporting biotechnology wrote President Clinton,

"If the FDA were to change its policy and require special labeling for biotech foods, such labeling could have the effect of misleading consumers into believing that biotech foods are either 'different' from conventional foods or present a risk or a potential risk. . . . Such special labeling of biotech foods could lead to the very kind of consumer confusion that labels are designed to prevent. . . . Changing the current policy to require special labeling could impact significantly consumers' perception of the safety of biotech foods and undermine the credibility the FDA currently enjoys. Furthermore, such a change in policy would have the effect of validating the charges and claims being advanced by opponents of modern biotechnology."[36]

The letter was signed by 38 organizations, including the American Crop Protection Association (a consortium of pesticide manufacturers), the American Meat Institute, the National Turkey Federation, the Biotechnology Industry Association, the United Egg Association, International Dairy Foods, and the National Chicken Council.

Advocates of genetic engineering don't always respond graciously to criticism. In 2000, biotech proponent Jack Kemp, the former Republican nominee for vice president, came up with a whole series of names for those calling for safety testing and labeling of genetically engineered foods. They are, he said, "ill-considered, anti-progress, left-wing, self-appointed . . . anti-technology activists."[37]

How is it, I have wondered, that the U.S. government could be so totally in the pocket of the biotech industry, and so asleep at the switch when protecting the public? How is it that, rather than require that the biotech industry prove that genetic engineering is necessary and safe, the government has seemed to view public resistance as something to be conquered? How is it that these products have been put on the market without public input or labeling? How is it that little recourse is left for someone who doesn't want to eat genetically modified organisms, new viruses, and bacteria, or vegetables containing genes from toads and fish?

It's shameful how often people have moved back and forth between high-level positions in government regulatory agencies like the FDA, the EPA, and the USDA and highly paid positions with biotech corporations like Monsanto and DuPont. Mickey Kantor, who was Secretary of the Department of Commerce and President Clinton's trade representative, became a member of Monsanto's board of directors. William Ruckelshaus, former Chief Administrator of the EPA, also joined Monsanto's board. Clayton Yeutter, former U.S. Secretary of Agriculture, became a member of the board of directors of Mycogen Corporation, owned by Dow AgroSciences. Marcia Hale, who was Assistant to the U.S. President and Director of Intergovernmental Affairs, left the White House to become Director of International Government Affairs for

Monsanto. Josh King, former Director of Production for the White House, became Director of Global Communication for Monsanto.[38]

The revolving door between government agencies and the biotech industry continued when George W. Bush became president in 2001.[39] The new second-in-command at the EPA, Linda Fisher, was Vice President for Government and Public Affairs at Monsanto. Bush's new Secretary of Defense, Donald Rumsfeld, was president of a company (Searle Pharmaceuticals) that was bought by Monsanto. The new Attorney General, John Ashcroft, received more money from Monsanto than any other Congressional candidate in the previous election, and was a leading advocate of policies to force Europe to accept genetically engineered foods. Bush's new Secretary of Health and Human Services, Tommy Thompson, had, while Governor of Wisconsin, used state funds to set up a $300,000,000 biotech zone, and was one of a handful of governors to launch a campaign, partially funded by Monsanto, to persuade Americans of the benefits of genetically modified crops.[40]

And most significantly, Bush's new Secretary of Agriculture, Ann Veneman, was a former board member of the biotech company Calgene, owned by Monsanto.

Shortly after Veneman took over, her predecessor, now-former Secretary of Agriculture Dan Glickman, made a startling revelation. In an interview with the *St. Louis Post-Dispatch*, he acknowledged that the climate in the government regarding genetically engineered foods had been so pervasively pro-biotech that even as the top agricultural official in the nation he had literally felt unable to speak or act in the public interest.

> "What I saw . . . was the attitude that the technology was good and that it was almost immoral to say that it wasn't good. . . . There was a lot of money that had been invested in this, and if you're against it, you're Luddites, you're stupid. There was rhetoric like that . . . here in this department. You felt like you were almost an alien, disloyal, by trying to present an open-minded view on some of the issues being raised. So I pretty much spouted the rhetoric that everybody else around here spouted. It was written into my speeches."[41]

Ironically, the very day Glickman was describing how controlled he had been by the overwhelmingly pro-biotech atmosphere at the Department of Agriculture, the *New York Times* was running a feature story revealing that the government had been playing into the hands of Monsanto ever since the Reagan administration:

> "In late 1986, four executives of the Monsanto Company, the leader in agricultural biotechnology, paid a visit to Vice President George Bush at the White House to make an unusual pitch. . . . In the weeks and months that followed, the White House complied, working behind the scenes to help Monsanto—long a political power with deep connections in Washington—get (what) it wanted.
>
> "It was an outcome that would be repeated, again and again, through three administrations. What Monsanto wished from Washington, Monsanto—and, by extension, the biotechnology industry—got. . . . Even longtime Washington hands said that the control this nascent industry exerted over its own regulatory destiny—through the EPA, the USDA, and ultimately the FDA—was astonishing.
>
> 'In this area, the U.S. government agencies have done exactly what big agribusiness has asked them to do and told them to do,' said Dr. Henry Miller, a senior research fellow at the Hoover Institute, who was responsible for biotechnology issues at the FDA from 1979 to 1994."[42]

Labeling It Like It Is

In 1995, very few genetically modified plants had yet been grown for commercial sale. Four years later, nearly 100 million acres of genetically modified crops were planted worldwide, more than 70 million of them in the United States. By 2000, more than half of the American soybean and cotton crops and one-third of the corn crop were genetically engineered. By then, too, much of the Canadian canola (rapeseed) crop was also transgenic.[43]

For this rapid change to have occurred with a minimum of resistance from consumers, the FDA had to insist that genetically engineered foods not be labeled. It could not have happened if there had been labeling. Polls have consistently found that 80 to 95 percent of the American public wants genetically engineered food to be labeled.[44]

American consumers also overwhelmingly support the labeling of milk produced with the genetically engineered bovine growth hormone, rBGH. But the FDA has said such labeling would unfairly stigmatize rBGH milk as less healthy. The FDA official responsible for this policy is Michael R. Taylor, whose occupation prior to joining the FDA was as a partner in the law firm representing Monsanto when it applied for FDA approval for rBGH. His employer after he left the FDA, by the way, was Monsanto.

Monsanto's track record in these matters tends to be a tad shady. During Canada's scientific review of Monsanto's application for approval of rBGH, Canadian health officials said Monsanto tried to bribe them, and government scientists testified that they were being pressured by higher-ups to approve rBGH against their better scientific judgment. Canada's policies have been almost as ardently pro-biotech as those of the United States, but in 1999, Canadian health authorities, after eight years of study, rejected Monsanto's application for approval of rBGH.[45] In so doing, Canada joined the European Union, Japan, Australia, and New Zealand, all of whom have banned rBGH because of scientific health concerns.

In the United States, however, milk produced with the genetically engineered hormone is not only legal, it is also not labeled. And it is not only not labeled, but Monsanto has fought to make it impossible to reveal, truthfully, when it's *not* in milk.

When several companies that produced milk without rBGH, including the Pure Milk Company of Waco, Texas, and Swiss Valley Farms of Davenport, Iowa, factually advertised their milk as rBGH-free, Monsanto's response was to sue these companies, forcing then to refrain from telling their customers the truth.[46]

Monsanto's actions and ensuing lawsuit represent a new twist in libel litigation. For the first time, telling the truth was contended to be objectionable. Monsanto claimed that a statement of actual truth could be false advertising, because actual facts could induce consumers to believe that Monsanto's product was less than exemplary, and thereby cost the company money.

Currently, neither milk made with rBGH nor any other genetically engineered food product in the United States, is labeled. Biologist Brian

Goodwin, who has been deeply involved in this controversy understands the consequences.

> "You would never allow a new drug to be produced without a clear label, without knowing what company produced it, without knowing exactly where it was produced and even under what conditions, what batch it came from and so on. Genetically modified foods ought to be put in the same category as drugs because of their potential harm. They're actually even more dangerous than drugs, because after all, we eat a lot more food during the course of our lifetime than we take drugs. Even if there are small effects, they can accumulate over years. And therefore people should have the right to say, 'I'm not going to eat genetically modified food because I have no confidence that this is going to be safe for the whole of my lifetime.'"[47]

As citizens of a democratic society, most of us assume that we have the right to decide what to put into our bodies. But in order to do that, we have to know what's in the things we eat. That means they have to be labeled. If you cannot identify which foods have been genetically altered, it is very difficult to avoid eating them.

But the people who do not want them labeled have their own point of view. In explaining why genetically modified food should not be labeled, Janet Bainbridge, head of the U.K. Advisory Committee on Novel Foods and Processes, displayed something less than complete respect for democratic choice. She said that "most people don't even know what a gene is. . . . Sometimes my young son wants to cross the road when it's dangerous. Sometimes you just have to tell people what's best for them."[48]

She may be right that some people don't know what a gene is, but I'll bet you most people know a reckless and self-serving industry when they see one. Certainly in England the public has risen up in protest against genetically engineered food. Even employees at Monsanto's own headquarters, apparently, are less than enamored at the prospect of ingesting their company's creations. In December 1999, a statement was posted in the cafeteria of the Monsanto Corporation's United Kingdom headquarters in High Wycombe, England, that truly gives me pause. It read as follows:

"In response to concern raised by our customers . . . we have decided to remove, as far as is practicable, genetically modified soy and maize (corn) from all food products served in our restaurant. We will continue to work with our suppliers to replace GM (genetically modified) soy and maize with non-GM ingredients. . . . We have taken the above steps to ensure that you, the customer, can feel confident in the food we serve."[49]

chapter 18

The Emperor's New Foods

In 1999, 87,000 bags of organic tortilla chips worth hundreds of thousands of dollars were destroyed after a routine analysis found transgenic DNA to be present in the product. The organic corn had been grown on a 7,000-acre farm in Texas, but had been contaminated by cross-pollination from neighboring farms that were growing genetically engineered corn.[1] You might think that after such an occurrence, the biotech industry would at least apologize. But that's not how these companies tend to respond. They have come up with a more profitable, less embarrassing idea. Monsanto has been suing farmers whose crops have been contaminated by cross-pollination, accusing them, believe it or not, of stealing a patented product.

In Saskatoon, Saskatchewan, Percy Schmeiser has grown canola (rapeseed) on his 1,400-acre farm for 40 years. In 1997, he began to notice something unusual. When he sprayed Monsanto's weedkiller Roundup around electricity poles, the herbicide killed all the weeds except for a thin scattering of canola plants. Schmeiser had been crossbreeding his own canola for more than 30 years, saving seed from each year's harvest as farmers have done for centuries, and at first he thought he might have accidentally created some kind of Frankenstein mutant. He mentioned his concerns to some of his neighbors.

The next thing he knew, private investigators hired by Monsanto arrived at his farm uninvited and took samples of his crops.[2]

Sure enough, some of the plants were genetically similar to Monsanto's Roundup Ready Canola. The company then accused Schmeiser of "stealing" its seeds and infringing its patent. Monsanto demanded compensation to the entire value of Schmeiser's 1998 crop, plus punitive damages, court costs, and his signature on a nondisclosure agreement that required him to stay silent about the affair.[3]

But in this case, Monsanto picked the wrong guy to try to intimidate. Schmeiser had been mayor of the town of Bruno for several years and a member of the Saskatchewan provincial parliament. He is a hardy mountaineer who has three times attempted to scale Mt. Everest. Not one to be bullied, Schmeiser turned around and countersued the corporate giant for nearly $10 million Canadian—for trespass, crop contamination, and defamation. Further, he accused Monsanto of "arrogant, high-handed, and shocking conduct and callous disregard for the environment."[4]

Schmeiser said he had never bought Monsanto's seed and didn't want to grow the corporation's genetically engineered varieties. He was not a criminal who wanted to profit from stolen technology, he said, but a victim of that technology invading his property and crops. The reality, according to Schmeiser, is that many of his neighbors are growing genetically engineered canola, and pollen from them is blowing everywhere. "It's in the ditches and the roadsides; it's in the shelterbelts; it's in the gardens; it's all over. . . . We're just touching the tip of the iceberg in contamination of fields by this Roundup genetic canola."[5]

On October 2, 2000, the 131st anniversary of Mahatma Gandhi's birth, Gandhi's family gave this Canadian farmer the prestigious Mahatma Gandhi award. An enormous crowd of 300,000 Indian farmers gathered to listen to and support Percy Schmeiser.

When I first learned that Monsanto was suing Percy Schmeiser because their crops had invaded his fields, I could hardly believe it. It seemed ludicrous. But then I remembered that this is the same Monsanto that sues dairies who dare to inform their customers that they don't use the corporation's genetically engineered bovine growth hormone.

I have a friend—I'm sure you know people like this—who needs at all times to be positive. She has the same smile on her face in every situation, and her voice seems to me to have the deep human resonance of saccharine. When I told her about Monsanto and how I felt about some of their intimidation tactics, she reprimanded me for being "too negative."

"I'm sure their intentions are good," she admonished me. "They just need to be loved."

I agree with her, actually, that the people at Monsanto, like all people, need to be loved. But I also think that when a corporation runs roughshod over questions of public health, freedom of choice, and ecological stability, and presents us with the grave risk of irreversible genetic pollution, they need something else as well.

They need to be stopped.

Leaky Genes

In Percy Schmeiser's fields, Monsanto's genetically engineered canola apparently cross-pollinated with his traditional varieties and passed on the genetically engineered trait that enables them to tolerate the company's herbicide. In time, however, it is inevitable that traits that have been engineered into commercially grown transgenic crops will transfer not only to neighbors' fields but to wild plants and weeds.

In 2000, scientists from the government-funded National Institute of Agricultural Botany announced the first genetically modified superweeds in Britain. Pollen from a genetically modified trial crop of canola (rapeseed) had crossed with a field of wild turnip. According to the *Independent*, "Some of the 'Frankenstein' plants, which had inherited their GM parents' herbicide-resistant genes, were able to breed."[6]

Since the advent of genetic engineering, scientists have warned of the risk that crops that were engineered to be resistant to herbicides would leak the genes that provide that resistance into the very weeds those herbicides are intended to kill. Until recently, however, we did not know when this might occur. In fact, it has happened sooner than almost anyone imagined.

In 1998, only two years after the commercialization of transgenic crops, Canadian farmers reported that weeds had indeed acquired the ability to tolerate herbicides, frustrating weed control efforts and confirming fears of genetic pollution. Herbicide-resistant genes had been transferred to weeds in the environment of the genetically modified crops, producing fertile superweeds that were resistant to the herbicide. By 2000, reports of weeds (particularly hemp weed and pig weed) that were developing resistance to Roundup were becoming increasingly common.[7]

As farmers are faced with increasing herbicide resistance in the weeds they confront, how will they cope? In many cases, with ever more sprayings of ever more toxic, and expensive, poisons.

The problem of genetically modified organisms transferring their genetic traits to new organisms is not limited to the plant kingdom. More than 50 laboratories around the world are currently conducting research into transgenic fish. These labs are splicing genes from chickens, humans, cattle, and rats—into carp, catfish, trout, and salmon.[8]

One of the serious problems this practice is likely to cause is called "the Trojan Fish Syndrome." When you engineer human growth genes (or other growth genes) into fish, the fish that result grow far larger than normal. That's the whole point of the practice. But there is also an unintended consequence. These enormous fish, which have growth genes from other species (sometimes including humans) in every cell of their bodies, upset the balance of Nature. Native fish are attracted to, and mate with, these gigantic fish. This gives the genetically engineered fish a selective advantage, and they create more offspring. But it turns out that the offspring of the genetically engineered fish have far higher mortality.[9]

What you have, says Joseph Mendelson, legal director of the Center for Food Safety, is "Darwin on his head. You have a selective advantage to the genetically engineered fish, as far as reproduction, but their offspring are dying. . . . Scientists found that putting 60 genetically engineered fish into a population of 60,000 native fish could render the entire species extinct in as little as forty years."[10]

Standard salmon weigh about 8 ounces at the age of 18 months. But scientists have now genetically engineered salmon that grow so fast that by 18 months they weigh 7 pounds. Many scientists say that if these genetically engineered salmon were to escape, populations of wild fish could be wiped out by breeding with them. Edwin Rhodes, aquaculture coordinator of the National Marine Fisheries Service, says, "We have to have absolute certainty that transgenic fish do not interact with wild stocks."[11]

But the enclosures in which farmed salmon are usually kept are net pens, and they are notorious for being torn by waves or by hungry wild fish.

How often do farmed salmon escape? Routinely, sometimes by the tens of thousands. Almost 1 million farmed salmon escape annually in Norway alone. In fact, in some parts of Norway today, there are five times as many escaped farmed salmon living in the wild as there are wild salmon.[12]

Meanwhile, one company that had engineered Chinook salmon that could grow up to 550 pounds was forced to suspend its research after leaked secret papers revealed that deformed heads and other severe abnormalities had occurred during the breeding program.[13]

Frankenfoods

Our situation today reminds me of the birth of the nuclear era, another time when humanity stood at the threshold of a new technology. When nuclear power was first introduced, there was tremendous excitement about its potential. The Monsanto Corporation, always thinking big, proposed a plutonium-powered coffeepot that would boil water for 100 years without refueling.[14]

Enraptured with the possibilities, we believed that nuclear energy was going to give us "unlimited energy" that was "too cheap to meter." But of course, that's not what happened. Instead, it has given us radioactive waste too toxic to dispose of, and too long-lived to store safely. If you take into account the long-term environmental costs, most of them not yet paid, it's given us energy too expensive to comprehend.

If we could do it over again, knowing what we know now, we would surely not allow our excitement about the possibilities of "the peaceful atom" to lead us to leap blindly ahead. If we could do it over again, knowing what we have learned, we would certainly be far more cautious.

Our challenge today with genetic engineering may be even more profound, because this technology acts on the blueprint of life itself. Medical biotechnology is one story, because it intentionally contains its creations; but agricultural biotechnology is something very different, because it intentionally releases its creations into the natural world. As new living organisms, bacteria, and viruses are released into the environment, they do things that even nuclear contamination cannot do. They reproduce, migrate, and mutate. They transfer their new characteristics to other organisms.

In the tightly controlled laboratories of medicine, scientists splicing genes and altering DNA may well find cures for dreaded diseases. But what holds so much promise under the totally regulated conditions of medical research presents entirely different implications in the open fields of the world's farms. Medical research advances through trial and error, and mistakes bring new insights and understanding. But when it comes to genetically altered life forms, once a mistake is made and released into the environment, there is no telling the damage it may do, damage that may then continue to reproduce and exist virtually forever.

The story of Frankenstein has occupied a prominent place in the imaginations and dreams of our culture for more than 100 years. It is the story of a mad scientist, infused with his own excitement, working in his laboratory to create a new life form, only to have it turn on him and on all humanity. Has the Frankenstein story lived so powerfully in our culture because it had a message for us, a warning that if we become too arrogant and too enthralled with our own scientific prowess, our own creations may be our undoing?

Our recent experiences, not only with nuclear power but also with CFCs (chlorofluorocarbon chemicals that destroy the ozone layer) strongly indicate the need for caution. But genetic engineering, possibly the most powerful technology humans have ever discovered, is now being deployed at a breakneck speed by the very same corporations that, historically, have produced one large-scale calamity after another.[15]

When Rachel Carson launched the environmental movement in the United States by publishing her classic book, *Silent Spring*, Monsanto responded by taking out full-page ads ridiculing her conclusions, attacking her integrity, and implying that failure to use pesticides would cause a plague of insects that would devastate the world. As it happened, we've taken Monsanto's route and built our entire agriculture around agro-chemicals and pesticides, with the result that the pests have developed resistance to the chemicals. Now, even as we assault our farmland with millions of pounds of poisons annually, bugs are eating as large a share of the world's food crops as they did in medieval times.[16]

Monsanto is also the company that brought us Agent Orange and PCBs, and told us repeatedly, before they were banned, that each was safe. Today, Monsanto still produces many pesticides that are banned in North America for export to countries whose laws are not as strict as ours. There they are used on fruits and vegetables, many of which are then, in a circle of poison, sold to the United States to be consumed by unsuspecting consumers. All non-organic fruits and vegetables from tropical countries such as Mexico are likely today to be carrying residues of pesticides that are banned, but are nevertheless manufactured, in the United States.

Monsanto has been convicted in U.S. courts of at least four major offenses, including neglect and widespread dissemination of misinformation and a $108 million liability finding in the case of the leukemia death of a Texas employee. The EPA ranks Monsanto's factories as among the largest generators of toxic emissions in the country.[17]

This is the company that is talking about consolidating, and controlling, the entire food chain. This is the company in whose hands, with barely a trace of governmental oversight, we are placing what may be the most awesome technology human beings have ever known.

Is THAT SO?

"Monsanto should not have to vouchsafe the safety of biotech food. Our interest is in selling as much of it as possible. Assuring its safety is the FDA's job."
—Phil Angell, Monsanto's Director of Corporate Communications,
New York Times, 1999[18]

"Ultimately, it is the food producer who is responsible for assuring safety."
—FDA Federal Register, Statement of Policy:
Foods Derived from New Plant Varieties

Pesticides in Every Cell

In 2000, what Monsanto calls "insect-resistant" crops made up roughly a quarter of the nearly 100 million acres planted in transgenics worldwide. (The other three-quarters of worldwide acreage were planted in herbicide-resistant crops, primarily Monsanto's Roundup Ready varieties.)[19]

Insect-resistant crops contain a gene from a naturally occurring soil organism, *Bacillus thuringiensis* (commonly known as Bt). By transferring the gene responsible for making Bt—a natural pesticide that kills many kinds of leaf-eating caterpillars—into corn and cotton, Monsanto and other companies have produced crops that are toxic to the European corn borer and the cotton bollworm. Every cell of every plant contains the Bt gene and produces the Bt toxin. Caterpillars that nibble, die.

But there's a problem. For many decades, Bt has played a crucial role in organic farming and other low-input sustainable farming practices. Farmers who have wanted to minimize their use of chemicals have relied on an occasional dusting of Bt to prevent a crop from being overrun with leaf-eating caterpillars. Because Bt has been used judiciously, insects have not developed resistance. But crops that have been genetically engineered to generate the Bt toxin produce it constantly, and in every cell. This means that insects are continually exposed to the toxin and are under constant pressure to develop resistance. When insects eat any part of these plants, the only insects that can survive are those that have developed resistance. Dow Chemical scientists, who have created their own line of Bt-containing crops, said in 1998 that Bt would lose its usefulness within 10 years, because so many insects would become resistant to the toxin.[20]

What will occur is entirely predictable and indisputable. Once insects become resistant, naturally occurring Bt will no longer be useful in organic farming. Genetically engineered Bt crops will destroy the usefulness of the natural pesticide that has for decades been a foundation of organic farming and a mainstay of other forms of low-pesticide farming.[21]

In 1999, the International Federation of Organic Agricultural Movements joined with the Center for Food Safety and Greenpeace to file a lawsuit charging that the EPA, in approving genetically engineered Bt cotton, corn, and potatoes, was permitting the "wanton destruction . . . of the worlds' most important biological pesticide."[22]

In an effort to slow the development of insect resistance, the EPA now requires farmers to surround their genetically engineered crops with non–Bt protected crops in what are called "refuge areas." Here some insects can safely feed without developing resistance. It is hoped that these insects will breed with those that have become Bt resistant, thereby diluting the evolved resistance. But Bt resistance is apparently a dominant trait, so these anti-resistance measures are, unfortunately, doomed to fail.

What's the value of these crops? In 1999, Bob Shapiro, Monsanto's CEO, said that cotton growers planting the company's insect-resistant variety of cotton used 80 percent fewer pesticides.[23] If this were as it seems, it would be a boon to our imperiled ecosystems and to humanity.

But, alas, there's more to the story. The plants Monsanto calls "insect-resistant" are actually "insecticide-producing." And the toxins in Bt plants are present in a more active form than naturally occurring Bt, so they harm a wider range of insects. Lacewings, for example, are beneficial insects that prey on crop pests. A 1998 Swiss study found that when lacewings were fed corn borers raised on Bt corn, many of the lacewings died.[24]

Ladybugs (also called ladybirds, lady beetles, and lady flies) are another beneficial insect. Like lacewings, they help control mosquitoes, and they are crucial to keeping aphid populations in check. But in 1997 a Scottish study reported in the *New Scientist* that when ladybugs were fed aphids that had been eating potatoes genetically engineered to be insect-resistant by incorporating the Bt gene, the ladybugs laid fewer eggs and lived only half as long.[25] By essentially breeding Bt resistant pests, and killing off those pests' natural predators, we are potentially doing incalculable harm to the future of agriculture.

Then there are bees. It's been calculated that in the state of New York, on a summer day, bees pollinate more than a trillion flowers. But one study found that when bees were exposed to the more active genetically engineered form of Bt, their ability to distinguish the different smells of flowers was impaired.[26]

You may have heard about the Monarch butterflies. In 1999, the scientific journal *Nature* published a study finding that the pollen from Bt corn killed the caterpillars of the Monarch butterfly. These creatures feed on milkweed, which often grows alongside and among corn. When pollen from Bt corn was scattered onto milkweed leaves, simulating the corn pollen that blows over milkweed plants every summer, the Monarch caterpillars that ate those leaves died.[27]

In 2000, the worldwide acreage planted in crops containing the Bt toxin was greater than the entire world's organic acreage. But as Monsanto bragged publicly about the benefits of these crops, still other pieces of the story were unfolding.

Naturally occurring forms of Bt are degraded by soil microbes, but the more active forms produced in Bt crops are far more hardy and remain in soil much longer, with much greater capacity to kill insects.[28] As farmers incorporate plant material from genetically engineered Bt crops into the ground after harvests, these toxins accumulate, posing serious dangers to the myriad forms of bacteria, fungi, and other micro-organisms that make up healthy soil ecosystems. We have yet to see what will happen as unprecedented quantities of this more active form of Bt build up in soils.

There's more. When corn and other food crops are genetically altered to incorporate the Bt toxin into their cells, those Bt toxins also wind up in our food supply. Do we have any idea what effect these toxins and gene products will have on the bacteria and other organisms (microflora) that live in the human digestive tract? Or what the effects on humans will be of the concentrated amounts of Bt that will accumulate in meat and dairy products high on the food chain?

The Bt toxin—in the form in which it naturally occurs in the bacteria that produce it—is considered relatively safe for humans. When produced by bacteria, the toxin exists in a "protoxic" form, which becomes dangerous to insects only after it has been shortened, or "activated," in the insect's digestive system. In marked contrast, however, some genetically engineered crops produce the toxin in its activated form.[29] Humans have little experience with exposure to this form of the toxin, which has up until now only existed inside the digestive systems of certain insects.

Furthermore, people eating genetically engineered Bt crops are exposed to amounts of the Bt toxin that are completely unprecedented. In the past, no one has ingested any form of the Bt toxin in large quantities.

But when the Bt toxin is incorporated into our common foods, we are exposed with every bite we eat. A pesticide engineered into every cell of a food source cannot simply be washed off before a meal.

When Monsanto's Bob Shapiro speaks about the marvels of Bt cotton, there is one other thing he doesn't mention. I can understand why he'd want to keep silent about it, because it raises serious concerns about everything he and his company stand for and are doing.

There is a very real risk that crops engineered to produce their own pesticide, such as Monsanto's Bt corn and cotton, will spread their genes into the plants of the surrounding fields or woods. This would cause something I am sure Bob Shapiro would never want to see—what Worldwatch Institute's Ed Ayres has called "one of the true nightmares of technology gone haywire—toxic chemicals that reproduce."[30]

We often think of insects as nuisances and believe that we'd be better off if they did not exist. But like the fungi in soil that assist plants in taking up nutrients, and like the bacteria in our own intestines that produce B vitamins, insects have a role to play in the greater scheme of things. If Bt crops weaken the populations of ladybugs and Monarch butterflies, lacewings, and bees, and damage innumerable other insects and microorganisms, we will have paid an incredible price for factory farms to have cheap corn for feeding livestock and for agribusiness hiring fewer employees to tend its cotton fields.

Each time the fabric of life becomes more unraveled, things become more tenuous for human life. Biosphere II, the $200 million experiment in the Arizona desert in which eight people were sealed inside a giant bubble, failed primarily because of problems in the mix of soil organisms, bacteria, and other microbes. The environment in the bubble of Biosphere II became increasingly untenable for human life.

Is it conceivable that in our haste to grow genetically engineered foods, we will cause a much larger experiment, Biosphere I, otherwise known as planet Earth, to become likewise jeopardized in its ability to sustain human life?

One thing's for sure. You'd have a hard time convincing the dead and dying Monarch butterflies, or the lacewings or the ladybugs, that crops genetically engineered to carry the Bt toxin are substantially equivalent to traditional varieties.

At the Grocery Store and Restaurant

Due to the lack of labeling, very few Americans realize how many of the foods for sale in U.S. grocery stores today contain genetically engineered ingredients. When I first learned that two-thirds of the foods sold in U.S. supermarkets now include genetically modified substances, I was flabbergasted.[31] When I first heard this high figure, I thought it must be a gross exaggeration. But I have since learned that it is all too true.

There are three reasons that the amount is so great and that the public has virtually no idea this is happening. The first is that more than half of the U.S. soybean crop and one-third of the U.S. corn crop are genetically engineered.[32] The second is that soy and corn are widely disseminated in processed foods. (Soy oil accounts for 80 percent of the vegetable oil consumed in the United States,[33] and various forms of corn syrup are the most widely used sweeteners.) And the third reason is that genetically altered foods are not labeled in the United States, so consumers have been eating increasing amounts of genetically engineered ingredients without even knowing it.

If salt is added to a bag of corn chips, for example, there must be a label to disclose that salt has been added. The label tells exactly how much sodium is in the product, permitting shoppers to make informed choices. But there is no requirement for the package to reveal whether the corn, itself, has been genetically engineered.

In 2001, the FDA put forth a new policy that did nothing to remedy this situation. In fact, under the new policy, not a single producer of genetically engineered foods would have to reveal that their products are genetically engineered. Instead, the agency created a "GE Free" voluntary labeling scheme which punishes food producers who do not use genetic engineering, by putting the burden on them to certify, test, and label their foods as "GE Free." Many companies, of course, cannot afford to undergo the considerable time, expense, and liability of testing, certifying, and labeling their foods as "GE Free."

How did FDA officials explain the agency's opposition to mandatory labeling of genetically engineered foods? Labeling, they said, was potentially misleading to consumers, since it might suggest that there was a reason for concern.

At the present time in the United States, the only sure way to avoid eating genetically engineered food is to eat organically grown food. No organically grown food is made from transgenic crops. But since it is not possible for most of us to eat only organic foods, the next best thing is to read labels carefully and to bear in mind which foods are most likely to contain genetically altered substances. Here's what to watch out for . . .

Products Made from Plants

- *Soybeans:* There are more acres of genetically engineered soybeans being grown than any other transgenic crop. And many processed and manufactured foods use ingredients that contain soybeans. You have to read labels carefully. Watch for soy flour, soy oil, lecithin (used as an emulsifier and stabilizer), soy protein isolates, and concentrates. Watch also for textured vegetable protein (TVP), any unidentified vegetable oil, and just about every form of margarine. The only soy products you can be sure are free from genetically modified substances are those made from organic soybeans, or ones that specifically say "GMO-free," or "Non-GMO."

- *Corn:* Corn accounts for the second largest transgenic acreage. Watch out for corn flour, corn starch, corn oil, corn sweeteners (including corn syrup, or high-fructose corn syrup). Many processed food products are made with corn ingredients. As with soy, only if such foods say "Organic," or "GMO-free," or "Non-GMO" can you be sure they do not contain genetically engineered ingredients.

- *Canola oil:* Most of the canola oil consumed in the United States comes from Canada (indeed, the *can-* in canola derives from the first three letters of *Canada*). Since much of Canada's canola (also called rapeseed) crop is genetically engineered,[34] and seeds from both kinds of plants are mixed together, it's almost certain that any product containing canola oil includes genetically altered substances, unless it's labeled GMO-free. The exceptions are organic canola oil, and a specialty product called "Super Canola," which, using traditional breeding methods, was developed to tolerate heat so that it can be used for frying without smoking up the kitchen.

- *Potatoes:* As of 2001, the only genetically engineered potato commercially available was the Burbank Russet, but you still have to look out for potato starch and potato flour.

- *Papaya:* Most non-organic papayas grown in Hawaii are genetically engineered.

- *Cottonseed oil:* Since more than half the U.S. cotton crop is transgenic, products containing cottonseed oil are almost certain to include genetically altered substances.

- *Squash:* Some crookneck squash and zucchini now in stores have been genetically altered.

- *Other foods:* There are many other varieties of genetically engineered plant foods that are under development. For a brand-name shopping guide to non-transgenic foods, visit *www.safe-food.org.*

WHAT WE KNOW

Global transgenic acreage accounted for, in 2000, by soybeans: 54 percent[35]

Global transgenic acreage accounted for, in 2000, by corn: 28 percent[36]

Global transgenic acreage accounted for, in 2000, by cotton: 9 percent[37]

Global transgenic acreage accounted for, in 2000, by canola: 9 percent[38]

Crop that Monsanto is hoping to put into large-scale production in 2003 or 2004: Roundup Ready wheat

Products Made from Animals

Ninety-five percent of the soy meal grown in the United States, and almost that high a percentage of corn, are used as livestock feed. The result is that virtually every non-organic meat, poultry, dairy, or egg product in the United States today contains genetically engineered substances.[39] Feedlots and factory farms in the southern United States seasonally add cotton silage to animal feed, which further increases the animals' exposure.

Roundup has been shown to build up in the hulls of soybeans, and the hulls are used as animal feed, so meat eaters in the United States today also have increased exposure to the herbicide in the animal products they consume.[40] Dr. Marc Lappé, the author of numerous landmark studies on the nutritional realities of genetically engineered soybeans, writes,

> "Use of herbicide tolerant crops virtually guarantees that beef, poultry and pork will have higher contamination levels of selected pesticides than such livestock had previously. Special tolerances for Roundup herbicide residues in silage were instituted to increase the utility of Roundup Ready soybeans in animal feed crops."[41]

Of the millions of acres of soybeans planted in the United States in 2000, more than half were planted in Roundup Ready soybeans. Feedlots and factory farmers were already buying most of these beans for animal feed. In the future, the consumer demand for non-GMO soy products will almost certainly increase, and the price of genetically engineered soy and corn will predictably drop to a lower tier than the price for traditional varieties. If that happens, we can predict that feedlots and factory farms will increase their use of genetically engineered soybeans and corn to cut costs, making meat and other animal products an increasing risk.

Indeed, if mandatory labeling were to become a reality, the direct human consumption of genetically engineered soybeans and corn would diminish dramatically, but people consuming U.S. meat, poultry, dairy, and egg products would still be unknowingly ingesting ever-increasing concentrations of genetically modified substances. Labeling would not protect people consuming meat and dairy products unless these products were also labeled with information about how the animals were fed.

In the United Kingdom, McDonald's has pledged not to use meat from animals fed genetically engineered food.[42] But in the United States, the meat industry has done quite the opposite. In late 2000, Dan Murphy, the editor of *Meat Marketing and Technology*, wrote an essay that showed just how ardently pro-biotechnology the U.S. meat industry has become and how blatantly hostile toward those who would question it:

"Most [U.S. meat] industry executives I've talked with will take a pretty hard-line stance against the anti-biotechnology activists. Who can blame them? The 'biotech is bad' position is based not on thoughtful, rational deliberation but on a visceral loathing of all things corporate and technological. . . . [The anti-genetic engineering movement is driven] by activists who've found a reason to live in fighting what they see as a psychological replacement for the terror we once felt about the atomic bomb."[43]

Meanwhile with about 25 percent of U.S. dairy products coming from cows injected with rBGH, most commercial milk, ice cream, yogurt, butter, and cheese sold in the United States now contains some quantity of genetically altered material.

It's not just the feed the animals are given that's transgenic. In some cases, the animals themselves are being genetically engineered. The goal is to produce cattle, pigs, and chickens that are "better suited" to the overcrowded and unsanitary conditions of factory farming. Agribusiness dreams of pigs as large as hippopotamuses but as docile as slugs, and featherless chickens that won't need to be plucked and never peck.

Human genes have been transplanted into pigs, but with little publicity, owing to concern about "public acceptance" of the idea. The pigs developed severe arthritis, had spinal deformities, and most were blind.[44]

This may seem like the stuff of horror movies, but it is rapidly becoming reality. Andy Kimbrell, Director of the International Center for Technology Assessment in Washington, D.C., explains what has, in fact, already happened.

"The USDA has, without telling the public, been allowing into slaughterhouses and into the food chain, animals that have been involved in experiments making them transgenic. These are animals that have foreign genes in every one of their cells, and that have been part of experiments by major . . . corporations. . . . These are animals with human genes; these are animals that have a variety of viruses in them. They did this without consulting Congress. They did this without making it public. These animals have been in the food chain now since 1995."[45]

If this is true, people eating meats and meat products in the United States today are not only exposing themselves without their knowledge or consent to higher than ever herbicide residues and genetically engineered substances. They may also be eating parts of animals that have had human genes engineered into their DNA.

Kimbrell, like many who share his concerns, is outraged:

> "We didn't get to vote on whether to take human genes and put them in animals, which they're doing through genetic engineering. . . . Do we really want unlimited genetic engineering of humans, of animals, of plants? Do we really want our generation and the generations to come after us to view the entire animal kingdom as so many machines to be reprogrammed, cloned, and patented?"[46]

chapter 19

The Turning of the Tide

A t the same time that genetically engineered food has flashed on the scene, another very different approach to food and farming has been developing as a major force in our world and our kitchens. Slowly and steadily, with the patience and persistence of a plant growing through the cycle of the seasons, the organic farming movement has been gaining strength. In recent years, organic agriculture has emerged as a major force in world food production.

> "Driven by rising consumer demand and growing dissatisfaction with conventional farming practices, the organic agriculture industry is soaring." (Worldwatch Institute, 2000)[1]

By the turn of the millennium, more than 17 million acres worldwide were planted with organic foods. Though this was less than a fifth of the area planted with transgenics, the number of acres dedicated to organic farming was 10 times what it had been only 10 years previously. And the market for organic food had swelled to $22 billion annually.[2]

Leading the global organic explosion was the European Union, where a phenomenal 35-fold expansion in organic acreage took place in the last 15 years of the twentieth century. In 1999, 3 percent of the European Union's total agricultural acreage, amounting to 10 million acres, was organic. In some countries, notably Sweden, Finland, Switzerland, and Italy, the organic acreage was even higher, running between 5 and 10 percent of total agricultural land. In Austria, fully 13 percent of the farmland was organic, and in some Austrian provinces the share was as high as 50 percent. In only the last four years of the twentieth century, the United Kingdom's organic area surged tenfold.[3]

At the turn of the millennium, Worldwatch Institute predicted that by 2010, 30 percent of the total farmed area in the European Union would be organic.[4]

Even Uganda was in on the organic expansion. In 1999, this one tiny African country was producing 10 percent of the world's organic cotton. And in Egypt, where tea drinking is a daily ritual, the country's best-selling brand had become Sekem's certified organic tea.[5]

In Canada, organic agriculture was also rising rapidly, though on a percentage basis it remained behind the standards set by many other countries. In 1999, 1.3 percent of Canada's cropland was organic. In the United States, organic acreage was also increasing rapidly, though it lagged even further behind international standards, amounting in 1999 to only 0.2 percent of the nation's overall cropland.[6]

Yet even with the United States and Canada running at the rear of the pack, retail sales of organic produce and products in North America were growing steadily at an impressive 20 percent a year, and by 1999 total organic sales were estimated at $10 billion.[7]

Why, you might wonder, has organic agriculture remained relatively rare in the United States, compared to other industrialized countries? For the same reason genetic engineering has become so big so fast—government support, or in the case of organics, the lack of it. In the 1990s, less than one-tenth of 1 percent of USDA research projects had any relevance to organic agriculture.

In fact, in 1997, the USDA attempted to set federal organic standards that would have completely destroyed the organic industry by allowing genetically engineered foods, as well as foods that had been irradiated and grown with heavy metal-laden sewage sludge, to be classified as organic. Consumers would have lost all trust in the organic label. The

Department of Agriculture had every intention of putting this heavily diluted standard into practice, even though it betrayed the organic tradition, offended the consumers who value organic food, and violated the recommendations of the Organic Standards Board that had been established by Congress to come up with a definition of *organic* for nationwide use.

But in one of the great moments in the history of citizen protest in the United States, consumers rose up and made their voices heard. They sent in postcards, they commented directly on the USDA's Web page, they wrote long and specific letters, they called their congressional representatives and asked for their support, and they wrote President Clinton. Natural foods companies and health food stores created flyers, posters, advertisements, Web sites, and letters. Messages were printed on cartons, and people were educated in a host of other ways. By the time the smoke cleared, the USDA had received more than 275,000 comments, virtually all of them vehemently opposing the agency's plan. As a direct consequence, the proposed standards, with the watered-down definition of *organic* were scuttled, and the path was forged for a new, legitimate, national organic standard.

This was crucial, because it was the establishment of a common European Union definition for *organic* in 1993 that had spurred the phenomenal growth of organics in Europe in subsequent years.[8] Once it was established, consumer awareness and trust in organics grew swiftly, and the door was opened for additional support, including subsidies in the early years of conversion and research on organic farming methods at agricultural universities.

On December 20, 2000, the USDA released the United States' first official organic standards. The regulations, which formally went into effect on February 19, 2001, were a major victory for the organic movement. The agrochemical and genetic engineering industries had fought them bitterly, and sought until the last moment to have a disclaimer on all organic labels saying that such food was no safer and no more nutritious than conventional food. But in the end the USDA refused their demands. Katherine DiMatteo, Executive Director of the Organic Trade Association, commented, "The USDA has delivered a strict organic standard that is a great boost to the organic industry."[9]

Keeping a Good Sense of Humus

Not everyone, however, has been pleased to see organic agriculture thriving in the United States. In 2000, the ABC television show *20/20* twice aired a program hosted by John Stossel that was harshly critical of organic foods. Relying heavily on the opinions of author Dennis Avery, the program did not mention that the title of Avery's most recent book was *Saving the Planet with Pesticides and Plastic*, nor that Avery's current employer was the Hudson Institute, an organization funded in part by chemical and genetic engineering companies including Monsanto, AgrEvo, Novartis, Dow, and Zeneca.

Avery denies that there is any link between pesticides and cancer or other illnesses. But organic food, he says, can kill you. According to Avery, "People who eat organic and natural foods are eight times as likely as the rest of the population to be attacked by a new strain of E. coli bacteria." This happens, he says, because organic food is grown with animal manure, a known carrier of the deadly microbe. How does he back this up? He says his data comes from Dr. Paul Mead, an epidemiologist at the Centers for Disease Control and Prevention (CDC).[10]

Mead, however, says nothing could be further from the truth. In fact, Mead says he has explicitly told Avery that CDC data *don't support* Avery's allegations.[11]

Additionally, Robert Tauxe, M.D., chief of the food-borne disease branch of the CDC, says that Avery's claims are "absolutely not true."[12]

The *20/20* program told the public that ABC tests had found no pesticide residues in either conventional or organic produce. But the scientists that performed the tests for ABC, Drs. Michael Doyle and Lester Crawford, told the *New York Times* that they had not tested any produce for pesticides on ABC's behalf. On the contrary, Dr. Crawford said he had tested only chickens, and had actually found pesticide residues on the conventional poultry but *not* on the organic poultry.[13]

The *20/20* program mentioned a young girl who became ill after eating lettuce that had been contaminated from sewage. The viewing public received the impression, because of the order of presentation, that the lettuce was organically grown. But in fact organic certification practices specifically prohibit the use of sewage sludge. It is commercial growers, not organic farmers, who can, and do, use sewage sludge to amend the soil.

John Stossel, co-anchor of ABC's *20/20*, and the host of the program that attacked organic food, publicly apologized on a subsequent episode of the national television show for falsifying evidence in the report and relying on fabricated laboratory tests.[14] He was reprimanded by ABC, and the show's producer was suspended for a month. Many "accuracy in journalism" groups said Stossel should have been fired.

What had been Stossel's motive? Unfortunately, his shows have often been slanted in favor of the chemical industry, food irradiation, and large-scale agribusiness, and he has had a long and troubling history of sacrificing accuracy to promote his far right-wing personal ideology. "I have come to believe that markets are magical and the best protectors of consumers," he once declared. "It is my job to explain the beauties of the free market."[15] Unfortunately, this enthusiasm for laissez-faire capitalism has too often led Stossel to neglect his job as a journalist—seeking truth and reporting it.[16] According to Jeff Cohen, the director of Fairness and Accuracy in Reporting (FAIR), "Stossel's clearly one of the most biased reporters in the business."

Even with Stossel's public apology, many who had seen the original program were left confused, with the mistaken idea that since organic farmers favor manure over agrochemicals, organic produce might carry a heightened risk of E. coli infection. Avery and Stossel had said precisely that on the program. But in fact both organic and conventional farms use manure. The difference is that organic farmers are not allowed, by organic certification standards, to use raw manure. They must first compost it, or else apply it to the soil long enough in advance of harvest so that any pathogenic microbes, including E. coli 0157:H7, are rendered harmless by the many soil organisms that can be found in the fertile soil of an organic farm. Conventional farmers, on the other hand, can apply raw, uncomposted manure far closer to the day of harvest.[17]

Ironically, according to USDA research, it is the commercial meat industry's practice of keeping cattle in feedlots and feeding them grain (not their natural diet) that is responsible for the heightened prevalence of E. coli 0157:H7 bacteria. When cattle are grain-fed, their intestinal tracts become far more acidic, which favors the generation of pathogenic E. coli bacteria. This does not happen when cattle are allowed to graze and eat hay, as they are in organic production. In fact, several months after the 20/20 program aired, the Food and Agriculture Organization (FAO) of the United Nations issued a report completely repudiating Avery and Stossel's statements that organic food is more apt to cause E. coli infections. "Cows mainly fed with hay generate less than 1 percent of the E. coli (compared to) grain-fed animals," said the report. "It can be concluded that organic farming potentially reduces the risk of E. coli infection."[18]

Do pesticides help protect against E. coli 0157:H7 and other pathogens? Do the agrochemicals designed to kill insects and weeds also kill pathogenic bacteria? No. In fact, according to research carried out at the University of Manitoba in Winnipeg, pesticide sprays actually encourage life-threatening bacteria to grow on crops. "Numbers (of E. coli 0157:H7) could increase one-thousandfold," says lead researcher Greg Blank, who found that the life-threatening microbes flourished in many pesticides.[19]

The advantages of organic agriculture are many, including reduced soil erosion, greatly improved soil health, far less contribution to global warming, and dramatically reduced water pollution. And there are nutritional advantages, too, according to a study published in the *Journal of Applied Nutrition* that analyzed the mineral content of organically and conventionally grown apples, potatoes, pears, wheat, and sweet corn over a two-year period. . .

What we know

Amount of minerals in organic food compared to conventional food:[20]

Calcium:	63 percent higher
Chromium:	78 percent higher
Iodine:	73 percent higher
Iron:	59 percent higher
Magnesium:	138 percent higher
Potassium:	125 percent higher
Selenium:	390 percent higher
Zinc:	60 percent higher

In dramatic contrast to genetic engineering, organic farming is an expression of what Aldo Leopold called "a land ethic," extending the concept of community to include all the species of life with which we share the planet. It upholds the understanding that, as Leopold put it, "a thing is right when it tends to preserve the integrity, stability, and beauty of the biotic community. It is wrong when it tends otherwise. . . . When we see the land as a community to which we belong, we may begin to use it with love and respect."

The difference is profound. In one case, the natural world is seen as a collection of resources for us to exploit. In the other, the natural world is affirmed as a living community to which we belong and to which we owe our lives. In one case, we seek our power from dominating nature, forcing it to divulge its secrets and conform to our will. In the other, our power comes from our ability to respond to and nurture life, to cooperate with, care for, and cherish natural systems. It's the difference between poisoning our food and water with pesticides and developing a sustainable and healthy agriculture based on fertile living soil. It's the difference between playing genetic roulette and developing truly healthier plant varieties through careful research and testing.

One approach kills unwanted insects with pesticides, meanwhile also killing beneficial insects and birds and provoking pests to develop resistance to the poisons so that ever more must be used. The other supports a healthy ecosystem in which birds thrive, because no insect ever develops resistance to a bird.

Earl Butz, the former secretary of agriculture, used to say that before the United States could consider organic farming, it would have to decide which 50 or 60 million Americans were going to be chosen to starve. His attitude exemplified the stance that government and agribusiness have taken in the past—that organic farming is a luxury that cannot provide enough food for our people.

But many studies have found yields from organic production to be comparable to conventional systems, especially over the long term. In fact, a recent study of grain and soybean production in the American Midwest found that organic systems were actually more profitable than conventional systems, not even counting the higher price organic food typically fetches. The reason was that organic farms growing grains and soybeans had lower input costs and greater yield stability in bad weather years.

In 1995, the Rodale Institute completed the first 14 years of extensive trials comparing organic versus chemical farming of corn. "Our results," the Institute said, "from the first 14 years show that comparable yields can be obtained without the use of chemical pesticides or fertilizers." In fact, the organic fields did better than the conventional ones during drought years.[21]

One of the most complete research projects ever undertaken to assess the feasibility of organic agriculture was conducted by the Center for the Study of Biological Systems at Washington University in St. Louis—the same city, ironically, where Monsanto is headquartered. The study matched a group of farms with similar soil conditions, crops, and acreage, half of which used the chemical approach, while half went organic. At the end of the study, the center's director concluded, "A five year average shows that the organic farms yielded, in dollars per acre, exactly the same returns. In terms of yield, the organic farms were down about 10 percent. The reason why the economics came out is that the savings in chemicals made up for the difference."[22]

You might think that a 10 percent decrease in yield would mean food shortages. But the vast majority of American agriculture doesn't grow food for people. It grows food for animals, whose flesh, milk, and eggs we then consume. With even a modest reduction in meat consumption, we would be able to convert our entire nation's agriculture to organic, thus sparing ourselves, our environment, and future generations the dangers of pesticides and genetic engineering, and feeding ourselves far healthier food in the bargain.

The Turning of the Tide

The citizen revolt that took place in the United States in the late 1990s, when the USDA tried to establish a definition of *organic* that would have included genetically modified organisms, irradiated food, and food grown with toxic sewage sludge, changed the course of American agriculture. But even more powerful, and even more historic, has been the uprising that has been taking place globally against genetically engineered food.

When Monsanto initiated a major advertising campaign to "encourage a positive understanding of biotechnology," the corporation hired

Stanley Greenburg, former polling advisor to Bill Clinton and Tony Blair, to advise the company on the progress of its efforts to develop public acceptance for genetic engineering. Some months later, Greenburg told Monsanto that the ad campaign "was, for the most part, overwhelmed by the society-wide collapse of support for genetic engineering in foods." There were, Greenburg said, "large forces at work that are making public acceptance problematic."[23]

What are these "large forces"? They are people, like you and me — concerned individuals, church groups, environmental groups, public health organizations, scientists, farmers, consumer organizations, chefs, food writers, and other citizens of planet Earth. One of Monsanto's executives complained, "These people work for nothing — How can you stop that?"[24]

Some have been angry. In Great Britain, India, and Ireland, farmer-led uprisings have burned and destroyed Monsanto's test plots. In India, Monsanto has had to grow genetically modified plants in greenhouses constructed of bullet-proof plastic.[25] In the southern Indian state of Karnataka, an organization of farmers has launched a campaign called "Operation Cremate Monsanto," uprooting and burning field trials of genetically engineered crops.[26]

The uprising has been spreading everywhere. In France, a band of 120 farmers broke into a storage facility of the biotech company Novartis and destroyed 30 tons of genetically modified corn. In the United States, Germany, and the Netherlands, genetically modified crops have been destroyed by angry citizens. Genetically engineered fields have been torched in New Zealand, Australia, Brazil, and Greece. (These actions have been condemned as violent, but it's important to note that no person has ever been harmed.)

In 1999, the seven largest grocery chains in six European countries (Tesco, Safeway, Sainsbury's, Iceland, Marks & Spencer, the Co-op, and Waitrose) made a public commitment to go "GMO (genetically modified organisms) free" and began contracting with growers to provide GM-free corn, potatoes, soybeans, and wheat. Like dominoes falling, other food companies followed. Days later, Unilever, a huge transnational corporation involved in every aspect of food distribution, and a company that had been one of the most aggressive supporters of genetic engineering, threw in the towel and joined the GM-free consortium.

The next day, the Swiss firm Nestlé followed suit. And the following day, another enormous food producer, Cadbury-Schweppes, joined the ranks of the GM-free.[27]

A spokesperson for the Tesco chain of supermarkets in England said, "We will remove GM ingredients where we can and label where we can't. In the short and medium term, I expect the number of products containing GM ingredients to decline steadily, quite possibly to zero."[28]

Meanwhile, Europe's largest bank, Deutsche Bank, was recommending that investors sell all holdings in companies involved in genetic engineering, declaring that "GMOs Are Dead." The bank's report predicted a two-tiered commodity market, in which transgenic crops would be sold for far lower prices than traditional varieties. No sooner was the ink dry on the bank's prophecy than Archer Daniels Midland, one of the world's largest grain distributors, began paying farmers 18 cents less per bushel for genetically modified soybeans than for the traditional product.[30]

At the same time, Japan's two largest breweries, the Kirin Brewery Company and Sapporo Breweries, were announcing that they would not use gene-altered corn in their beer.[31] Food producers, beverage companies, and restaurants all over the world were going GMO-free.

While this was happening, thousands of organizations throughout the world, including the 115,000 physician-strong British Medical Association, were demanding a moratorium on all genetically engineered crops. In every nation, groups were adding their voices to the demand, including COAG, which represents 200,000 Spanish farmers.

The governor of Brazil's major soybean growing state (Rio Grande del Sul) declared the entire state a GMO-free zone. The Supreme Court of India banned the testing of GM crops. The governments of France, Italy, Denmark, Greece, and Luxembourg announced that they would block any attempt to approve new varieties of genetically engineered crops in the European Union. Japan, South Korea, Australia, and Mexico joined the European Community in requiring the mandatory labeling of genetically engineered food.

Trying to stem the tide, the biotech industry funded a survey and then announced, as loudly as they could, that "two-thirds to three-quarters of U.S. consumers are positive about food biotechnology." This was strange, since only a short time before a *Time* magazine poll had found

81 percent of Americans want genetically engineered foods to be labeled; and a poll of U.S. consumers by the Swiss drug firm Novartis had found more than 90 percent of the public want labeling.[32]

What accounted for the discrepancy? It was subsequently discovered that the poll that found Americans in favor of biotech had been loaded with language designed to bias the answers. Questions included "How likely would you be to buy a variety of produce, like tomatoes or potatoes, if it had been modified by biotechnology to taste better or fresher?" And, "How likely would you be to buy a variety of produce if it had been modified by biotechnology to be protected from insect damage and required fewer pesticides?" The survey, noted a communications professor from the University of Southern California, was "so biased with leading questions favoring positive responses that any results are meaningless." A professor from UCLA added that the questions "only talk about the food tasting better, being fresher, protecting food from insect damage, and providing benefits." The results would have been utterly different, he said, if other factors had been mentioned.[33]

Trying to overcome mounting problems with public acceptance, the industry began developing a second generation of genetically modified crops that would, they said, have health benefits, including oils that would make healthier margarines and shortenings, and vegetables with longer shelf lives. But some critics were pointing out that these same benefits can be achieved through conventional breeding methods.[34] And others, noting that no technological fix can substitute for a healthy diet, were saying that these new foods were more marketing gimmicks than genuine steps toward increased health.

Monsanto spoke of bananas containing vaccines as evidence that genetic engineering could hold the key to solving many of the world's most intractable health problems. But one critic, molecular biologist Dr. D. P. Witsky, wasn't impressed. "Vaccine-toting bananas sound great," she said, "until you peel back the image. How will the masses of poor and hungry people, those most vulnerable to infectious diseases, become suddenly able to afford these genetically prepared vaccine snacks? If these bananas look like other bananas, what is to prevent people from accidentally overdosing? What will prevent their genetic leakage into food banana crops? How will unsuspecting farmers and consumers be protected?"[35]

Faced with increasing public distrust, one industry executive came up with a bright idea. "Drop the term GMOs," he said enthusiastically, "and replace it with GIFTS—genetically improved foods through science."

The biotech industry was trying everything it could think of, but the tide was turning. A Canadian writer, Gwynne Dyer, described what was happening: "The strategy for the high-speed introduction (of genetically modified crops) throughout the world is shaping up as one of the great public-relations disasters of all time. Public suspicion outside North America is reaching crippling proportions, and the reason is not at all mysterious. It is because the biotech firms literally tried to shove the stuff down peoples' throats without giving them either choice or information."[36]

As the highly heralded success of agricultural biotechnology was floundering throughout the world, the impact finally reached the United States, home of Monsanto and the country that grows three-quarters of the world's transgenic crops. By 1999, the third-largest corn purveyor in the United States, A. E. Staley Co., of Decatur, Illinois, was declaring that it would no longer accept genetically modified corn varieties that were not approved by the European Union.[37] And even USDA Secretary Dan Glickman, long a fervent supporter of genetically modified foods, who prior to his appointment to President Clinton's cabinet had worked for the law firm that represented Monsanto, was now comparing agricultural biotechnology to another severely wounded industry—nuclear power.[38] As he left office in 2001, Glickman even began advising biotech companies to consider labeling genetically modified foods.[39]

With each passing month, public resistance continued to gain strength and stature. In 2000, the *Wall Street Journal* announced that investors were losing all confidence in agricultural biotechnology. "With the controversy over genetically modified foods spreading across the globe and taking a toll on the stocks of companies with agricultural-biotechnology businesses," said the daily chronicler of the business world, "it's hard to see those companies as a good investment, even in the long term."[40]

The *Journal* had a point. In 1996, the United States had sold $3 billion worth of corn and soybeans to Europe. But in the next few years, as the consumer backlash in Europe gained momentum, those exports shrank to $1 billion.[41] In 1998, 2 million tons of American corn were shipped to Europe, but only a year later the figure had plummeted to 137,000 tons.[42] It was hard to argue with a drop, in only one year, of more than 93 percent. Monsanto's stock, which sold for $50 a share in February 1999, had lost more than half of its value by the end of 2000, even though the Dow Jones increased in value by nearly 15 percent during the same period.

As a result of its debacle with agricultural biotechnology, Monsanto, far and away the world leader in genetically engineered crops, the company whose seeds were planted on more than four-fifths of the world's transgenic acreage, could no longer sustain itself as an independent company, and was taken over by Pharmacia, a New Jersey drug company.[43]

While this was happening, farmers in the United States were becoming increasingly worried about liability issues. A coalition of 30 U.S. farm groups, including the National Family Farm Coalition and the American Corn Growers Association, was warning American farmers that "inadequate testing of gene-altered seeds could make farmers vulnerable to massive liability" from damage caused by transgenic crops. And American soy farmers were filing a multibillion-dollar lawsuit against the biotech industry, alleging that companies such as Monsanto had "forced genetically modified seeds onto the market . . . without sufficient testing for safety to human health and the environment."[44]

Meanwhile, Aventis, the company that created a transgenic Bt corn variety named Starlink, was spending hundreds of millions of dollars trying to clean up the mess when 9 million bushels of the genetically engineered corn, deemed unfit for human consumption by the FDA, got mixed into the U.S. corn supply. Three hundred different kinds of taco shells, tortilla chips, and tostados had to be recalled from U.S. grocery stores. A major law firm filed a national class-action lawsuit against Aventis on behalf of all U.S. farmers.

By late 2000, even those consumers who had been assuming biotech companies knew what they were doing were losing faith. One-third of Americans were saying that U.S. farmers should not be allowed to grow gene-altered crops at all.[45]

Meanwhile, fast-food chains, including McDonald's and Burger King, were telling their suppliers they didn't want any more genetically altered potatoes.[46] A spokesperson for the J. M. Simplot Company of Boise, Idaho, a major potato supplier, was saying that "virtually all the (fast food) chains have told us they prefer to take non-genetically modified potatoes." Proctor and Gamble, maker of Pringle's potato chips, was phasing out genetically engineered potatoes. Frito-Lay, which markets Lay's and Ruffle's brands of potato chips, was telling its farmers not to plant genetically engineered potatoes.[47]

The message that consumers did not want to eat "frankenfoods" was getting to more and more food companies. Frito-Lay was telling its corn farmers to abandon genetically engineered varieties of corn for use in its Doritos, Tostitos, and Fritos.[48] Gerber was pledging to get all genetically altered ingredients out of its baby foods, doing so even though it is owned by Novartis, one of the world's largest biotech firms. Chains of natural food stores in the United States, including Wild Oats and Whole Foods Markets, were banning genetically modified ingredients from their house brands, and were asking their suppliers to do the same. Starbucks, one of the largest milk users in the country, was eliminating all genetically engineered ingredients, including dairy products that contain rBGH, from their nearly 3,000 stores in the United States.

If genetic engineering had been railroaded in, now the freight train was hitting a brick wall. Transgenic acreage, which had multiplied by a factor of 20 in the final three years of the twentieth century, suddenly was going nowhere. In 2000, the acreage devoted to genetically engineered corn dropped by 25 percent. And Pope Paul II, who had never before opposed biotechnology, was now saying that genetically engineered foods was contrary to God's will.[49]

"At each point in this project we keep thinking that we have reached the low point and that public thinking will stabilize," Monsanto was told by those the company hired to advise it on the sticky issue of consumer acceptance. "But we apparently have not reached that point. The latest survey shows a steady decline over the year, which may have accelerated in the most recent period."[50]

Giving new meaning to the word *denial*, Monsanto's CEO Bob Shapiro proclaimed, "This (genetically engineered food) is the single most successful introduction of technology in the history of agriculture, including the plow."[51]

That would have been news to the European Commission, which was voting 407 to 2 to ban the import of American genetically engineered corn. And to the *New York Times*, which was reporting that "in Europe, the public sentiment against genetically engineered food [has] reached a groundswell so great that the cultivation and sale of such food there has all but stopped."[52]

As hard as Monsanto and the other biotech companies were trying to prevent it, the world was waking up. In 1999, U.K. Prime Minister Tony Blair said he had "no hesitation" about eating genetically engineered food. But only a year later the prime minister, long one of biotech's most diehard supporters, and whose election was financially supported by Monsanto, was saying "there's no doubt that there is potential for harm, both in terms of human safety and in the diversity of our environment, from genetically modified food and crops."[53]

Most important, despite vehement U.S. opposition, 130 nations were signing the landmark Cartagena Protocol on Biosafety, giving nations the right to refuse entry to genetically altered seeds, crops, animals, and microbes. The treaty placed the burden on the producers of genetically modified foods to demonstrate safety before such foods are widely deployed, emphatically repudiating the prevailing U.S. practice of requiring critics to prove that transgenics are dangerous. It was the first time nations had ever agreed on an attempt to prevent environmental problems before they begin. The world was saying it had had enough of the "Deploy now, ask questions later" approach that placed industry aspirations above public interest and safety.[54]

In the United States, the nonprofit group Mothers for Natural Law was presenting to Congress a petition that had been signed by half a million people calling for the mandatory labeling of genetically engineered food. In 2000, safety and labeling bills to curtail the biotech industry were being introduced by U.S. Representative Dennis Kucinich and 55 bipartisan co-sponsors in the House and by Barbara Boxer and Daniel Moynihan in the Senate. And *Time* magazine was exclaiming that the Campaign to Label Genetically Engineered Foods (1-425-771-4049; *www.thecampaign.org*) was growing at "warp speed."[55]

The movement was gathering strength with every passing day. In 2001, the large and powerful Consumer Federation of America, an association of 270 pro-consumer groups including the American Association of Retired People and Consumers Union, was issuing a 258-page report calling for the mandatory labeling of genetically engineered food. And Congressman Kucinich and Senator Boxer were reintroducing legislation to require labeling into the new 107th Congress.

All over the world, people were calling for their governments to protect human welfare and the environment, rather than putting corporate profits over public health. People everywhere were insisting on a society that restores the Earth, not one that destroys it.

In the early years of the new millennium, it remained to be seen whether they would get what they were asking for. . . .

chapter 20 Conclusion

Our Food,
Our Future

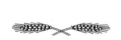It is amazing how rapidly things are chang-
ing in our world today. When I look back
a few years to the late 1980s, when I wrote
Diet for a New America, I see how swiftly history is being made.

At that time, not a single genetically engineered seed had yet been
commercially planted, and organic agriculture was primarily seen as a
stubborn and outdated refusal to utilize the benefits of technology.

Meanwhile, Americans were eating veal without the slightest awareness of the misery that was on their plates, and hardly anyone had heard
the phrase "factory farm." Even in Europe, no laws had yet been passed
limiting the degree of confinement or level of abuse to which livestock
could be subjected. Most people still pictured animals being raised on
farms with barnyards and pastures, with Lassie and Timmy running
around.

In the late 1980s, as well, the public was almost completely unaware
that there might be any connection between hamburgers and rainforest destruction, or between the production of modern meat and other forms of
ecological ruin. Only a few scientists were talking about global warming,
and they were debating whether there was anything to the "hypothesis."

Mad Cow disease and E. coli 0157:H7 were not even known to exist. Patients with cardiovascular disease were still being fed bacon and eggs for breakfast in hospitals. And Dean Ornish was just beginning to do the work that would come to revolutionize the treatment of heart disease.

It was only a few years ago that vegetarians were relegated to the margins of society, and had not yet been recognized as being on the leading edge of movements toward health, ecological sustainability, and social justice.

But by late 1999, *Time* magazine, a forum not particularly known for challenging conventional wisdom, ran a two-page feature article by Ed Ayres of Worldwatch Institute that documented the horrendous environmental and health impacts of modern meat production and predicted the demise of a meat-based culture. A month later, *New York Times* business columnist Daniel Akst wrote, "You've noticed that scientists believe fatty foods kill people, and that fast-food outlets are selling cheeseburgers with both hands. . . . [It] makes perfect sense for 'victims' of fast-food to sue, and the sooner the better." Akst continued, "Far-fetched? Why? The same line of reasoning underlies the litigation that has succeeded spectacularly against the tobacco companies."

When you see how much has occurred in such a short span of time, it is hard not to stagger. We are experiencing a rate of change that is historically unprecedented. Never before have human beings dealt with anything like the speed of transformation that we live with today.

The next 10 or 15 years will likely bring even vaster changes, and I often wonder what life will be like a decade or two from now. I reflect on what the future will bring us, not only as individuals, but as a country, as a species, and as a planet.

Will genetic engineering take over completely, so that all our foods will become transgenic, as Monsanto is hoping? Or will organic food and agriculture prevail and become the standard?

What will be the plight of the world's least fortunate? Will we give up on the eternal prayer to end the great sorrow of human starvation, and wall ourselves off ever more from our fellow human beings? Or will we finally do something about this ancient scourge and find out what magnificent treasures we have in each other?

In the years to come, will we suffer from increasing ecological havoc, with ever more devastating storms and extreme weather events, with hundreds of millions of people driven from their homes by rising seas and terrifying "acts of God"? Or will we shift to solar, hydrogen, and wind as sources of energy, move toward low-petroleum input agriculture, and plant enough trees to return the atmosphere and the climate to stability?

Will the web of life continue to unravel, with ever more species driven to extinction? Or will we save wilderness and wildlife habitat, realizing that our lives are as dependent on the interconnected functioning of other species for survival as our brains are dependent on the interconnected functioning of our hearts and arteries?

Will a pound of meat still sell in the supermarket for only a few dollars a pound, despite requiring astronomical quantities of water, energy, grain, and land for its production? Or will we stop subsidizing polluting industries and begin instituting environmental taxes so that the true ecological costs of production come to be incorporated into the price of all the things we buy and sell?

Will we look at the natural world and other life forms as commodities having value only insofar as we can convert them into revenue? Or will we live with reverence for life on this planet, seeing it as a community of which we are a part and to which we owe our lives?

Will we continue to house animals destined for human consumption in conditions that violate their biological natures and frustrate their every instinct and need? Or will we widen the circle of our compassion to include these creatures who draw breath from the same source we do?

Will we eat ever more un-natural food, and watch our rates of obesity, heart disease, cancer, and diabetes continue to skyrocket? Or will we begin to feed ourselves and our children life-giving food with which we and they can build truly healthy and vibrant bodies?

Will our children think that a balanced diet is a Big Mac in each hand? Or will they know where their food came from, and want to eat healthy food because their parents, whom they love and admire, have shown them the value of doing so?

Will all our food be irradiated, and will we wash our hands, plates, and cutlery before each meal with chemical disinfectants? Or will we address the problem of food-borne disease at its source—the feedlots,

factory farms, and slaughterhouses where pathogens originate and proliferate?

Will we become even more alienated from the natural world as our
food becomes even more processed, refined, and adulterated? Or will
our cities be full of urban and rooftop gardens, with ever more people
celebrating the pleasures of food that is wholesome, fresh, and full of vitality?

This Moment on Earth

So much is at stake in our times. Whether we like it or not, and whether
we accept it or not, the choices we make, individually and collectively,
in the coming years will make an incredible amount of difference, perhaps more so than at any other time in the history of life on this planet.
It is not just the quality of our personal lives and health that depends,
now, on the choices we make. The destiny of life on Earth is up for
grabs. And we are each part of how it will turn out.

I am thinking, now, about some of the truly wonderful people I have
had the privilege and pleasure of working closely with, who have died
during the past few years. I'm remembering Cesar Chavez, John
Denver, Raul Julia, Linda McCartney, Helen Nearing, David Brower,
Donella Meadows, Danaan Parry, Cleveland Amory, and River
Phoenix—people who stood for, worked for, and dedicated their lives to
the creation of a thriving, sustainable, and compassionate world.

Though each has passed on, their love and commitment are still very
much with me. I miss them and I'm sad they are gone, and yet they give
me strength. To me, they are heroes.

These people have taught me that there are two things you need to
know if you want to live a life of great meaning and magnificence. The
first thing you must not forget is that heroic people don't always conform
to what is popular at a given time. You must be willing to be out of step
with public opinion. This was true of the founders of the United States—
most colonists were content with dependence on England. It was true of
Abraham Lincoln—most Northerners didn't want blacks to be free or
equal. It was true of Susan B. Anthony—even most women at the time

weren't in favor of women voting. And it is true today. If you are going to be a voice for the future, you can't be a creature of the current fads.

The other thing that you must never forget, if you want to be a bringer of the dawn, is that it's no use trying to be perfect. The people I have known who have moved the world were all flawed human beings, like you and me. But they didn't let that stop them. They knew that it is part of our glory as human beings that, even with our imperfections and wounds, we can still help heal and cherish each other and our beautiful planet.

In the years to come, other dedicated people will also leave us. Some, like the people I've mentioned, will be well known and recognized as influential. Most, though, will have lived relatively anonymous lives, making choices and working without public recognition, serving the greater healing for which we all pray as well as they could, given the circumstances of their lives. There is no calculating the debt humanity owes those who labor without receiving much validation or affirmation for their efforts, who bring faith even where there seems to be only doubt, and who bring love even where there seems to be only indifference or hate.

When each of us comes to the end of our lives, what will matter is not what our social standing was, or whether the world thought we were important or influential. What will matter, what in fact always matters, are the values we uphold and the principles and possibilities we stand for. What will matter then, and what matters now, are the quality of the love we share with the world and the statements we make with our choices and our lives.

Far too often, our culture today tells us a tremendous lie. It tells us that we don't, as individuals, make a difference unless we happen to be one of the "rich and famous." But nothing could be further from the truth.

Your life does matter. It always matters whether you reach out in friendship or lash out in anger. It always matters whether you live with compassion and awareness or whether you succumb to distractions and trivia. It always matters how you treat other people, how you treat animals, and how you treat yourself. It always matters what you do. It always matters what you say. And it always matters what you eat.

When you choose to affirm the dignity inherent in life and to uphold the beauty, the magic, and the mystery of the living Earth, something happens. It happens whether or not anyone else recognizes your efforts, and it happens regardless of how wounded and flawed you are. What happens is you join the long lineage of human beings who have stood for and helped to bring about a future worthy of all the tears and prayers our species has known. Your life becomes a statement of human possibility. Your life becomes an instrument through which a healthier, more compassionate, and more sustainable future will come to be.

Cesar Chavez, John Denver, Raul Julia, Linda McCartney, Helen Nearing, David Brower, Donella Meadows, Danaan Parry, Cleveland Amory, River Phoenix, and many others like them have left us. But every day, new heroes are being born. They are born at every age and at every stage of life. They are the people who hear the call of the future and seek, with their lives, to answer it. Perhaps you know someone like this. Perhaps you are one of them.

Thank you for doing what you can to bring hope where there has been despair and light where there has been darkness. Thank you for listening to life. Thank you for acting on its behalf.

May all be fed. May all be healed. May all be loved.

Resource Guide

Vegetarian Community, Online

VegSource Interactive

A tremendous Web site, providing valuable information and support on the Internet. VegSource is an online magazine with cutting-edge articles on nearly every topic discussed in *The Food Revolution* and thousands of healthy recipes, book reviews, and articles on the environment and compassion by many of the top experts in the field of vegetarian living. You can read up on scientific research and lifestyle issues, and you will find wonderful, free, personal support from award-winning chefs, top medical doctors, and bestselling authors. VegSource also offers hundreds of active discussion boards on a wide range of topics. You can join right in and become part of this bustling online community. VegSource is operated by a husband-and-wife team, Jeff and Sabrina Nelson, who are close personal friends of John Robbins, and provide a wonderful resource for the vegetarian community. Check it out and you'll see why hundreds of thousands of people call it home. www.Vegsource.com

Food and Healing

EarthSave

EarthSave was founded in 1989 by John Robbins to channel the tremendous response to his book, *Diet for a New America,* into sustained and positive action. With nearly 40 chapters in the United States, and many others throughout the world, the organization promotes food choices that are healthy for people and for the planet, helping countless numbers to shift toward plant-based diets and to take compassionate action for all life on Earth. The organization's programs are essentially educational, working internationally, nationally, and through local chapters to get the word out and to help people discover alternatives to the Standard American Diet. 20555 Devonshire Blvd., Suite 105, Chatsworth, CA 91311; 818-407-0289; www.earthsave.org; info@earthsave.org

Center for Science in the Public Interest (CSPI)

Educates the public as well as policy makers about the critical importance of food safety, and publishes the *Nutrition Action Healthletter.* 1875 Connecticut Ave., NW, Ste. 300, Washington, DC 20009; 202-332-9110; www.cspinet.org; cspi@cspinet.org

Citizens for Health

Empowers consumers to make informed health choices; areas of focus include dietary supplements, complementary and alternative medicine, food and water safety. P. O. Box 2260, Boulder, CO 80306; 800-357-2211; www.citizens.org; citizens4health@gmail.com

Physicians Committee for Responsible Medicine

Promotes preventive medicine, encourages higher standards for ethics and effectiveness in research, advocates broader access to medical services, offers Vegetarian Starter Kit and numerous publications including *Good Medicine,* a quarterly magazine. 5100 Wisconsin Ave., NW, Ste. 400, Washington, DC 20016; 202-686-2210; www.pcrm.org; pcrm@pcrm.org

Public Citizen

Founded by Ralph Nader, fights for safer drugs and medical devices, cleaner energy sources and environment, fair trade, and a more open and democratic government. 1600 20th St., NW, Washington, D.C. 20009; 202-588-1000; www.citizen.org; member@citizen.org

Safe Tables Our Priority (STOP)

Supports victims of food-borne illness, provides public education on the dangers in food, and does policy advocacy for safe food and public health. 3149 Dundee Road, #276, Northbrook, IL 60062; 800-350-STOP; www.safetables.org

Our Fellow Creatures

Animal Place Sanctuary

Provides homes for animals rescued from slaughter and educates the public about factory farms. 17314 McCourtney Ave., Grass Valley, CA 95949; 530-477-1757; www.animalplace.org; info@animalplace.org

Humane Society Veterinary Medical Association

Works on a variety of animal protection issues, particularly those that focus on veterinary medical ethics. Information for membership: 2100 L St., NW, Washington, DC 20037; 301-258-1478; info@hsvma.org. Information for advocacy: P. O. Box 208, Davis, CA 95617-0208; 530-759-8106; www.hsvma.org; advocacy@hsvma.org

Endangered Species Coalition

Works to protect and recover at-risk species by defending and supporting the Endangered Species Act; invites and encourages public participation in decisions affecting the fate of endangered species. P.O. Box 65195, Washington, DC 20035; 240-353-2765; www.stopextinction.org

Farm Animal Reform Movement (FARM)

Promotes vegetarianism and advocates for the well-being of farm animals through national grassroots educational campaigns, massive media blitzes, and participation in government decision-making processes. 10101 Ashburton Lane, Bethesda, MD 20817; 888-FARM-USA; www.farmusa.org; info@farmusa.org

Farm Sanctuary

Provides refuge for animals rescued from factory farms, stockyards, and slaughterhouses; wages campaigns to stop cruelty to farm animals, hosts conferences, and operates a bed and breakfast for visitors to the sanctuary. National office and New York shelter: P. O. Box

150, Watkins Glen, NY 14891; 607-583-2225. California shelter: P. O. Box 1065, Orland, CA 95963; 530-865-4622; www.farmsanctuary.org

Food Animal Concerns Trust (FACT)
Promotes more humane, safe, and sustainable methods of raising livestock and poultry; runs Food Safety and On-Farm programs. P. O. Box 14599, 411 W. Fullerton Parkway #1402 W, Chicago, IL 60614; 773-525-4952; www.foodanimalconcerns.org

Friends of Animals
Works to protect animals from cruelty, abuse, and institutionalized exploitation. 777 Post Road, Darien, CT 06820; 203-656-1522; www.friendsofanimals.org; info@friendsofanimals.org

The Fund for Animals
Protects wildlife and domestic animals through education, legislation, litigation, and hands-on care at several sanctuaries. 200 West 57th St., Ste. 705, New York, NY 10019; 888-405-FUND; www.fundforanimals.org; info@fundforanimals.org

Humane Farming Association
Works to stop animal abuse in factory farming and slaughterhouses with anti-cruelty investigations and exposés, national media and ad campaigns, direct hands-on emergency care and refuge for abused farm animals, consumer awareness programs, state and federal legislation, and youth humane education. P. O. Box 3577, San Rafael, CA 94912; 415-771-CALF; www.hfa.org; hfa@hfa.org

Humane Society of the United States (HSUS)
Promotes the humane treatment of animals and fosters respect, understanding, and compassion for all creatures and the environment. 2100 L St., NW, Washington, DC 20037; 202-452-1100; www.humanesociety.org; membership@humanesociety.org

People for the Ethical Treatment of Animals (PETA)
Works to expose and stop animal cruelty in factory farms, laboratories, the fur trade, and the entertainment industry; activities include public education, cruelty investigations, research, animal rescue, legislation, special events, celebrity involvement, and dramatic direct action. 501 Front St., Norfolk, VA 23510; 757-622-PETA; www.peta.org

PETA's GoVeg Campaign

Provides Vegetarian Starter Kit with information, tips, and recipes for new vegetarians; provides fact sheets, photographs, and other resources for activists. 501 Front St., Norfolk, VA 23510; 757-622-PETA; www.goveg.com

Poplar Spring Animal Sanctuary

Provides permanent, loving homes for abused and abandoned farm animals and rehabilitated wildlife. P. O. Box 507, Poolesville, MD 20837; 301-428-8128; www.animalsanctuary.org; info@animalsanctuary.org

Tribe of Heart

Makes use of storytelling, visual media, and the arts to present a vision of a compassionate future; creators of *Witness,* a powerful documentary about the fur industry. P. O. Box 149, Ithaca, NY 14851; 607-275-0806; www.tribeofheart.org

United Poultry Concerns

Promotes the compassionate and respectful treatment of domestic fowl through investigations and education, operating a chicken sanctuary, and publishing *Poultry Press,* a quarterly newsletter. P. O. Box 150, Machipongo, VA 23405-0150, 757-678-7875; www.upc-online.org

Our Food, Our World

Circle of Life Foundation

Founded by Julia Butterfly Hill; strives to inspire, support, and network individuals, organizations, and communities working for environmental and social solutions through public education, research, media, and outreach; P. O. Box 6783, Albany, CA 94706; 707-923-9522; www.circleoflifefoundation.org

Earth Island Institute

Develops and supports projects that counteract threats to biological and cultural diversity and that promote preservation and restoration of the Earth; publishes the "tree free" *Earth Island Journal.* 2150 Allston Way, Suite 460, Berkeley, CA 94704; 510-859-9100; earthislandinstitute.net

Friends of the Earth
Works to protect the planet from environmental degradation, preserve biological, cultural, and ethnic diversity, and empower citizens to have an influential voice in decisions affecting the quality of their environment and their lives. 1100 15th Street NW, 11th floor, Washington, DC 20005; 877-843-8687; www.foe.org

Global Resource Action Center for the Environment (GRACE)
Works to link the research, policy, and grassroots communities to preserve the future of the planet and protect the quality of the environment. 215 Lexington Ave., Suite 1001, New York, NY 10016; 212-726-9161; www.gracelinks.org

GRACE Factory Farm Project
Helps rural communities around the country oppose the spread of new factory farms and helps close down existing ones which threaten health and well-being; addresses the impacts of industrial animal production on diet, the environment, and human and animal health. 215 Lexington Ave, Suite 1001, New York, NY 10016; 212-726-9161; www.factoryfarm.org

Greenpeace
Campaigns and educates on behalf of our threatened environment, forests, climate, oceans, and species. 702 H St., NW, Ste. 300, Washington, DC 20001; 202-462-1177; www.greenpeace.org/usa; info@wdc.greenpeace.org

The Natural Step
Serves businesses, communities, academia, government, and individuals in redesigning their activities to be more ecologically and economically sustainable. 133 SW Second Ave., Suite 302, Portland, OR 97204; 503-241-1140; www.naturalstepusa.org

Rainforest Action Network
Works to protect the Earth's rainforests and support the rights of their inhabitants through education, grassroots organizing, and nonviolent direct action. 221 Pine St., Fifth Floor, San Francisco, CA 94104; 415-398-4404; www.ran.org; answers@ran.org

Rainforest Foundation

Strives to help rainforest communities in 18 countries to protect their ancestral territories from exploitive development. 180 Varick St., Suite 528, New York, NY 10014; 212-431-9098; www.rainforestfoundation.org

Redefining Progress

Generates and refines innovative policies and ideas that balance economic well-being, the environment, and social equity to improve quality of life for current and future generations. 1904 Franklin St., Suite 600, Oakland, CA 94612; 510-444-3041; www.rprogress.org

Ruckus Society

Provides training in the skills of nonviolent civil disobedience to help environmental and human rights organizations achieve their goals. P.O. Box 28741, Oakland, CA 94604; 510-931-6339; www.ruckus.org; ruckus@ruckus.org

Sierra Club

Works to protect the wilderness, promote responsible use of the Earth's resources, and educate and enlist humanity to protect and restore the natural and human environment. 85 Second St., 2nd Fl., San Francisco, CA 94105-3441; 415-977-5500; www.sierraclub.org; information@sierraclub.org

Union of Concerned Scientists (UCS)

Works to affect government in areas of health, agriculture, arms control, energy and global resources, transportation, and biotechnology through campaigns, education, and advocacy. 2 Brattle Sq., Cambridge, MA 02238; 617-547-5552; www.ucsusa.org

Worldwatch Institute

Produces superb reports on the state of the planet, including the outstanding monthly magazine *WorldWatch*. 1776 Massachusetts Ave., NW, Washington, DC 20036; 202-452-1999; www.worldwatch.org

Reversing the Spread of Hunger

Food First (Institute for Food and Development Policy)
Founded by Frances Moore Lappé; highlights root causes and value-based solutions to world hunger and poverty; provides a wide variety of resources to policy makers, activists, the media, students, researchers, and the public. 398 60th St., Oakland, CA 94618; 510-654-4400; www.foodfirst.org; info@foodfirst.org

Food Not Bombs
Feeds hot, vegetarian meals prepared with surplus food collected from supermarkets, restaurants, and natural food stores to hungry people in more than 175 cities; protests war and poverty worldwide. P. O. Box 424, Arroyo Seco, NM 87514; 575-770-3377; www.foodnotbombs.net; menu@foodnotbombs.net

The Hunger Project
Works toward the sustainable end of hunger worldwide through mobilizing grassroots action and local leadership, and empowering women in their communities. 5 Union Square West, New York, NY 10003; 212-251-9100; www.thp.org

Genetic Engineering

Alliance for Bio-Integrity
Integrates the perspectives of both science and religion to preserve the safety of our food, the health of our environment, and the harmony of our relationship with nature through education, responsible action, and litigation. 2040 Pearl Lane #2, Fairfield, Iowa 52556; 206-888-4852; www.biointegrity.org; info@biointegrity.org

The Center for Food Safety (CFS)
Provides leadership in legal, scientific, and grassroots efforts to address the increasing concerns about the impacts of our food production systems on human health, animal welfare, and the environment. 660 Pennsylvania Ave SE, #302, Washington, DC 20003; 202-547-9359; www.truefoodnow.org

The Council for Responsible Genetics
Fosters public debate about the social, ethical, and environmental implications of the new genetic technologies and advocates for socially responsible use of these technologies. 5 Upland Rd., Ste. 3, Cambridge, MA 02140; 617-868-0870; www.councilforresponsiblegenetics.org; crg@gene-watch.org

Rural Advancement Foundation International (RAFI)
Works to promote sustainable agriculture, strengthen family farms and rural communities, protect diversity of plants, animals, and people in agriculture, and ensure responsible use of new technologies. P. O. Box 640, Pittsboro, NC 27312; 919-542-1396; www.rafiusa.org

Organic Foods

Community Alliance with Family Farmers
Promotes community agriculture through campaigns, farm tours, and publications, including the *National Organic Directory*. P. O. Box 363, Davis, CA 95617; 530-756-8518; www.caff.org

Environmental Working Group
Provides research, reports, articles, technical assistance, and Internet resources to public interest groups and concerned citizens who are campaigning to protect the environment. 1436 U St. NW, Suite 100, Washington, DC 20009; 202-667-6982; www.ewg.org

Organic Consumers Association
Dedicated to building a healthy, safe, and sustainable system of food production and consumption; a global clearinghouse for information and grassroots technical assistance. 6771 South Silver Hill Dr., Finland, MN 55603; 218-226-4164; www.organicconsumers.org

Organic Farming Research Foundation
Fosters the improvement and widespread adoption of organic farming practices by sponsoring and disseminating research and educating the public and decision makers about organic farming issues. P. O. Box 440, Santa Cruz, CA 95061; 831-426-6606; www.ofrf.org; info@ofrf.org

Pesticide Action Network, North America (PANNA)
Advances alternatives to pesticides worldwide through research, policy development, education, media, demonstration of alternatives, and advocacy campaigns. 49 Powell St., Ste. 500, San Francisco, CA 94102; 415-981-1771; www.panna.org; panna@panna.org

Vegetarian Societies

International Vegetarian Union (IVU)
Promotes vegetarianism throughout the world by supporting and connecting national and regional groups, and holding the International Vegetarian Congress. Contact IVU for a listing of international vegetarian organizations. www.ivu.org

North American Vegetarian Society (NAVS)
Dedicated to promoting the vegetarian way of life by sponsoring regional and national conferences and campaigns, distributing educational materials, and publishing *Vegetarian Voice*. Contact NAVS for a listing of vegetarian organizations in North America. P. O. Box 72, Dolgeville, NY 13329; 518-568-7970; www.navs-online.org

Notes

Introduction to the 10th Anniversary Edition

i. Andrew Weil, *Why Our Health Matters: A Vision of Medicine That Can Transform Our Future.* Hudson Street Press, New York, 2009, pg 7.

ii. Dan Lothian, "Health Crisis: A Bankruptcy Every 30 Seconds," CNNMoney.com, March 5, 2009.

iii. "Starbucks Pays More for Health Insurance than for Coffee," Health Care For All, Sept 22, 2005. http://blog.hcfama.org/?p=369.

iv. Andrew Weil, *Why Our Health Matters: A Vision of Medicine That Can Transform Our Future.* Hudson Street Press, New York, 2009, pg 53–54.

v. John Abramson, *Overdo$ed America: The Broken Promise of American Medicine.* Harper Perennial, New York, 2005, pg 47.

vi. Dolecek TA, McCarthy BJ, Joslin CE, et al. Prediagnosis food patterns are associated with length of survival from epithelial ovarian cancer. *J Am Diet Assoc.* 2010;110:369-382.

vii. Butler LM, Wu AH, Wang R, Koh WP, Yuan JM, Yu MC. A vegetable-fruit-soy dietary pattern protects against breast cancer among postmenopausal Singapore Chinese women. *Am J Clin Nutr.* Published ahead of print February 24, 2010. doi: 10.3945/ajcn.2009.2857

viii. Zhang Q, Ma G, Greenfield H, et al. The association between dietary protein intake and bone mass accretion in pubertal girls with low calcium intakes. *Br J Nutr.* 2010;103:714-723.

ix. Sinha R, Park Y, Graubard BI, et al. Meat and meat-related compounds and risk of prostate cancer in a large prospective cohort study in the United States. *Am J Epidemiol.* Advance access published October 6, 2009. DOI: 10.1093/aje/kwp280.

x. Schimazu T, Inoue M, Sasazuki S, et al. Isoflavone intake and risk of lung cancer: a prospective cohort study in Japan. *Am J Clin Nutr.* Published ahead of print January 13, 2010. doi:10.3945/ajcn.2009.2816.

xi. Dod HS, Bhardwaj R, Sajja V, et al. Effect of intensive lifestyle changes on endothelia function on inflammatory markers of atherosclerosis. *Am J Cardiol.* 2010;105:362–367.

xii. Vincent C, Boerlin P, Daignault D, et al. Food reservoir for Escherichia coli causing urinary tract infections. *Emerg Infect Dis.* 2010;16:88–95.

xiii. Sluijs I, Beulens JWJ, Van Der A DL, Spijkerman AMW, Grobbee DE, Van Der Shouw YT. Dietary intake of total, animal, and vegetable protein and risk of type 2 diabetes in the European Prospective Investigation into Cancer and Nutrition (EPIC)-NL study. *Diabetes Care.* 2010; 33:43–48.

xiv. Shu XO, Zheng Y, Cai H, et al. Soy food intake and breast cancer survival. *JAMA.* 2009;302:2437–2443.

xv. Beezhold BL, Johnston CS, Daigle DR. Restriction of flesh foods in omnivores improves mood: a pilot randomized controlled trial. Poster presented at: American Public Health Association's 137th Annual Meeting and Exposition; November 9, 2009: Philadelphia, PA.

xvi. Brekke HK, Ludvigsson J. Daily vegetable intake during pregnancy negatively associated to islet autoimmunity in the offspring—The ABIS study. *Pediatr Diabetes.* Advanced access published September 16, 2009. DOI: 10.1111/j.1399-5448.2009.00563.x.

xvii. Aune D, Ursin G, Veierod MB. Meat consumption and the risk of type 2 diabetes: a systematic review and meta-analysis of cohort studies. *Diabetologia.* 2009;52:2277–2287.

xviii. Koh WP, Wu AH, Wang R, et al. Gender-specific associations between soy and risk of hip fracture in the Singapore Chinese Health Study. *Am J Epidemiol.* 2009;170:901–909.

xix. Kathy Freston, "Vegetarian is the new Prius," Huffington Post, Jan 18, 2007.

xx. *Livestock's Long Shadow: Environmental Issues and Options*, Food and Agriculture Organization (FAO) of the United Nations, Rome, 2006.

xxi. Gidon Eshel and Pamela Martin, "Diet, Energy and Global Warming," *Earth Interactions*, Vol 10, 2006.

xxii. Ezra Klein, "The Meat of the Problem," *The Washington Post*, July 29, 2009. See also Mike Tidwell, "The Low-Carbon Diet," *Audubon magazine*, Jan 2009.

xxiii. Nathan Fiala, "How Meat Contributes to Global Warming: Producing beef for the table has a suprising environmental cost: it releases prodigious amounts of heat-trapping gases," *Scientific American*, Feb 4, 2009. See also Christopher L. Weber and H. Scott Matthews, "Food-Miles and the Relative Climate Impacts of Food choices in the United States," *Environmental Science & Technology*, April 16, 2008. And Bryan Walsh, "Meat: Making Global Warming Worse," Time magazine, Sept 10, 2008. And Jim Motavelli, "The Meat of the Matter: Animals Raised for Food are Warming the Planet Faster than Cars," E Magazine, July/Aug 2008. And Julliette Jowit, "UN Says Eat Less Meat to Curb Global Warming," *The Observer*, Sept 7, 2008.

xxiv. Robert Goodland and Jeff Anhang, "Livestock and Climate Change," *World Watch* Nov/Dec 2009.

chapter 2 Healthy Heart, Healthy Life

1. Messina, Virginia, and Messina, Mark, *The Dietitian's Guide to Vegetarian Diets: Issues and Applications* (Gaithersburg, MD: Aspen Publishers, 1996), p. 58.
2. "Myths and Facts about Beef Production," National Cattlemen's Beef Association, displayed on the Web site of the National Cattlemen's Beef Association in 2001.
3. "Position of American Dietetic Association on Vegetarian Diets," *Journal of the American Dietetic Association* 97 (1997):1317–21.
4. American Heart Association, Heart Attack and Angina Statistics, 1999.
5. Roberts, William, "Atherosclerotic Risk Factors: Are There Ten or Is There Only One?", *American Journal of Cardiology* 64 (1989):552.
6. Personal communication with author.
7. Liebman, B., "Where's the Ground Beef Labeling?", *Nutrition Action*, June 1997.
8. "Here's the Beef," *Nutrition Action*, September 1999.
9. Murphy, Dan, "Food Fascists on the Attack Again," October 27, 2000; www.meatingplace.com.
10. Law, M. R., Wald, N. J., Wu, T., et al., "Systematic Underestimation of Association between Serum Cholesterol Concentration and Ischaemic Heart Disease . . . ," *British Medical Journal* 308 (1994):363–6.
11. Resnicow, K., Barone, J., Engle, A., et al., "Diet and Serum Lipids in Vegan Vegetarians: A Model for Risk Reduction," *Journal of the American Dietetic Association* 91 (1991):447–53. See also West, R. O., et al., "Diet and Serum Cholesterol Levels: A Comparison between Vegetarians and Nonvegetarians . . . ," *American Journal of Clinical Nutrition* 21 (1968):853–62; Sacks, F. M., Ornish, D., et al., "Plasma Lipoprotein Levels in Vegetarians: The Effect of Ingestion of Fats from Dairy Products," *Journal of the American Medical Association* 254 (1985):1337–41; Messina and Messina, *The Dietitian's Guide to Vegetarian Diets*.
12. Phillips, R., et al., "Coronary Heart Disease Mortality among Seventh-Day Adventists with Differing Dietary Habits," *American Journal of Clinical Nutrition* 31 (1978):S191–8; Burr, M., et al., "Vegetarianism, Dietary Fiber, and Mortality," *American Journal of Clinical Nutrition* 36 (1982):873–7; Burr, M., et al., "Heart Disease in British Vegetarians," *American Journal of Clinical Nutrition* 48 (1988):830–2; Thorogood, M., et al., "Risk of Death from Cancer and Ischaemic Heart Disease in Meat and Non-meat Eaters," *British Medical Journal* 308 (1994):1666–71; Berkel, J., et al., "Mortality Pattern and Life Expectancy of Seventh-Day Adventists in the Netherlands," *International Journal of Epidemiology* 12 (1983):455–9; Chang-Claude, J., et al., "Mortality Pattern of German Vegetarians after 11 Years of Followup," *Epidemiology* 3 (1992):395–401.
13. Resnicow, et al., "Diet and Serum Lipids in Vegan Vegetarians." See also Messina and Messina, *The Dietitian's Guide to Vegetarian Diets*.
14. Anderson, J. W., et al., "Meta-Analysis of the Effects of Soy Protein Intake on Serum Lipids," *New England Journal of Medicine* 333 (1995):276–82. See

also Carroll, K. K., "Dietary Protein in Relation to Plasma Cholesterol Levels and Atherosclerosis," *Nutrition Review* 36 (1978):1–5.

15. Ibid.

16. "Myths and Facts about Beef Production."

17. Barnard, Neal, *The Power of Your Plate* (Summertown, TN: Book Publishing Company, 1990), pp. 25–6.

18. National Cattlemen's Association, "Fact Sheet" Retort to the PBS Documentary, *Diet for a New America*, 1991.

19. Walles, C., "Hold the Eggs and Butter: Cholesterol Is Proved Deadly and Our Diets May Never Be the Same," *Time*, March 26, 1984, p. 62.

20. "Dairy Farmers of Canada Response to *Becoming Vegetarian*," Dairy Bureau of Canada, 1996.

21. Messina and Messina, *The Dietitian's Guide Vegetarian Diets*, p. 18.

22. Ibid.

23. Ibid.

24. McDougall, John, *The McDougall Program for a Healthy Heart* (New York: Dutton, 1996), p. 134.

25. McDougall, *The McDougall Program*, pp. 66–7; see also Fisher, M., et al., "The Effect of Vegetarian Diets on Plasma Lipid and Platelet Levels," *Archives of Internal Medicine* 146 (1986):1193–7; Sacks, et al., "Plasma Lipoprotein Levels in Vegetarians":1337–41.

26. Ibid.

27. Barnard, *The Power of Your Plate*, p. 15.

28. Holerton, Gene, *The Beef-Eater's Guide to Modern Meat* (Los Angeles: Holerton Publishing, 1998), p. 6.

29. Barnard, *The Power of Your Plate*, pp. 33–4.

30. Davidson, M., et al., "Comparison of the Effects of Lean Red Meat vs. Lean White Meat on Serum Lipid Levels . . . ," "*Archives of Internal Medicine* 159 (1999):1331–8. See also Barnard, Neal, Letter to the Editor, *Archives of Internal Medicine*, February 14, 2000.

31. Ornish, Dean, "Can Lifestyle Changes Reverse Coronary Heart Disease?" *Lancet* 336 (1990):129–33; Ornish, Dean, et al., "Intensive Lifestyle Changes for Reversal of Coronary Heart Disease," *Journal of the American Medical Association* 280 (1998):2001–7; Thorogood, M., et al., "Plasma Lipids and Lipoprotein Cholesterol Concentrations in People with Different Diets in Britain," *British Medical Journal* 295 (1987):351–3.

32. Barnard, Neal, *Food for Life* (New York: Harmony/Crown Publishers, 1993), p. 30.

33. Ibid.

34. Castelli, W., "Epidemiology of Coronary Heart Disease," *American Journal of Medicine* 76(2A) (1984):4–12.

35. Cheeke, Peter, *Contemporary Issues in Animal Agriculture*, 2nd ed. (Danville, IL: Interstate Publishers, 1999), p. 47.

36. *Nutrition Action*, June 1999.

37. O'Connor, G. A., "A Regional Prospective Study of In-Hospital Mortality Associated with Coronary Artery Bypass Grafting," *Journal of the American Medical Association* 266 (1991):803; Hannan, E., "The Decline in Coronary Artery

Bypass Graft Mortality . . . ," *Journal of the American Medical Association* 273 (1995):209; Williams, S., "Differences in Mortality from Coronary Artery Bypass Surgery at Five Teaching Hospitals," *Journal of the American Medical Association* 266 (1991):810; McDonald, C., "CABG Surgical Mortality in Different Centers," *Journal of the American Medical Association* 267 (1992):932; Steinbrook, R., "Hospital Death Rates for Five Surgeries Vary," *Los Angeles Times*, March 27, 1988; Shortell, S., "The Effects of Regulation, Competition, and Ownership on Mortality Rates among Hospital Inpatients," *New England Journal of Medicine* 318 (1988):1100; Kirklin, J., "Summary of a Consensus Concerning Death and Ischemic Events after Coronary Bypass Grafting," *Circulation* 79 Sup 1) (1989):81.

38. Hill, J., "Neuropathological Manifestations of Cardiac Surgery," *Annals of Thoracic Surgery* 7 (1969):409; Editorial, "Brain Damage after Open-Heart Surgery," *Lancet* 1 (1982):1161; Henriksen, L., "Evidence Suggestive of Diffuse Brain Damage Following Cardiac Operations," *Lancet* 1 (1984):816; Editorial, "Brain Damage and Open Heart Surgery," *Lancet* 2 (1989):364; Murkin, J., "Anesthesia, the Brain, and Cardiopulmonary Bypass," *Annals of Thoracic Surgery* 56 (1993):1461; McDougall, *The McDougall Program*, pp. 206–7.

39. *Nutrition Action*, June 1999.

40. McDougall, *The McDougall Program*, p. 211.

41. Ibid.

42. Parisi, A., "A Comparison of Angioplasty with Medical Treatment of Single Vessel Coronary Artery Disease," *New England Journal of Medicine* 326 (1992):10; Graboys, T., "Results of a Second-Opinion Trial among Patients Recommended for Coronary Angioplasty," *Journal of the American Medical Association* 268 (1992):2537; Graboys, T., "Second-Opinion Trial in Patients Recommended for Coronary Angiography," *Journal of the American Medical Association* 269 (1993):1504; McGivney, S., "Angioplasty vs. Medical Therapy for Single-Vessel Coronary Artery Disease," *New England Journal of Medicine* 326 (1992):1632.

43. McDougall, *The McDougall Program*, p. 210.

44. Ornish, et al., "Intensive Lifestyle Changes."

45. Ornish, Dean, "Can Lifestyle Changes Reverse Coronary Heart Disease?"

46. Ibid.

47. Ornish, et al., "Intensive Lifestyle Changes."

48. Ibid.

49. Ornish, Dean, comments in Millennium Lecture Series Symposium on the Great Nutrition Debate, Jefferson Auditorium, U.S. Department of Agriculture, February 24, 2000.

50. *Nutrition Action*, June 1999.

51. Esselstyn, C. B., Jr., "Updating a 12–Year Experience with Arrest and Reversal Therapy for Coronary Heart Disease," *American Journal of Cardiology* 84 (1999):339–41.

52. Ibid.

53. Ibid.

54. Esselstyn, Caldwell, "Making the Change," www.heartattackproof.com/morethan04_change.htm.
55. "Heart Disease Programme Wins Plaudits," BBC News, February 14, 2000; see also Worldwatch Institute, *State of the World 2000* (New York: W. W. Norton, 2000), p. 77.
56. Dass, Ram, *Still Here* (New York: Riverhead Books, 2000), p. 186.
57. McDougall, *The McDougall Program*, p. 216.
58. Sacks, F. M., et al., "Low Blood Pressure in Vegetarians: Effects of Specific Foods and Nutrients," *American Journal of Clinical Nutrition* 48 (1988):795–800.
59. Ibid.
60. Ophir O., et al., "Low Blood Pressure in Vegetarians . . . ," *American Journal of Clinical Nutrition* 37 (1983):755–62; see also Melby, C. L., et al., "Blood Pressure in Vegetarians and Non-Vegetarians: A Cross-Sectional Analysis," *Nutrition Research* 5 (1985):1077–82; Melby, C. L., et al., "Relation between Vegetarian/Non-Vegetarian Diets and Blood Pressure . . . ," *American Journal of Public Health*, 79 (1989):1283–8.
61. Ophir, et al., "Low Blood Pressure in Vegetarians."
62. Lindahl, O., et al., "A Vegan Regimen with Reduced Medication in the Treatment of Hypertension," *British Journal of Nutrition* 52 (1984):11–20; Margetts, B. M., et al., "Vegetarian Diet in Mild Hypertension: A Randomised Controlled Trial," *British Medical Journal* 293 (1986):1468–71; Rouse, I. L., et al., "Blood Pressure Lowering Effect of a Vegetarian Diet: Controlled Trial . . . ," *Lancet* 1 (1983):5–10.
63. McDougall, *The McDougall Program*, pp. 222–3.
64. Ibid, p. 213.
66. Personal communication with author.
67. Gregory, Dick, *Callus on My Soul* (Marietta, GA: Longstreet Press, 2000), p. 301.

chapter 3 Preventing Cancer

1. Wilber, Ken, *Grace and Grit* (Boston: Shambhala, 1991), pp. 251–4.
2. Ibid.
3. Cited in Moss, Ralph, *Questioning Chemotherapy* (Brooklyn: Equinox, 1995), p. 20.
4. Cairns, John, "The Treatment of Diseases and the War Against Cancer," *Scientific American* (Nov 1985), pp. 51–9.
5. Bailar, John, and Smith, Elaine, "Progress Against Cancer?" *New England Journal of Medicine* 314 (1986):1226–33.
6. World Cancer Research Fund and American Institute for Cancer Research, *Food, Nutrition and the Prevention of Cancer: A Global Perspective*, 1997.
7. Ibid, p. 509.
8. Ibid, pp. 456–7.
9. National Cattlemen's Association, "Fact Sheet" Retort to the PBS Documentary, *Diet for a New America*, 1991.

10. Barnard, Neal, *The Power of Your Plate* (Summertown, TN: Book Publishing Company, 1990), p. 26.

11. Key, T. J. A., et al., "Dietary Habits and Mortality in 11,000 Vegetarians and Health Conscious People: Results of a 17–Year Follow Up," *British Medical Journal* 313 (1996):775–9; see also Key, T., et al., "Mortality in Vegetarians and Nonvegetarians: Detailed Findings from a Collaborative Analysis of 5 Prospective Studies," *American Journal of Clinical Nutrition* 70 (Sup) (1999):516S–24S; and Frentzel-Beyme, R., et al., "Vegetarian Diets and Colon Cancer: The German Experience," *American Journal of Clinical Nutrition* 59 (Sup) (1994):1143S–52S.

12. Chang-Claude, J., et al., "Mortality Pattern of German Vegetarians after 11 Years of Follow-Up," *Epidemiology* 3 (1992):395–401; Thorogood, M., et al., "Risk of Death from Cancer and Ischaemic Heart Disease in Meat and Non-Meat Eaters," *British Medical Journal* 308 (1994):1667–70.

13. "Cancer Society: Back Off the Red Meat, Alcohol," CNN, September 17, 1996.

14. Cummings, J., et al., *British Medical Journal* 317 (1998):1636–40; see also "Low-Meat/High-Vegetable Diets Cut Cancer Risk," Reuters, December 11, 1998.

15. Fisher, B., et al., "Tamoxifen for Prevention of Breast Cancer . . . ," *Journal of the National Cancer Institute* 18 (1998):1371–88.

16. "Breast Cancer Prevention," *Rachel's Environment and Health Weekly*, December 24, 1998, p. 2.

17. "Breast Cancer Breakthrough," *New York Times* editorial, April 8, 1998, A24.

18. "The Truth about Breast Cancer," *Rachel's Environment and Health Weekly*, November 6, 1997, p. 2.

19. Paulsen, Monte, cited in Hightower, Jim, *There's Nothing in the Middle of the Road but Yellow Stripes and Dead Armadillos*, (New York: Harper Collins, 1997), pp. 215–6.

20. Hightower, *Nothing in the Middle of the Road*, p. 215.

21. Proctor, Robert, *Cancer Wars: How Politics Shapes What We Know and Don't Know about Cancer* (New York: Basic Books,1995), pp. 255, 257.

22. "Stepping Off the Toxic Treadmill," Worldwatch Paper #153, November 30, 2000.

23. Becher, Heiko, et al., "Quantitative Cancer Risk Assessment for Dioxins Using an Occasional Cohort," *Environmental Health Perspectives* 106 (Sup 2) (1998): 663–70.

24. Courtney, Diane, Testimony before Senate Commerce Committee Subcommittee on the Environment, August 9, 1974.

25. "FDA Launches Study on Dioxin in Fish, Dairy Foods," *Food Chemical News*, February 27, 1995, cited in "Dioxin in Chicken and Eggs," *Rachel's Environment and Health Weekly*, July 17, 1997, p. 2.

26. "Hormone Mimics Hit Home," *Consumer Reports* (June 1998), p. 53.

27. According to independent laboratory tests cited by Michael Gough, who chaired the U.S. Department of Health and Human Services advisory panel

on the effects of dioxin-contaminated Agent Orange on U.S. Air Force personnel in Vietnam; see www.junkscience.com/nov99/benjerry.htm.

28. "'Unsafe' levels of dioxin in gourmet ice cream; more dioxin in Ben & Jerry's than gasoline refinery effluent, researchers report," August 17, 2000; for further information, see note 27.

29. Thune, I., et al., "Physical Activity and the Risk of Breast Cancer," *New England Journal of Medicine* 336 (1997):1269–75.

30. Decarli, A., et al., "Macronutrients, Energy Intake and Breast Cancer Risk . . . ," *Epidemiology* 8 (1997):425–28; see also Wynder, E., et al., "Breast Cancer: Weighing the Evidence for a Promoting Role of Dietary Fat," *Journal of the National Cancer Institute* 89 (1997):766–75; Nicholson, A., "Diet and the Prevention and Treatment of Breast Cancer," *Alternative Therapies* 2 (1996):32–8; and Outwater, J., et al., "Dairy Products and Breast Cancer . . . ," *Medical Hypotheses* 48 (1997):453–61.

31. Ronco, E., et al., "Meat, Fat, and Risk of Breast Cancer: A Case Control Study from Uruguay," *International Journal of Cancer* 65 (1996):328–31.

32. Hirayama, T., "Epidemiology of Breast Cancer with Special Reference to the Role of Diet," *Preventive Medicine* 7 (1978):173–95.

33. Huang, Z., et al., *Journal of the American Medical Association* (1997), cited in "Weight Gain Increases Risk of Breast Cancer," Associated Press, November 4, 1997.

34. Barnard, N. D., et al., "Beliefs about Dietary Factors in Breast Cancer among American Women, 1991–1995," *Preventive Medicine* 26 (1997):109–13.

35. Ibid.

36. Ibid.

37. Hirayama, T., "Diet and Cancer," *Nutrition and Cancer* 1 (1979a):67–81. See also Colditz, G. A., et al., "Diet and Lung Cancer: A Review of the Epidemiologic Evidence in Humans," *Archives of Internal Medicine* 147 (1987):157–60; and *International Journal of Cancer* 78 (1998):430–6, cited in "Fruits, Carrots May Reduce Lung Cancer Risk," Reuters, November 25, 1999.

38. Cited in "Fruits, Carrots May Reduce Lung Cancer Risk."

39. Ibid.

40. Key, "Dietary Habits and Mortality."

41. Ibid.

42. Frentzel-Beyme, "Vegetarian Diets and Colon Cancer."

43. "12 Myths about Beef: A Dozen of the Most Popular Misconceptions about America's Most Popular Meat," National Cattlemen's Association, American Angus Association, West Salem, OH, publication date unknown; distributed by the National Cattlemen's Association, 1993.

44. Health Professionals Follow-up Study, reported in "Dairy Products Linked to Prostate Cancer," Associated Press, April 5, 2000.

45. Jacobsen, B. K., et al., "Does High Soy Milk Intake Reduce Prostate Cancer Incidence?" *Cancer Causes, Control* 9 (1998):553–7.

46. Cook, N., et al., "Beta-Carotene Supplementation for Patients with Low Baseline Levels and Decreased Risk of Total and Prostate Carcinoma," *Cancer* 86 (1999):1783–92; see also Zhang, S., et al., "Dietary Carotenoids and Vitamins

A, C, and E and Risk of Breast Cancer," *Journal of the National Cancer Institute* 86 (1999):1783–92.

47. Giovannucci E., et al., "Tomatoes, Tomato-Based Products, Lycopene, and Cancer: Review of the Epidemiologic Literature," *Journal of the National Cancer Institute*, 91 (1999):317–31; see also Giovannucci, *Journal of the National Cancer Institute*, 87 (1995):1767–76.

48. *Journal of the National Cancer Institute* 92 (2000):61–8, cited in "Vegetables Lower Prostate Cancer Risk," *Loma Linda University Vegetarian Nutrition and Health Letter*, March 2000.

49. Physicians Committee for Responsible Medicine Cancer Awareness Survey, 1999, reported in *Good Medicine* (Autumn 1999), 7.

50. "12 Myths about Beef."

51. Willet, Walter, et al., "Relation of Meat, Fat, and Fiber Intake to the Risk of Colon Cancer . . . ," *New England Journal of Medicine* December 13, 1990; Willet quoted in Kolata, Gina, "Animal Fat Is Tied to Colon Cancer," *New York Times*, December 13, 1990.

52. American Association of Endocrine Surgeons Presidential Address: Beyond Surgery, Caldwell Esselstyn, San Jose, CA, April 15, 1991; www.heartattackproof.com/address01.

53. Singh, P. N., et al., "Dietary Risk Factors for Colon Cancer in a Low-Risk Population," *American Journal of Epidemiology* 148 (1998):761–74.

54. Ibid.

55. Ibid.

56. Ibid.

57. O'Keefe, S. J., et al., "Rarity of Colon Cancer in Africans Is Associated with Low Animal Product Consumption, Not Fiber," *American Journal of Gastroenterology* 94 (1999):1373–80.

58. Ibid.

59. Reported in *Good Medicine* (Autumn 1999), p. 7.

60. Cheeke, Peter, *Contemporary Issues in Animal Agriculture,* 2nd ed. (Danville, IL: Interstate Publishers, 1999), p. 50.

61. Holerton, Gene, *The Beef-Eater's Guide to Modern Meat* (Los Angeles: Holerton Publishing, 1998), p. 77.

62. Quoted in "Behavior More Key Than Genes in Cancer," Reuters, January 21, 2000.

63. "12 Myths about Beef."

chapter 4 The Great American Diet Roller Coaster

1. Brown, Lester, "Obesity Epidemic Threatens Health in Exercise-Deprived Countries," Worldwatch Institute, December 19, 2000.

2. Allison, D., et al., "Annual Deaths Attributable to Obesity in the United States," *Journal of the American Medical Association* 16 (1999):1530–8.

3. Root, Marty, "Obesity and Health: A Hard Look at the Data," New Century Nutrition, 2000.

4. Ibid.

5. Ibid.

6. Ibid.

7. Mokdad, A., et al., "The Spread of the Obesity Epidemic in the United States," *Journal of the American Medical Association* 282 (1999):1519–22.

8. Wyatt, C., et al., "Dietary Intake of Sodium, Potassium, and Blood Pressure in Lacto-Ovo Vegetarians," *Nutrition Research* 15 (1995):819–30; see also Kahn, H. S., et al., "Stable Behaviors Associated with Adults'10–Year Change in Body Mass Index and Likelihood of Gain at the Waist," *American Journal of Public Health* 87 (1997):747–54; and Key, T., et al., "Prevalence of Obesity Is Low in People Who Do Not Eat Meat," *British Medical Journal* 313 (1996):816–7.

9. Author's estimate after extensive consultation with physicians and dietitians who are familiar with the vegan community.

10. Hardinge, M. G., et al., "Nutritional Studies of Vegetarians," *Journal of Clinical Nutrition* 2 (1954):73–82; Freeland-Graves, J. H., et al., "Zinc Status of Vegetarians," *Journal of the American Dietetic Association* 77 (1980):655–61; Key, et al., "Obesity Is Low."

11. Troiano, R., et al., "Overweight Children and Adolescents . . . ," *Pediatrics* 101 (1998):497–504; Troiano, R., "Overweight Prevalence and Trends for Children and Adolescents," *Archives of Pediatric and Adolescent Medicine* 149 (1995):1085–91.

12. Author's estimate based on lengthy discussions with many physicians and dietitians who are familiar with the vegetarian and vegan communities.

13. Munoz, K., et al., "Food Intakes of U.S. Children and Adolescents Compared with Recommendations," *Pediatrics* (September 1997):323–9. See also, "Few Young People Eat Wisely, Study Shows," *New York Times*, September 3, 1997, A-12.

14. Author's estimate based on lengthy discussions with many physicians and dietitians familiar who are with the vegetarian and vegan communities.

15. Berkeley Farms butter served in Marie Callender restaurants in Santa Cruz, California.

16. Burger King Corporation, "Nutritional Information," 2000.

17. Burger King, "Nutritional Information."

18. Mangels, Reed, "Guide to Burgers and Dogs," *Vegetarian Journal* (May/June 2000).

19. Worldwatch Institute, *State of the World 2000* (New York: W. W. Norton, 2000), p. xviii.

20. Roth, Geneen, *Feeding The Hungry Heart* (New York: The Bobbs-Merrill Company, 1982), pp. 1–2.

21. "Demand for Meat Diet Fattens Prices," *Meat Industry Insights*, October 26, 1999.

22. Atkins, Robert, *Dr. Atkins' New Diet Revolution* (New York: Avon Books, 1999), front and back cover.

23. Dr. Atkins' Web site (2000): www.atkinsdiet.com/faq.

24. American Institute for Cancer Research, "Fad Diets Versus Dietary Guidelines" (1999), www.aicr.org/faddiets.

25. Ibid.

26. Weil, Andrew, *Eating Well for Optimum Health* (New York, NY: Alfred Knopf, 2000), p. 55.

27. American Institute for Cancer Research, "Fad Diets."

28. *Journal of the American Dietetic Association* 77 (1980):264, cited in McDougall, J., "Americans Are Getting Fatter—and Dying from It," EarthSave (2000), www.earthsave.org/news/hiprotein.htm.

29. *International Journal of Obesity Related Metabolic Disorders* 19 (1995):811.

30. Millennium Lecture Series Symposium on the Great Nutrition Debate, Jefferson Auditorium, U.S. Department of Agriculture, February 24, 2000.

31. Cited in McDougall, "Americans Are Getting Fatter."

32. This was brought forth by Dr. Dean Ornish at the Great Nutrition Debate, U.S. Department of Agriculture, February 24, 2000. Dr. Westman was present and spoke, but did not dispute this finding.

33. Great Nutrition Debate, February 24, 2000.

34. Lawrence, Jean, "High Fat, Low Carbs, What's the Harm," *CBS Healthwatch, Medscape*, Dec 1999.

35. Hellmich, Nanci, "Success of Atkins Diet Is in the Calories," *USA Today*, Nov 8, 2000.

36. Great Nutrition Debate, February 24, 2000.

37. Ibid.

38. Atwood, Charles, "Enter the 'Zone': A Giant Leap Backwards" (1998) www.vegsource/attwood/zone.htm.

39. Sears, Barry, *Enter the Zone* (New York: Harper/Collins, 1995).

40. From Barry Sears' Web site (2000): www.zonediet.com/site/Tools/FAQs/FAQsHome.nsf.

41. Putnam, Judy, and Gerber, Shirley, "Trends in U.S. Food Supply 1970–97," in *America's Eating Habits: Changes and Consequences* (n.d.), USDA, Economic Research Service, Food and Rural Economics Division, Agriculture Information Bulletin No. 750.

42. Data from USDA's CNPP *Nut. Insights* #5 (1998) at www.usda.gov/fcs/cnpp.htm, and NHANES III, Phase 1.

43. Sears, *Enter the Zone.*

44. Ibid., p. 97.

45. Raymond, Jennifer, "Caution: Approaching the Zone" (1998) www.cyberveg.org/navs/voice/zone.html.

46. Barry Sears' Web site (2000): www.zonediet.com/site/Tools/FAQs/FAQsHome.nsf.

47. Ibid.

48. Lindner, Lawrence, "Eating Right," *Washington Post*, May 9, 2000, Z18.

49. Sears, *Enter the Zone*, p. 259.

50. Ibid., p. 30.

51. Liebman, Bonnie, "Carbo-Phobia: Zoning Out on the New Diet Books," *Nutrition Action* (July/Augst 1996).

52. Sears, *Enter the Zone*, p. 102.

53. Ibid., p. 206.

54. Liebman, "Carbo-Phobia."
55. Sears, *Enter the Zone*, pp. 3, 96, back cover.
56. Ibid., p. 73.
57. Barry Sears' Web site (2000):
    www.zonediet.com/site/Tools/FAQs/FAQsHome.nsf.
58. Liebman, "Carbo-Phobia."
59. Sears, *Enter the Zone*, pp. 67, 69.
60. Havala, S., et al., "Position of the American Dietetic Association: Vegetarian
    Diets," *Journal of the American Dietetic Association* 93 (1993): 1317–9.
61. Quoted in Melina, Vesanto, et al., *Becoming Vegetarian* (MacMillan Canada,
    1994), p. 37. For harmful effects of unnecessarily high intake of animal pro-
    tein, see McCarty, M. F., "Vegan Proteins May Reduce Risk of Cancer, Obe-
    sity, and Cardiovascular Disease . . . ," *Medical Hypotheses* (December 1999),
    pp. 53, 459–85; Feskanich, D., et al., "Protein Consumption and Bone Frac-
    tures in Women," *American Journal of Epidemiology* 143 (1996):472–9.
62. Durning, Alan and Brough, Holly, "Taking Stock: Animal Farming and the
    Environment," Worldwatch Paper #103 (July 1991), p. 28.
63. Bell, G., *Textbook of Physiology and Biochemistry*, 4th ed. (New York:
    Williams and Wilkins, Ballentine, 1954), pp. 167–70.
64. "Protein Requirements," Food and Agriculture Organization, World Health
    Organization Expert Group, United Nations Conference, Rome, 1965.
65. Food and Nutrition Board, *Recommended Daily Allowances* (Washington DC:
    National Academy of Sciences, n.d.).
66. As per numerous WHO publications.
67. Messina, Virginia, and Messina, Mark, *The Dietitian's Guide to Vegetarian
    Diets* (Gaithersburg, MD: Aspen Publishers, 1996), pp. 102, 46–8.
68. Sears, *Enter the Zone*, p. 47.
69. Ibid., p. 73.
70. D'Adamo, Peter, *Eat Right for Your Type* (New York: Putnam, 1996).
71. "Eating According to Your Blood Type: A Bloody Bad Idea," *Tufts University
    Health and Nutrition Letter*, August 1997.
72. D'Adamo, *Eat Right for Your Type*, p. 101.
73. Peter D'Adamo's Web site (2000): www.dadamo.com/lr4yt.
74. Red Cross data, 2000.
75. Peter D'Adamo's Web site (2000): www.dadamo.com/forum/board-add/index.
76. Personal communication with author. See also Gould, et al., "Changes in My-
    ocardial Perfusion Abnormalities by Positron Emission Topography after
    Long-Term, Intense Risk Factor Modification," *Journal of the American Medi-
    cal Association* 274 (1995):894–901.
77. Peter D'Adamo's Web site (2000): www.dadamo.com/forum/board-add/index.
78. D'Adamo, *Eat Right for Your Type*, p. 55.
79. "The Blood Type Diet: Latest Diet Scam" (2000); www.vegsource.com/arti-
    cles/blood_hype.
80. D'Adamo, *Eat Right for Your Type*, pp. 6–7.
81. Quoted in Barnard, Neal, *The Power of Your Plate*, (Summertown, TN: Book
    Publishing Company, 1990), p. 170.

82. Ibid., p. 169.

83. "The Blood Type Diet."

84. "Eating According to Your Blood Type."

85. Personal communication with author.

86. D'Adamo, *Eat Right for Your Type*, front cover.

87. Stare, Fredrick, and Whelan, Elizabeth, *Fad-Free Nutrition* (Alameda, CA: Hunter House Publishers, 1998), pp. 209–11.

88. List compiled by author from various sources, including Havala, Suzanne, *The Complete Idiot's Guide to Being Vegetarian* (New York: Alpha Books/Macmillan General Reference, 1999), pp. 26–9, 130; Avery-Grant, Anika, *The Vegetarian Female* (Garden City, NY: Avery Publishing, 1999); Dorfman, Lisa, *The Vegetarian Sports Nutrition Guide* (New York: John Wiley & Sons, 2000).

chapter 5 A Healthy Plant-Based Diet

1. Based on USDA figures for nutrients contained in wheat flour (whole grain) and wheat flour (white, all-purpose, unenriched). See www.nal.usda.gov/fnic/foodcomp/contact.html.

2. Ibid.

3. Gardner, Gary, and Halweil, Brian, "Escaping Hunger, Escaping Excess," *WorldWatch*, July/August 2000, p. 29.

4. Ibid., p. 33.

5. Letter to the Secretaries of the U.S. Department of Health and Human Services and the U.S. Department of Agriculture signed by Dr. George Blackburn of Harvard Medical School, Dr. Kelly Brownell of Yale University, Dr. Marion Nestle of New York University, Dr. Walter Willett of the Harvard School of Public Health, the American Public Health Association, the American School Health Association, C. Everett Koop's "Shape Up America!" Organization, the Society for Nutrition Education, and 39 other professors and health groups, cited in "Sugar Consumption Off the Charts," Center for Science in the Public Interest news release, December 30, 1998.

6. Gardner and Halweil, "Escaping Hunger," p. 26.

7. Ibid., p. 30.

8. Quoted in Suzuki, David, *The Sacred Balance* (Vancouver, BC: Greystone Books, 1997), p. 21.

9. "California's 'All Organic' School Lunches," *Meat Industry Insights*, August 19, 1999.

10. Ibid.

11. Nathan, I., et al., "A Longitudinal Study of the Growth of Matched Pairs of Vegetarian and Omnivorous Children . . .," *European Journal of Clinical Nutrition* 51 (1997):20–5; O'Connell, J. M., et al., "Growth of Vegetarian Children: The Farm Study," *Pediatrics* 84 (1989):475–89; Sanders, T. A. B., "Growth and Development of British Vegan Children," *American Journal of Clinical Nutrition* 48 (1988):822–5.

12. Craig, W., "Iron Status of Vegetarians," *American Journal of Clinical Nutrition* 59 (Sup) (1994): 1233S–37S; Messina, Virginia, and Messina, Mark, *The Dietitian's Guide to Vegetarian Diets: Issues and Applications* (Gaithersburg, MD: Aspen Publishers, 1996).

13. "Meat's Nutrients and Cognitive Development," Facts from the Meat Board: Nutrition, National Live Stock and Meat Board, 1995, p. 4.

14. Dwyer, J. T., et al., "Mental Age and I.Q. of Predominately Vegetarian Children," *Journal of the American Dietetic Association*, 76 (1980):142–7.

15. Statement on National Cattlemen's Beef Association Web site in 2000.

16. Murphy, Dan, "Great Debate Builds the Rationale for Eating Meat," www.meatingplace.com, August 11, 2000.

17. McMurray, M., "Changes in Lipid and Lipoprotein Levels and Body Weight in the Tarahumara Indians after Consumption of an Affluent Diet," *New England Journal of Medicine* 325 (1991):1704.

18. Ibid.

19. Ibid.

20. Fishwick, Marshall, ed., *Ronald Revisited: The World of Ronald McDonald* (Bowling Green, OH: Bowling Green University Popular Press, 1983), p. 118.

21. Barnard, Neal, *The Power of Your Plate* (Summertown, TN: Book Publishing Company, 1990), p. 20.

22. Schlosser, Eric, *Fast Food Nation* (New York: Houghton Mifflin, 2001), p. 49.

23. Ibid., p. 50.

24. Ibid.

25. Coleman, Jennifer, "Soft Drink Firms Defend Contracts with School Districts," *Santa Cruz Sentinel*, September 27, 2000, C-2.

26. Hill, Julia Butterfly, *The Legacy of Luna: The Story of a Tree, a Woman, and the Struggle to Save the Redwoods* (San Francisco: HarperSanFrancisco, 2000).

27. Personal communication with author.

28. Collins, Karen, "What Kind of Carbohydrate," American Institute for Cancer Research, November 26, 2000.

29. Simopoulos, Artemis, and Robinson, Jo, *The Omega Diet: The Livesaving Nutritional Program Based on the Diet of the Island of Crete* (New York: Harper Perennial, 1999), p. 29.

30. Havala, Suzanne, *Being Vegetarian For Dummies* (New York: Hungry Minds, 2001).

31. Melina, Vesanto, et al., *Becoming Vegetarian: The Complete Guide to Adopting a Healthy Vegetarian Diet* (Summertown, TN: Book Publishing Company, 1995); Davis, Brenda, and Melina, Vesanto, *Becoming Vegan: The Complete Guide to Adopting a Healthy Plant-Based Diet* (Summertown, TN: Book Publishing Company, 2000).

32. Hu, Frank, et al., "Frequent Nut Consumption and Risk of Coronary Heart Disease in Women: Prospective Cohort Study," *British Medical Journal*, 317:14 (1998):1341–5.

33. Personal communication with author.

34. Weil, Andrew, *Eating Well for Optimum Health* (New York: Alfred A. Knopf, 2000), p. 117.

35. American Heart Association, *Heart And Stroke Facts: 1995 Statistical Supplement* (Dallas, TX: American Heart Association National Center, 1994).

36. Gardner, Gary, and Halweil, Brian, "Underfed and Overfed," Worldwatch paper #150, March 2000, p. 33.

37. "The Politics of Meat and Dairy," *EarthSave News*, www.earthsave.org/news/polsmd.htm

38. "Dietary News," *Rachel's Environment and Health Weekly*, January 2, 1997.

39. "Dietary News."

40. Halweil, Brian, "United States Leads World Meat Stampede," Worldwatch Issues Paper, July 2, 1998.

41. Ibid.

chapter 6 Got BS?

1. Physicians Committee for Responsible Medicine, "The 'Milk Mustache' Ads Are All Wet," *Good Medicine*, Spring 1999, p. 8. In fact, African American men have been excluded from most research studies on osteoporosis because of their better bone density.

2. Ibid.

3. Ibid.

4. Feskanich D, et al., "Milk, Dietary Calcium, and Bone Fractures in Women . . . " *American Journal of Public Health* 87 (1997):992–7.

5. Lloyd, T., "Adult Female Hip Bone Density Reflects Teenage Sports-Exercise Patterns, But Not Teenage Calcium Intake," *Pediatrics* 106: 1 (July 2000):40–4.

6. "Doctors Denounce Milk Ads Starring Marc Anthony, Britney Spears, Others, as Deceptive; Group Petitions FTC to Investigate Health Claims," U.S. Newswire, July 25, 2000.

7. Flatz, G., "Genetics of Lactose Digestion in Humans," in Harris, H. and Hirschhorn, K., eds., *Advances in Human Genetics* (New York: Plenum Publishers, 1987); Cuatrecasas, P., et al., "Lactase Deficiency in the Adult: A Common Occurrence," *Lancet* 1 (1965):14–8; Bayless, T., et al., "A Racial Difference in Incidence of Lactase Deficiency . . .," *Journal of the American Medical Association* 197 (1966):968–72; Mishkin, S., "Dairy Sensitivity, Lactose Malabsorption . . . ," *American Journal of Clinical Nutrition* 65 (1997): 564–7; Scrimshaw, N., et al., "The Acceptability of Milk and Milk Products in Populations with a High Prevalence of Lactose Intolerance," *American Journal of Clinical Nutrition* 48 (1988):1083–5.

8. *Wall Street Journal*, February 23, 1999.

9. "Dairy Farmers of Canada Response to *Becoming Vegetarian*," Dairy Bureau of Canada, 1996.

10. Davis, Brenda, et al., "The Rebuttal: to the Dairy Farmer's of Canada Response to *Becoming Vegetarian*," Fall 1996; www.nutrispeak.com/becoming.htm.

11. "Dairy Farmers of Canada Response."

12. Weaver, C. M., et al., "Dietary Calcium: Adequacy of a Vegetarian Diet," *American Journal of Clinical Nutrition* 59(Sup)(1994):1238S–41S.

13. *Bowes and Church's Food Value of Portions Commonly Used*, 17th edition, ed. by J. Pennington (Philadelphia: Lippincott Williams and Wilkins, 1998). See also Weaver, C., et al., "Absorbability of Calcium from Common Beans," *Journal of Food Science* 58 (1993): 1401–3, and Davis, et al., "Rebuttal."

14. "Dairy Farmers of Canada Response."

15. Quoted in Davis, et al., "Rebuttal."

16. "Dairy Farmers of Canada Response."

17. Davis, et al., "Rebuttal." See also, Weaver, et al., "Dietary Calcium"; Hardinge, M., et al., "Nutritional Studies of Vegetarians," *American Journal of Clinical Nutrition* 2 (1954):73–82; Freeland-Graves, J., et al., "Zinc Status of Vegetarians," *Journal of the American Dietetic Association* 77 (1980):S655–61; Calkins, B., et al., "Diet, Nutrition Intake and Metabolism in Populations . . .," *American Journal of Clinical Nutrition* 1 (1982):131; Carlson, E., et al., "A Comparative Evaluation of Vegan, Vegetarian, and Omnivore Diets," *Journal of Plant Foods* 6 (1985): 89–100; Janelle, K. et al., "Nutrient Intakes and Eating Behavior Scores of Vegetarian and Nonvegetarian Women," *Journal of the American Dietetic Association* 95 (1995):180–5.

18. Nordin, B., "Calcium Requirement Is a Sliding Scale," *American Journal of Clinical Nutrition* 71 (June 2000):1381–3.

19. Cumming, R. G., et al., "Case-Control Study of Risk Factors for Hip Fractures in the Elderly," *American Journal of Epidemiology* 139 (1994):493–503.

20. Recker, R., "The Effect Of Milk Supplements on Calcium Metabolism, Bone Metabolism, and Calcium Balance," *American Journal of Clinical Nutrition* 41 (1985):254.

21. Ibid.

22. Sebastian, Anthony, quoted in untitled article by Douglas Fox in U.S. News online, U.S. News and World Report, Inc., October 30, 2000.

23. McDougall, John, *McDougall's Medicine* (Piscataway NJ: New Century Publishers, 1985), p. 67.

24. Ibid.

25. Abelow, B. J., et al., "Cross-cultural Association Between Dietary Animal Protein and Hip Fracture: A Hypothesis," *Calif Tissue Int* 50 (1992):14–8.

26. Ibid.

27. Campbell, T. C., et al., "Diet and Health in Rural China: Lessons Learned and Unlearned," *Nutrition Today* 34:3 (1999):116–23.

28. Ibid.

29. Statement by Connie Weaver, Ph.D., of Purdue University, at the Physicians Committee for Responsible Medicine's Summit on the Dietary Guidelines 2000, Georgetown University Medical Center, September 1998.

30. Ibid.

31. Havala, Suzanne, *The Complete Idiot's Guide to Being Vegetarian* (New York: Alpha Books/Macmillan General Reference, 1999), p. 43.

32. Quoted in *Vegetarian Times*, June 2000, p. 20.

33. "Dairy Farmers of Canada Response."

34. Davis, et al., "Rebuttal."
35. Draper, A., et al., "The Energy and Nutrient Intakes of Different Types of Vegetarian . . .," *British Journal of Nutrition* 69 (1993):3–19; Carlson, et al., "Vegan, Vegetarian and Omnivore Diets"; Hughes, et al., "Riboflavin Levels in the Diet and Breast Milk of Vegans and Omnivores," *Proceedings of Nutritional Science* 38 (1979):95A; Janelle, et al., "Nutrient Intakes and Eating Behavior Scores," 180–6.
36. Davis, et al., "Rebuttal."
37. Ibid.
38. Ibid.
39. Anderson J. W., et al., "Meta-Analysis of the Effects of Soy Protein Intake on Serum Lipids," *New England Journal of Medicine* 333 (1995):276–82; Sirtori, C. R., et al., "Double-Blind Study of the Addition of High-Protein Soya Milk vs. Cow's Milk to the Diet of Patients . . . ," *British Journal of Nutrition* 82 (1999):91–6.
40. Jacobsen, B. K., et al., "Does High Soy Milk Intake Reduce Prostate Cancer Incidence?" *Cancer Causes, Control* 9 (1998):553–7.
41. "Soymilk Makes the Grade with Federal Diet Panel," Physician's Committee for Responsible Medicine news release, February 11, 2000.
42. Begley, Sharon, "The End of Antibiotics," *Newsweek*, March 28, 1994, pp. 47–51.
43. Iacono G., et al., "Intolerance of Cow's Milk and Chronic Constipation in Children," *New England Journal of Medicine* 339 (1998):110–4.
44. "U.S. Public Wrong About Dairy in Rest of World," *The Dairy Express*, October 29, 1999, p. 6.
45. Ibid.

chapter 7 Unsafe On Any Plate

1. Suzuki, D., and Dressel, H., *From Naked Ape to Superspecies* (Toronto, Stoddart Publishing, 1999), pp. 9–10.
2. Ibid.
3. Ibid., p. 12.
4. Suzuki, David, *The Sacred Balance: Rediscovering Our Place in Nature* (Vancouver, BC: Greystone Books, 1997), p. 128.
5. Margulin, Lynn, and Sagan, Dorion, *Microcosmos: Four Billion Years of Microbial Evolution* (New York: Simon and Schuster, 1986), cited in Fox, Nicols, *Spoiled: The Dangerous Truth about a Food Chain Gone Haywire* (New York: Basic Books/HarperCollins, 1997), p. 10.
6. Suzuki and Dressel, *Naked Ape*, p. 17.
7. Presentation by Professor John Hermon-Taylor, medical researcher at St. George's Medical School, London, to the Medical Journalists Association at the Royal Society of Medicine, London, January 24, 2000; reported in "Micro-Organisms in Milk Cause Crohn's Disease," Environment News Service, London, January 27, 2000.

8. Stephenson, Jean, "When Microbes Are on the Menu," *Harvard Health Letter*, December 1994.
9. "Sara Lee Fourth Quarter Net Falls on Meat Recall," *Meat Industry Insights*, August 7, 1999.
10. "Apples Don't Do Drugs," Letter to the Editor, *WorldWatch*, March/April 1998, p. 6.
11. Sifry, Micah, "How Money in Politics Hurts You," *Dollars and Sense*, July/August 2000, p. 18.
12. Fox, *Spoiled*, p. 256.
13. Public Citizen Foundation, "A Citizen's Guide to Fighting Food Irradiation," (2000), p. 13.
14. Ibid., pp. 13–6.
15. Murphy, Dan, "Rip Job on Irradiation Sad Spin-Off of Activists' Publicity Push," www.meatingplace.com, October 6, 2000.
16. "Irradiation Fact Sheet—January 2000," National Cattlemen's Beef Association.
17. "Consumers and Companies Battle Over Meat Labels," *Meat Industry Insights*, May 29, 1999. And "Battle Over Labels for Irradiated Beef," *Meat Industry Insights*, June 4, 1999. And "USDA Finally Approves Rules for Meat Irradiation," *Meat Industry Insights*, December 17, 1999. For amount of radiation involved, see Gibbs, Gary, *The Food That Would Last Forever* (Garden City Park, NY: Avery Publishing, 1993), p. 10.
18. Gillette, Becky, "Try Our Nukeburgers," *E*, July/August 2000, p. 40.
19. Quoted in Sassoon, R., "The Irradiation Controversy," *Food Safety Issues* 39, August 20, 2000, p. 27.
20. Quoted in Gillette, "Nukeburgers," p. 41.
21. "USDA Approves Rules for Meat Irradiation." See also "Microbiologists Battle E. Coli," *Meat Industry Insights*, October 26, 1999.
22. Fox, *Spoiled*, p. 346.
23. Women who consume hamburgers, beef, and bacon well done have almost five times the risk of breast cancer as women who consume these meats rare or medium-done. Zheng, W., et al., "Well-Done Meat Intake and the Risk of Breast Cancer," *Journal of the National Cancer Institute* 90 (1998):1724–9; see also accompanying editorial, "Dietary Mutagens and the Risk of Breast Cancer," *Journal of the National Cancer Institute* 90 (1998):1687–9.
24. Fox, *Spoiled*.
25. Ibid., p. 216.
26. Eisnitz, Gail, *Slaughterhouse: The Shocking Story of Greed, Neglect, and Inhumane Treatment inside the U.S. Meat Industry* (Amherst, NY: Prometheus Books,1997), pp. 37–9.
27. "Deadly E. Coli Bug May Affect Half of Cattle," *Meat Industry Insights*, November 15, 1999.
28. "USDA May Tighten E. Coli Controls," *Meat Industry Insights*, November 15, 1999.
29. Karleff, Ian, "Canadian Scientists Test E. Coli Vaccine on Source," Reuters News Service, August 10, 2000.

30. Fox, *Spoiled*, p. 10.
31. Ibid., p. 178.
32. Kaldor, J., and Speed, B., "Guillain-Barre' Syndrome and Campylobacter Jejuni: A Serological Study," *British Medical Journal* 288 (1984):1867–70; Kuroki, A., et al., "Guillain-Barre' Syndrome Associated with Campylobacter Infection," in *Microbial Ecology in Health and Disease* (New York: Wiley, 1994).
33. CDC estimate, cited in Fox, *Spoiled*, p. 191.
34. "*Consumer Reports* Finds 71 Percent of Store-Bought Chicken Contains Harmful Bacteria," Consumers Union press release, February 23, 1998. See also "Safety Last—The Politics of E. Coli and Other Food-Borne Killers," statement of Charles Lewis, Chairman and Executive Director, Center for Public Integrity, February 26, 1998.
35. "How Hazardous Is Your Turkey?" Center for Science in the Public Interest news release, November 19, 1998.
36. "Biological Control Could Reduce Food Safety Problems of Poultry," *Science Report*, University of Wisconsin, Madison, December 10, 1990.
37. Ibid.
38. Behar, Richard, and Kramer, Michael, "Something Smells Fowl," *Time*, October 17, 1994, pp. 42–5.
39. Fox, *Spoiled*, p. 194.
40. Behar and Kramer, "Something Smells Fowl."
41. Fox, *Spoiled*, p. 197.
42. Ibid., p. 179.
43. Barnard, Neal, *The Power of Your Plate* (Summertown, TN: Book Publishing Company, 1990), p. 104.
44. Ibid.
45. Ibid.
46. Ibid., p. 165.
47. St. Louis, M., et al., "The Emergence of Grade A Eggs as a Major Source of Salmonella Enteritis Infections," *Journal of the American Medical Association* 25 (1988):2105.
48. Fox, *Spoiled*, p. 18.
49. Quoted in Simmons, R., "Eggs a Health Risk?" *Food Safety Issues* 39, September 24, 2000, p. 29.
50. Caroline Smith DeWaal, quoted in "House Modifies Planned Egg Safety Rules," Associated Press, May 5, 2000.
51. Vorman, Julie, "US Groups Seek Food Safety Warning Label on Meat," Reuters News Service, January 13, 2000.
52. "CDC Says Deadly E. Coli Cases Up Sharply in 1998," *Meat Industry Insights*, March 12, 1999.
53. According to Mike Doyle, food safety expert at the University of Georgia. See, "USDA Targets Deadly Bacteria in Hot Dots and Meat," *Meat Industry Insights*, May 26, 1999.
54. Center for Science in the Public Interest, "Protect Your Unborn Baby," 2000.
55. Vorman, "Food Safety Warning Label on Meat."

56. Ibid.
57. Ibid.
58. Bjerklie, "World's Safest Meat Supply?"
59. Ibid.
60. Fox, *Spoiled*, p. 213.
61. Ibid., p. 214.
62. Bjerklie, "World's Safest Meat Supply?"
63. Ibid.
64. Ibid.
65. Ibid.

chapter 8 Policing the Pathogens

1. "Safety Last—The Politics of E. Coli and Other Food-Borne Killers," Statement of Charles Lewis, Chairman and Executive Director, The Center for Public Integrity, February 26, 1998.
2. Fabi, Randy, "Millions of Pounds of Turkey Recalled for Listeria," Reuters News Service, December 15, 2000.
3. Fauber, John, "Recalls of Tainted Meat This Year Are Highest Ever," *Milwaukee Journal Sentinel*, August 18, 2000.
4. Ibid.
5. "Safety Last."
6. Personal communication with author.
7. "Safety Last."
8. "Myths and Facts about Beef Production—Hormones and Antibiotics," National Cattlemen's Beef Association, displayed on the Web site of the National Cattlemen's Beef Association in 2000.
9. Bjerklie, Steve, "Starting Over," *Meat Processing* (March 1999), p. 90.
10. Personal communication with author.
11. "Industry Forum," *Meat and Poultry* (March 1998).
12. "Safety Last."
13. Gay, Lance, "Meat from Diseased Animals Approved for Consumers," Scripps Howard News Service, July 14, 2000.
14. Vorman, Julie, "Feces, Vomit on Raw Meat a Growing Risk," Reuters News Service, September 6, 2000.
15. "Agricultural Inspectors Killed at Sausage Factory," *Santa Cruz Sentinel*, June 22, 2000, A-6.
16. Fisher, Jeffrey, *The Plague Makers* (New York: Simon and Schuster, 1994), p. 15.
17. Ibid., p. 30.
18. Ibid., p. 31.
19. Institute of Medicine, "Human Health Risks from the Subtherapeutic Use of Penicillin or Tetracyclines in Animal Feed" (Washington, DC: National Academy Press, 1989).
20. Institute of Medicine, "Emerging Infections: Microbial Threats to Health in the United States" (Washington, DC: National Academy Press, 1992).

21. "World Health Organization Meeting on the Medical Impact of the Use of Antimicrobial Drugs in Food Animals, Berlin, Germany, October 4 1997," WHO Press Release, October 20, 1997. See also, "Bill Summary for H.R. 3266—Preservation of Essential Antibiotics for Human Diseases Act of 1999," Sponsor Sherrod Brown. Original cosponsors: Henry Waxman, Louise Slaughter.

22. *Science* 279 (1998):996–7.

23. Glynn, K., et al., "Emergence of Multidrug-Resistant Salmonella Enterica Serotype Typhimurium DT104 Infections in the United States," *New England Journal of Medicine* 338 (1998):1333–8.

24. Smith, Kirk, et al., "Quinolone-Resistant Campylobacter Jejuni Infections in Minnesota, 1992–1998," *New England Journal of Medicine* 340 (1999):1525–32.

25. "Hidden Costs of Animal Factories," *Rachel's Environment and Health Weekly*, March 9, 2000.

26. Grady, D., "A Move to Limit Antibiotic Use in Animal Feed," *New York Times*, March 8, 1999, A1.

27. Mellon, Margaret, "If Antibiotics Are to Work as Medicine, They Shouldn't Be Used to Fatten Chicken," Humane Society of the United States, 1999.

28. Centers for Disease Control and Prevention, "Emergence of Fluoro-quinolone-Resistant Campylobacter in the United States," *The C.A.U.S.E.* 2 (January 1998).

29. Grady, "Limit Antibiotic Use."

30. "Are Antibiotics in Feed a Menace or a Miracle?" *Annals of Meat, Poultry, and Seafood* (April 1999).

31. Fox, Nicols, *Spoiled: The Dangerous Truth About a Food Chain Gone Haywire* (New York: Basic Books/HarperCollins, 1997), p. 11.

32. Grady, D., "Scientists see higher use of antibiotics on farms," *New York Times*, January 28, 2001.

33. Ibid.

34. Ibid.

35. "The Consequences for Food Safety of the Use of Fluoroquinolones in Food Animals," Editorial, *New England Journal of Medicine* (May 20, 1999).

36. Ibid.

37. Lieberman, Patricia, in "Ban the Use of Certain Antibiotics to Fatten Farm Animals, Groups Ask," Center for Science in the Public Interest news release, March 9, 1999.

38. Ibid.

39. "Fact Sheet—June 1998," National Cattlemen's Beef Association.

40. Grady, "Limit Antibiotic Use."

41. "Factsheet—January 2000," National Cattlemen's Beef Association.

42. "The Bad Seed," *Rachel's Environment and Health Weekly*, September 2, 1999.

43. "Myths and Facts about Beef Production."

44. "European Scientists Say U.S. Beef Unsafe," *Santa Cruz Sentinel*, May 4, 1999, A-8.

45. Carter, Janelle, "U.S. Will Use Tariff to Ram Beef Down Europe's Throat," *Associated Press*, May 15, 1999.
46. "European Union Says Beef Hormone Can Cause Cancer," *Meat Industry Insights* (May 3, 1999).
47. Balter, Michael, "Scientific Cross-Claims Fly in Continuing Beef War," *Science*, May 28, 1999, pp. 1453–5.
48. Center for Science in the Public Interest, "U.S. Sold Beef with Cancer-Causing Hormone to Swiss," February 2, 2000.
49. Personal communication with author.
50. "Mad Cow Disease, Parts One and Two," *Rachel's Environment and Health Weekly*, July 9 and July 16, 1998.
51. Scott, Michael, et al., "Compelling Transgenic Evidence for Transmission of Bovine Spongiform Encephalopathy Prions in Humans," *Proceedings of the National Academy of Sciences* 151 (December 21, 1999):37–42.
52. Lemonick, Michael "Can It Happen Here?", *Time*, January 22, 2001.
53. Hansen, Michael, "The Reasons Why FDA's Feed Rule Won't Protect Us from BSE," *Genetic Engineering News* (July 1997), pp. 4, 40. See also, Altman, Lawrence, "FDA Proposal Would Ban Using Animal Tissue in Feed," *New York Times*, January 3, 1997, A14.
54. Darnton, John, "Britain Ties Deadly Brain Disease to Cow Ailment," *New York Times*, March 21, 1996, A1.
55. Cited in "Deaths from CJD . . . , " John von Radowitz, Medical Correspondent, PA News, January 20, 2000.
56. "Frequent Travelers to UK Banned from Donating Blood," *Journal of the American Veterinary Medical Association* (October 1, 1999).
57. Lipsky, Joshua, "Study Claims BSE-Infected French Cows Entered Food Supply," December 18, 2000, www.meatingplace.com.
58. Castle, Stephen and Woolf, Marie, "EU Wants Slaughter of 2m Cattle to Curb BSE," *The Independent*, November 30, 2000.
59. Lipsky, Joshua, "BSE-Contaminated Feed Sent to 70 Countries," www.meatingplace.com, February 6, 2001.
60. "Oprah Causes Beef Industry Flap," *Meat Processing* (June 1996), p. 8.
61. Quoted in Rampton, Sheldon, and Stauber, John, *Mad Cow U.S.A.: Could the Nightmare Happen Here?* (Monroe, ME: Common Courage Press, 1997), p. 21.
62. Petition by Paul F. Engler and Cactus Feeders, Inc. against Oprah Winfrey, Harpo Productions, Howard Lyman, and Cannon Communications, U.S. District Court, Texas, Northern District, May 28, 1996.
63. United States Court of Appeals for the Fifth Circuit, No. 98–10391.
64. Rampton, Sheldon, and Stauber, John, "One Hundred Percent All Beef Baloney: Lessons From the Oprah Trial," *PR Watch* 5:1 (First Quarter 1998).
65. "Summary of the Facts: CJD, BSE, and vCJD," National Cattlemen's Beef Association, 1999.
66. Rampton and Stauber, "One Hundred Percent All Beef Baloney."

67. Rampton and Stauber, *Mad Cow U.S.A.?* See also Institute of Food Science and Technology (UK), "Bovine Spongiform Encephalopathy (BSE)": Part 1/6, Part 1 of a 6-part position paper, 2000, www.easynet.co.uk/ifst/hottop5.htm.

68. "Feed makers violating rules meant to keep mad cow disease away: FDA" Associated Press, January 11, 2001.

69. Murphy, Dan, "Mad Cow made to order for activists; can industry react to their rhetoric?" www.meatingplace.com, January 26, 2001.

70. Cheng, Beverly, "Is the United States doing enough to prevent BSE?" www.meatingplace.com, January 19, 2001.

71. Boller, Francois, et al., "Diagnosis of Dementia: Clinicopathologic Correlations," *Neurology* (January 1989):76–79.

72. Manuelidis, E. E., et al., "Suggested Links between Different Types of Dementias: Creutzfeld-Jakob Disease, Alzheimer Disease, and Retroviral CNS Infections," *Alzheimer Disease and Associated Disorders* 3:1–2 (1989):s 100–9; see also Mulvihill, Keith, "Similarity Seen in Alzheimer's and Mad Cow Disease Proteins," Reuter's Health Information, August 26, 2000, and "Mad Cow, Alzheimer's Proteins Are Similar, Study Says," Reuters Science Headlines, August 23, 2000.

73. Estimate from Alzheimer's Association, Chicago, IL, 2000.

chapter 10 Old McDonald Had a Factory.

1. Duncan, I., "Can the Psychologist Measure Stress?" *New Scientist*, October 18, 1973.

2. *Animal Agriculture: Myths and Facts* (Arlington, VA: Animal Industry Foundation, 1989), p. 10.

3. Cheeke, Peter, *Contemporary Issues in Animal Agriculture*, 2nd ed. (Danville, IL: Interstate Publishers, 1999), p. 248.

4. "Bringing Home the Bacon: A Look Inside the Pork Industry," Humane Farming Association, 2000.

5. Ibid.

6. "Facts from the Meat Board: The Animal Welfare/Rights Challenge," Meat Science Department, National Live Stock and Meat Board, 1991.

7. Rollin, Bernard, *Farm Animal Welfare: Social, Bioethical and Research Issues* (Ames, IA: Iowa State University Press, 1995), p. 23.

8. Hall, M., "Heating Systems for Swine Buildings," *Hog Farm Management* (Dec 1975), p. 16.

9. Harrison, Ruth, *Animal Machines* (London: Vincent Stuart Ltd., 1964), p. 3.

10. Robbins, John, *Diet for a New America: How Your Food Choices Affect Your Health, Happiness, and the Future of Life on Earth* (Sausalito, CA: H. J. Kramer, 1987), p. xiv.

11. Smith, Gary, "A Perspective of John Robbins' *Diet for a New America*," in Cross, H. Russel, and Byers, Floyd M., eds., *Current Issues in Food Production: A Scientific Response to John Robbins' Diet For A New America*, sup-

ported by the National Cattlemen's Association (Englewood, CO: National Cattlemen's Association, 1990).

12. Personal communication with author, August 2000.

13. "The Dangers of Factory Farming," Consumer Alert, Humane Farming Association, 2000.

14. Bjerklie, Steve, "Who Really Has the World's Safest Meat Supply?" *Meat and Poultry* (August 1995).

15. Holerton, Gene, *The Beef-Eater's Guide to Modern Meat* (Los Angeles, CA: Holerton Publishing, 1998), p. 19.

16. Cheeke, *Animal Agriculture*, p. 258.

17. "British Vegetarians Win Some vs. McDonald's," *Meat Industry Insights*, April 1, 1999.

18. Wolfson, David, "McLibel," *Animal Law* 5 (1999).

19. Wolfson, David, *Beyond the Law: Agribusiness and the Systemic Abuse of Animals Raised for Food or Food Production*, Farm Sanctuary (1999), p. 7.

20. Letter dated July 29, 1997, from Bruce G. Friedrich, Vegetarian Campaign Coordinator, PETA.

21. In discussion among Bob Langert (McDonald's), Temple Grandin, and Steven Jay Gross (PETA), March 23, 1999.

22. *Animal Agriculture*, p. 13.

23. In discussion among Bob Langert (McDonald's), Temple Grandin, and Steven Jay Gross (PETA), June 22, 1999.

24. In discussion among Bob Langert (McDonald's), Temple Grandin, and Steven Jay Gross (PETA), December 11, 1998.

25. See August 30, 1999, letter from Steve Gross (PETA) to Jack Greenburg (CEO, McDonald's) and October 18, 1999, letter from Bruce Friedrich (PETA) to Jack Greenburg.

26. Mentioned in discussion among Bob Langert (McDonald's), Temple Grandin, and Steven Jay Gross (PETA), June 22, 1999.

27. Letter of August 12, 1999, from Steve Gross (PETA).

chapter 11 Misery on the Menu

1. Rollin, Bernard, *Farm Animal Welfare: Social, Bioethical and Research Issues* (Ames, IA: Iowa State University Press, 1995), pp. 109–10.

2. *Animal Agriculture: Myths and Facts* (Arlington VA: Animal Industry Foundation, 1989), p. 11.

3. "Our Farmers Care," Wisconsin Agri-Business Foundation, 1989, p. 15.

4. "The Truth about Veal," Veal Committee, National Cattlemen's Beef Association, 1989.

5. Ibid.

6. Welfare of Calves Regulations No. 2021 (U.K. 1987), cited in Wolfson, David, *Beyond the Law: Agribusiness and the Systemic Abuse of Animals Raised for Food or Food Production*, Farm Sanctuary (1999), p. 38.

7. Davis, Brenda, and Melina, Vesanto, *Becoming Vegan* (Summertown, TN: Book Publishing Co., 2000), p. 7.

8. "Campaign Update," *Humane Farming Association* XV: 1 (Spring 2000).

9. Ibid.
10. Personal communication with author, October 13, 2000.
11. Rollin, *Farm Animal Welfare*, p. 118.
12. Wolfson, *Beyond the Law*.
13. Quoted in Davis, Karen, *Poisoned Chicken, Poisoned Eggs* (Summertown, TN: Book Publishing Company, 1996), p. 99.
14. *Animal Agriculture*, p. 13.
15. Kaufman, Marc, "Cracks in the Egg Industry," *Washington Post*, April 30, 2000.
16. Ibid.
17. Ibid.
18. Ibid.
19. "Influence of Disease on Egg Quality," *Egg Industry*, June 1999. See also "Salmonella Control and Molting of Egg-Laying Flocks—Are They Compatible?", University of Florida Cooperative Extension Service, Fact Sheet VM92, July 1994; Kaufman, "Cracks in the Egg Industry."
20. Quoted in Kaufman, "Cracks in the Egg Industry."
21. Ibid.
22. USDA's National Statistics Service, referenced in "Facts about the Poultry Industry," Animal Protection Institute.
23. Rollin, *Farm Animal Welfare*, p. 133.
24. Quoted in "Birds Exploited for Meat," Farm Sanctuary, May 26, 1997.
25. David Martin, quoted in "Birds Exploited for Meat."
26. Davis and Melina, *Becoming Vegan*, p. 7.
27. Montgomery, David, "Not Quite a Slice of Poultry Heaven," *Washington Post*, November 24, 2000, B-1.
28. Wales, Rick, "Techno Turkeys," *Washington Post*, November 12, 1997, H-1.
29. Bjerklie, Steve, "Fowl Play," *Sonoma County Independent/ Metro Active*, May 15, 1997.
30. Ibid.
31. "Watch Out for Confusing Labels," Food Animals Concern Trust, FACT ACTS, Summer 2000, p. 5.
32. "The Rougher They Look, The Better They Lay," *Poultry Press* 2:4.
33. Ibid.
34. "How Hogs Are Raised Today," Pork Producers Council Web site, www.nppc.org/how.hogs.are.raised.
35. "A View Inside a U.S. Factory Hog Farm," *Humane Farming Association* XV:1 (Spring 2000).
36. Wolfson, *Beyond the Law*.
37. *National Hog Farmer*, November 15, 1993.
38. *Animal Agriculture*, p. 9.
39. Kilman, Scott, "Iowans Can Handle Pig Smells, But This Is Something Else," *Wall Street Journal*, May 4, 1996, A1.
40. Mason, Jim, "Assault and Battery," *Animals' Voice* 4:2 (April/May 1991):33.
41. Ibid.
42. "The Meat of the Matter," *Economist*, January 21, 1995.
43. Davis and Melina, *Becoming Vegan*, p. 7.

chapter 12 Eating with Conscience

1. Mason, Jim, "Assault and Battery," *Animals' Voice* 4:2 (April/May 1991):33.
2. Rollin, Bernard, *Farm Animal Welfare: Social, Bioethical and Research Issues* (Ames, IA: Iowa State University Press, 1995), pp. 103–4.
3. Ibid.
4. Adcock, Melanie, "The Dairy Cow: America's 'Foster Mother,'" Humane Society of the United States; www.hsus.org/programs/farm/dairy.
5. Ibid.
6. *World Farming Newsletter*, 1983, cited in Sheldrake, Rupert, *Dogs That Know When Their Owners Are Coming Home* (New York: Crown, 1999), pp. 224–5.
7. Sheldrake, *Dogs That Know*, p. 225.
8. "Cow's Long March," *Soviet Weekly*, January 24, 1987, cited in Sheldrake, *Dogs That Know*, p. 225.
9. *Animal Agriculture: Myths and Facts*, Animal Industry Foundation, Arlington VA, 1989, p. 17.
10. Schlosser, Eric, *Fast Food Nation* (Boston: Houghton Mifflin, 2001), p. 202.
11. Research by Eli Lilly and Co. and Flanco Products Co., reported in "The Dangers of Factory Farming," Humane Farming Association, 2000.
12. Cheeke, Peter, *Contemporary Issues in Animal Agriculture*, 2nd ed. (Danville, IL: Interstate Publishers, 1999), pp. 76, 278.
13. *Animal Agriculture*, p. 9.
14. *Feedstuffs*, July 6, 1998.
15. Ibid.
16. *Feedstuffs*, October 6, 1997, p. 2.
17. Schrimper, R., "U.S. Poultry Processing Employment and Hourly Earnings," *Journal of Applied Poultry Research* 6 (1997):81–9.
18. Eisnitz, Gail, *Slaughterhouse: The Shocking Story of Greed, Neglect, and Inhumane Treatment inside the U.S. Meat Industry* (Amherst, NY: Prometheus Books, 1997), p. 245.
19. Figures published by the National Turkey Federation, cited in Wolfson, David, *Beyond the Law: Agribusiness and the Systemic Abuse of Animals Raised for Food or Food Production*, Farm Sanctuary (1999).
20. Figures from *Drover's Journal* (July 1997), cited in Wolfson, *Beyond the Law*.
21. Wolfson, *Beyond the Law*.
22. *Feedstuffs*, October 6, 1997.
23. Silverstein, Ken, "Meat Factories," *Sierra*, www.sierraclub.org/sierra/199901/cafo.
24. Meadows, D., "How Campaign Reform Could Clean Up a Lot of Hog Manure," *Tidepool/Global Citizen*, January 20, 2000.
25. Eisnitz, *Slaughterhouse*.
26. "World's Largest Meat-Packer Caught Red Handed," Humane Farming Association, July/August 2000 newsletter.
27. Affidavit #3, cited in letter to Christine Gregoire, Attorney General, Washington State, from Humane Farming Association Director Bradley S. Miller.
28. Affidavit #9, Ibid.
29. Affidavit #6, Ibid.

30. Quoted in "He's Been Skinned All the Way to the Top, His Legs Have Been Cut Off . . . and He's Still Conscious," full-page ad taken out by the Humane Farming Association and published in Seattle newspapers.
31. Quoted in "World's Largest Meat-Packer Caught Red Handed."
32. Quoted in Case, David, "Tompaine.com Investigation: Food That's Not Safe to Eat," June 23, 2000.
33. Ibid.
34. Ibid.
35. Ibid.
36. Eisnitz, *Slaughterhouse*, p. 82.
37. "What Humans Owe to Animals," *Economist*, August 19, 1995.
38. Ibid.
39. Rollin, *Farm Animal Welfare*, p. 55.
40. Wolfson, *Beyond the Law*, p. 10.
41. Justice Roger Bell, McLibel Verdict, Section 8, June 19, 1997.
42. Wolfson, *Beyond the Law*, pp. 48, 51.
43. Ibid.
44. Ibid. See also "Swedish Animal Protection," cited in Swedish Ministry of Agriculture press release May 27, 1998.
45. Ibid., p. 40.
46. Ibid., 1999.
47. "Europe Urged to Stop Factory Farming to End Mad Cow," Reuters News Service, London, December 4, 2000.
48. Murphy, Dan. "EU proposes new animal welfare rules for pigs," www.meatingplace.com, January18, 2001
49. Wolfson, *Beyond the Law*, p. 11.
50. Bauston, G., "Agribusiness Wise to Consider Animal Welfare," *Feedstuffs*, October 25, 1999.

chapter 13 Choices for a Healthy Environment

1. Durning, Alan, and Brough, Holly, "Taking Stock: Animal Farming and the Environment," Worldwatch Paper 103, July 1991, p. 11.
2. Kieckhefer, E. W., "Drumming Up Support to Save Farms," United Press International, December 10, 2000.
3. Cheeke, Peter, *Contemporary Issues in Animal Agriculture,* 2nd ed. (Danville, IL: Interstate Publishers, 1999), p. 19.
4. "A Water Secure World: Vision for Water, Life, and the Environment," reported in Mittelstaedt, Martin, "World Water Use to Soar to Crisis Levels, Study Says," *The Globe and Mail,* March 14, 2000.
5. "Myths and Facts about Beef Production: Water Use," National Cattlemen's Beef Association, displayed on the Web site of the National Cattlemen's Beef Association in 2000.
6. Borgstrom, Georg, "Impacts on Demand for and Quality of Land and Water," Presentation to the 1981 annual meeting of the American Association for the Advancement of Science.

7. "Water Inputs in California Food Production," Water Education Foundation, Sacramento, CA.
8. Schulbach, Herb, et al., in *Soil and Water* 38 (Fall 1978).
9. *Audubon,* December 1999.
10. Ayres, Ed, *God's Last Offer* (New York/London: Four Walls Eight Windows, 1999), pp. 102–3.
11. Ayres, Ed, "Will We Still Eat Meat? Maybe Not, If We Wake Up to What the Mass Production of Animal Flesh Is Doing to Our Health, and the Planet's," *Time,* November 8, 1999.
12. "Myths and Facts about Beef Production."
13. Suzuki, David, *The Sacred Balance: Rediscovering Our Place in Nature* (Vancouver, BC: Greystone Books, 1997), p. 66.
14. "The Browning of America," *Newsweek,* February 22, 1981, p. 26.
15. Lang, John, "Environmentalists Rap Factory Farms for Manure Production," Scripps Howard News Service, June 9, 1998.
16. Ayres, *God's Last Offer,* p. 36.
17. Ryan, John, and Durning, Alan, *Stuff: The Secret Lives of Everyday Things* (Seattle: Northwest Environment Watch, 1997), p. 55.
18. Ayres, "Will We Still Eat Meat?"
19. Quoted in "The Environmental Consequences of Eating Meat," People for the Ethical Treatment of Animals, April 24, 1998.
20. *Feedstuffs,* July 3, 1995.
21. Williams, Ted, "Assembly Line Swine," *Audubon,* March/April 1998, p. 27. See also "Environmental and Health Consequences of Animal Factories," Natural Resources Defense Council report, 1998.
22. Ibid.
23. Ibid.
24. Facts and Data, Waste Pollution and the Environment, GRACE Factory Farm Project, www.gracelinks.org/factoryfarm/facts, 2000.
25. "Environmental and Health Consequences of Animal Factories."
26. "Most Commonly Asked Questions about Pork Production and the Environment," National Pork Producers Council.
27. "Group's Surprising Beef with Meat Industry: Study Ranks Production of Beef, Poultry and Pork as Second to Automobiles in Ecological Cost," *San Francisco Chronicle,* April 27, 1999; see also Brower, Michael, and Leon, Warren, *The Consumer's Guide to Effective Environmental Choices: Practical Advice from the Union of Concerned Scientists* (New York: Three Rivers Press/Crown Publishers, 1999).
28. Burkholder, J. M., et al., "Insidious Effects of Toxic Estuarine Dinoflagellate on Fish Survival and Human Health," *Journal of Toxicology and Environmental Health* 46 (1995):501–22; Chesapeake Bay Foundation, "Facts about Pfiesteria Piscicida in the Chesapeake Bay," 1997.
29. Burkholder, "Insidious Effects of Toxic Estuarine Dinoflagellate"; Burkholder, J. M., "Pfiesteria Piscicida and Other Toxic Pfiesteria-Like Dinoflagellates," North Carolina State University, 1997; Chesapeake Bay Foundation, "Facts about Pfiesteria Piscicida."

30. Silverstein, Ken, "Meat Factories," *Sierra,* www.sierraclub.org/sierra/199901/cafo; Burkholder, "Insidious Effects of Toxic Estuarine Dinoflagellate"; Burkholder, "Pfiesteria Piscicida and Other Toxic Pfiesteria-Like Dinoflagellates"; Chesapeake Bay Foundation, "Facts about Pfiesteria Piscicida."

31. Quoted in Silverstein, "Meat Factories."

32. Robinson, Ann, and Marks, Robbin, "Restoring the Big River: A Clean Water Act Blueprint for Mississippi," Izaak Walton League, Minneapolis, MN, and the Natural Resources Defense Council, Washington, DC (February 1994), p. 13. See also Lovejoy, S. B., "Sources and Quantities of Nutrients Entering the Gulf of Mexico from Surface Waters of the U.S.," EPA/800–R-92–002.

33. Silverstein, "Meat Factories."

34. Quoted in Lang, "Environmentalists Rap Factory Farms."

35. "Are Pork Operations Getting Blamed Again?" *Poultry Inc.* (September 1999), p. 38.

36. U.S. General Accounting Office, Briefing Report to the Committee on Agriculture, Nutrition and Forestry, U.S. Senate, "Animal Agriculture, Information on Waste Management and Water Quality Issues," GAO/RCED 95–200BR, Washington, DC, 1995, pp. 58–61.

37. Ibid.

38. According to Ken Midkiff of Sierra's Missouri chapter, quoted in Lang, "Environmentalists Rap Factory Farms."

39. Woolf, Jim, "Have Hogs Caused Milford Maladies?" *Salt Lake Tribune,* January 26, 2000.

40. Ibid.

41. "The State of the Planet, Climap," *Blue,* April/May 2000, p. 67.

42. "Group's Surprising Beef with Meat Industry"; see also Brower and Leon, *The Consumer's Guide to Effective Environmental Choices.*

43. Cone, Marla, "State Dairy Farms Try to Clean Up Their Act," *Los Angeles Times,* April 28, 1998.

44. Diringer, Elliot, "In Central Valley, Defiant Dairies Foul the Water," *San Francisco Chronicle,* July 7, 1997. See also Mayell, Hillary, "Chickens and Pigs and Cows . . .," Environmental News Network, August 28, 1998; and Silverstein, "Meat Factories."

45. "How States Fail to Prevent Pollution from Livestock Waste," ch. 4, Natural Resources Defense Council report, 1998, California.

46. Cone, "State Dairy Farms Try to Clean Up Their Act."

47. Letson, David, and Gjollehon, Noel, "Confined Animal Production and the Manure Problem," *Choices* (3rd Quarter 1996), p. 18.

48. "How States Fail to Prevent Pollution from Livestock Waste."

49. "Myths and Facts about Beef Production."

50. Quoted in "How States Fail to Prevent Pollution from Livestock Waste."

51. "Wow That Cow—How Cattle Enrich Our Lives, and Enhance the Planet," National Cattlemen's Beef Association; "This Earth Day, Celebrate Mother Nature's Recycling Machine," advertisement produced for the Beef Promotion and Research Board by the National Cattlemen's Association.

52. Williams, Ted, "He's Going to Have an Accident," *Audubon,* March/April 1991, pp. 30–9.
53. "Corporations on the Dole," *WorldWatch,* Januray/February 1996, p. 39.
54. Arizona State Land Department, 1998 annual report.
55. "Ranchers Benefit from State Land Give-Away," in the Tax-Payer's Guide to Welfare Ranching in the Southwest, New West Research and the Southwest Center for Biological Diversity, 2000 www.new-west-research.org/Taxpayers_ Guide/Welfare_Ranching.
56. Ibid.
57. Ibid.
58. "Who Pays: A Distributional Analysis of the Tax Systems in All 50 States," Citizens for Tax Justice, 1996.
59. "The Status of Women in the States," report by the Institute for Women's Policy Research, 1998.
60. "Wow That Cow."
61. U.S. Department of the Interior, Bureau of Land Management, "State of the Public Rangelands . . .," Washington, DC, 1990. See also Durning and Brough, "Taking Stock," pp. 20–4.
62. Quoted in Wuerthner, George, "The Price Is Wrong," *Sierra,* September/ October 1990, p. 39.
63. Wilkinson, Todd, "In a Battle over Cattle, Both Sides Await Grazing Ruling," *Christian Science Monitor,* May 1, 2000.
64. Abbey, Edward, *One Life at a Time Please* (New York: Henry Holt, 1988), pp. 13–4.

chapter 14 Once Upon a Planet

1. Sussman, Art, *Dr. Art's Guide to Planet Earth* (White River Junction, VT: Chelsea Green, 2000), p. 67.
2. "Livestock and Environment," Agriculture 21, Agriculture Department, Food and Agriculture Organization, United Nations.
3. Myers, Norman, *The Primary Source: Tropical Forests and Our Future* (New York and London, W. W. Norton, 1984), pp. 127, 142.
4. Denslow, Julie, and Padoch, Christine, *People of the Tropical Rainforest* (Berkeley, CA: University of California Press, 1988), p. 169.
5. "Seven Things You Can Do to Save the Rainforest," Rainforest Action Network Factsheet, 2000, www.ran.org/ran/info_center/factsheets/.
6. Raven, Peter, *We're Killing Our World: The Global Ecosystem in Crisis* (IL: MacArthur Foundation, 1987), p. 8.
7. Gore, Al, *Earth In Balance: Ecology and the Human Spirit* (New York: Plume, 1993), p. 23.
8. Denslow and Padoch, *People of the Tropical Rainforest,* p. 169.
9. "The Price of Beef," *WorldWatch,* July/August 1994, p. 39.
10. Ibid.
11. Ibid.

12. Belk, K., et al., "Deforestation and Meat Production," in Cross, H. Russel and Byers, Floyd M., eds. *Current Issues in Food Production: A Scientific Response to John Robbins' Diet* for a New America, *Supported by the National Cattlemen's Association* (Englewood, CO: National Cattlemen's Association, 1990), 2.2.

13. Ensminger, M. E., *Animal Science,* 9th ed. (Danville, IL: Interstate Publishers, 1991), p. 244.

14. Ayres, Ed, *God's Last Offer* (New York/London: Four Walls Eight Windows Publishers, 1999), p. 16.

15. Ibid., p. 12.

16. Quoted in Suzuki, David, and Dressel, Holly, *From Naked Ape to Superspecies* (Toronto: Stoddart Publishing, 1999), p. 59.

17. Suzuki and Dressel, *From Naked Ape to Superspecies,* p. 59.

18. Quoted in Suzuki and Dressel, *From Naked Ape to Superspecies,* p. 60.

19. Quoted in Gelbspan, Ross, "Reality Check: The Global Warming Debate Is Over . . .," *E,* September/October 2000, p. 24.

20. Sagan, Carl, *Billions and Billions* (New York: Random House, 1997), p. 108.

21. Gelbspan, "Reality Check," p. 25.

22. Brown, Lester, "OPEC Has World over a Barrel Again," Worldwatch Institute Alert 8, September 8, 2000.

23. Brown, Lester, "Climate Change Has World Skating on Thin Ice," Worldwatch Institute Issue Alert 7, August 29, 2000.

24. Motavalli, Jim, "Feeling Hot, Hot, Hot," *E,* September/October 2000, p. 4.

25. Ayres, *God's Last Offer,* p. 52.

26. Ibid., pp. 48–49.

27. Quoted in Keys, David, "Global Warming Creates Unstable Earth," UK Independent News, August 7, 2000.

28. Dunn, Seth, "Weather Damages Drop," *Vital Signs 2000,* Worldwatch Institute, p. 77.

29. Ibid.

30. Ibid.

31. Ibid.

32. Ibid.

33. Ibid.

34. Ibid.

35. Ibid.

36. Ibid.

37. Ryan, John, and Durning, Alan, *Stuff: The Secret Lives of Everyday Things* (Seattle: Northwest Environment Watch, 1997), p. 55.

38. Ibid.

39. Pimentel, David, and Pimentel, Marcia, *Food, Energy and Society* (1979), p. 59; and Pimentel, et al., "Energy and Land Constraints in Food Protein Production," *Science,* November 21, 1975; cited in Lappé, Frances Moore, *Diet for a Small Planet,* 20th anniversary ed. (New York: Ballantine Books, 1991), pp. 74–5.

40. Ibid.

41. David Pimentel at Cornell University gave the figure of 78 calories of fossil fuel to produce 1 calorie of protein from beef in *Food, Energy and Society*, p. 59; and in Pimentel, et al., "Energy and Land Constraints in Food Protein Production", *Science*, November 21, 1975. This figure was also cited in Lappé, *Diet for a Small Planet*, pp. 74–5. More recently, however, Pimentel has updated the figure to 54 calories.

42. "The Price of Beef," *WorldWatch*, July/August 1994, p. 39.

43. Ibid.

44. Heitschmidt, R. K., et al., "Ecosystems, Sustainability, and Animal Agriculture," *Journal of Animal Science* 74 (1996):1395–1405.

45. "Myths and Facts about Beef Production: Energy Use," National Cattlemen's Beef Association, displayed on the Web site of the National Cattlemen's Beef Association in 2000.

46. "The Price of Beef," p. 39.

47. Ciborowski, P., "Sources, Sinks, Trends and Opportunities," in Abrahamson, D., ed., *The Challenge of Global Warming* (Washington, DC: Island Press, 1989); see also Khalil, M., and Rasmussen, R., "Sources, Sinks, and Seasonal Cycles of Atmospheric Methane," *Journal of Geophysical Research* 88 (1983):5131–44.

48. Halweil, Brian, "United States Leads World Meat Stampede," Worldwatch Issues Paper, July 2, 1998.

49. "Myths and Facts about Beef Production: Methane Production," National Cattlemen's Beef Association, displayed on the Web site of the National Cattlemen's Beef Association in 2000.

50. Durning, Alan, and Brough, Holly, "Taking Stock: Animal Farming and the Environment," Worldwatch Paper 103, July 1991.

51. "Group's Surprising Beef with Meat Industry: Study Ranks Production of Beef, Poultry and Pork as Second to Automobiles in Ecological Cost," *San Francisco Chronicle*, April 27, 1999; see also Brower, Michael, and Leon, Warren, *The Consumer's Guide to Effective Environmental Choices: Practical Advice from the Union of Concerned Scientists* (New York: Three Rivers Press/Crown Publishers, 1999).

52. "Myths and Facts about Beef Production: Methane Production."

53. Booth, W., "Action Urged against Global Warming: Scientists Appeal for Curbs on Gases," *Washington Post*, February 2, 1990.

54. Ayres, *God's Last Offer*, p. 27.

55. Quoted in Suzuki and Dressel, *From Naked Ape to Superspecies*, p. 13.

56. Ibid.

57. Worldwatch Institute, *State of the World 2000* (New York/London: W. W. Norton, 2000).

58. "Livestock and Environment."

59. Wuerthner, George, "The Price Is Wrong," *Sierra*, September/October 1990, pp. 40–1. Also, Bogo, Jennifer, "Where's the Beef?", *E*, November/December 1999, p. 49.

60. Wuerthner, "The Price Is Wrong." See also, Ferguson, Denzel, and Ferguson, Nancy, *Sacred Cows at the Public Trough* (Bend, OR: Maverick Publications, 1983), p. 116.

61. Wilkinson, Todd, "In a Battle over Cattle, Both Sides Await Grazing Ruling," *Christian Science Monitor,* May 1, 2000.
62. "Property Rights," Position Paper, National Cattlemen's Beef Association, January 2000.
63. Durning and Brough, "Taking Stock," p. 27.
64. "Cattle Lose in Battle for Species Protection," Environmental News Network, October 9, 1997. (The study was prompted by a lawsuit filed by the Southwest Center for Biological Diversity.)
65. "Group's Surprising Beef with Meat Industry"; see also Brower and Leon, *The Consumer's Guide to Effective Environmental Choices.*
66. Suzuki, David, *The Sacred Balance: Rediscovering Our Place in Nature* (Vancouver BC: Greystone Books, 1997), pp. 4–5.
67. Ayres, *God's Last Offer,* p. 171.
68. The words in this paragraph were written by Neal Rogin, in a document summarizing six months of ongoing discussions that had taken place among a small group of dedicated people, including Neal, myself, Vicki Robin, Tom Burt, Lynn Twist, Richard Rathbun, Joe Kresse, Catherine Parrish, Catherine Grey, Mathis Wackernagel, Ocean Robbins, and Tracy Howard.

chapter 15 Reversing the Spread of Hunger

1. Brown, Lester, "Facing Reality at the World Food Summit," Worldwatch Press Release, November 1, 1996.
2. Ibid.
3. "Forty Percent of World's Farmland Degraded," World Wire, May 22, 2000; and "Soil Loss Threatens Food Prospects," BBC News Online, May 22, 2000.
4. Gardner, Gary, and Halweil, Brian, "Underfed and Overfed: The Global Epidemic of Malnutrition," Worldwatch Paper 150, Worldwatch Institute, 2000.
5. "12 Myths and Facts about Beef Production: A Dozen of the Most Popular Misconceptions about America's Most Popular Meat," National Cattlemen's Association, American Angus Association, West Salem, OH, publication date unknown; distributed by the National Cattlemen's Association in 1993.
6. Halweil, Brian, "United States Leads World Meat Stampede," Worldwatch Issues Paper, July 2, 1998.
7. Ensminger, M. E., *Animal Science,* 9th ed. (Danville, IL: Interstate Publishers, 1991), p. 20.
8. Halweil, "United States Leads World Meat Stampede."
9. Brown, "Facing Reality."
10. Brown, L., "China's Water Shortage Could Shake World Grain Markets," Worldwatch Press Release, April 22, 1998; "Falling Water Tables in China May Soon Raise Food Prices Everywhere," Worldwatch, May 2, 2000.
11. Brown, L., and Halweil, B., "Populations Outrunning Water Supply as World Hits 6 Billion," Worldwatch News Release, September 23, 1999.
12. Durning, Alan, and Brough, Holly, "Taking Stock: Animal Farming and the Environment," Worldwatch Paper 103, July 1991, p. 29.

13. Halweil, "United States Leads World Meat Stampede."
14. Shiva, Vandana, *Stolen Harvest: The Hijacking of the Global Food Supply* (Cambridge, MA: South End Press, 2000), p. 13.
15. Durning and Brough, "Taking Stock," p. 31.
16. "Emerging Water Shortages," Worldwatch News Release, July 17, 1999.
17. Brown, L., "Food Security Deteriorating in the Nineties," Worldwatch Press Briefing, March 6, 1997.
18. Ayres, Ed, *God's Last Offer* (New York/London: Four Walls Eight Windows, 1999), p. 102.
19. Durning and Brough, "Taking Stock," p. 31.
20. DeWalt, B., "The Cattle Are Eating the Forest," *Bulletin of the Atomic Scientist* 39:1 (January 1983):22; and Shane, D., *Hoofprints on the Forest: Cattle Ranching and the Destruction of Latin America's Tropical Forests* (Philadelphia: Institute for the Study of Human Issues, 1986), p. 78.
21. DeWalt, B., "The Cattle Are Eating the Forest."
22. Policy Alternatives for the Caribbean and Central America, *Changing Course: Blueprint for Peace in Central America and the Caribbean* (Washington, DC: Institute for Policy Studies, 1984).
23. Caulfield, Catherine, "A Reporter at Large: The Rain Forests," *New Yorker,* January 14, 1985. See also Myers, Norman, *The Primary Source* (New York: W. W. Norton, 1983), p. 133.
24. Gray, Mike, *Drug Crazy* (New York: Random House, 1998), p. 134.
25. DeWalt, B., "Mexico's Second Green Revolution," *Mexican Studies*1:1 (Winter 1985):30; Barkin, D., and DeWalt, B., "Sorghum, the Internationalization of Capital, and the Mexican Food Crisis," Paper presented at the American Anthropological Association Meeting, Denver, CO, November 16, 1984, p. 16; see also Halweil, "United States Leads World Meat Stampede."
26. Myers, *Primary Source,* p. 133.
27. Durning and Brough, "Taking Stock," p. 32.
28. Size of Brazil's commercial cattle herd from "Virus-Free Brazil Beef Headed for US in 2000," *Meat Industry Insights,* November 3, 1999.
29. "Myths and Facts about Beef Production."
30. Gardner and Halweil, "Underfed and Overfed."
31. Ibid.
32. Ibid.
33. Worldwatch Institute, *State of the World 2000* (New York: W. W. Norton, 2000), p. 61.
34. Ibid.
35. Ayres, *God's Last Offer,* p. 73.
36. "Ending Malnutrition by 2020: An Agenda for Change in the Millennium," released March 20, 2000.
37. Durning and Brough, "Taking Stock," p. 15.
38. Pimentel, David, and Hall, Carl, eds., *Food and Natural Resources* (San Diego, CA: Academic Press, 1989), p. 80.
39. Ibid.

40. "Cattle Feeding," in "Myths and Facts about Beef Production."
41. Ibid.
42. "Claims and Responses Regarding Cattle Production: A Response to Claims Made in *Diet for a New America,*" National Cattlemen's Association Fact Sheet, (Englewood, CO: National Cattlemen's Association, 1990).
43. 1993/1994 World Maize Facts and Trends (Mexico City: CIMMYT), pp. 50, 52; see also Ensminger, *Animal Science,* p. 23.
44. Ibid.
45. 1992 Census of Agriculture, Table 0A, U.S. Dept of Commerce, Bureau of the Census.
46. Ibid.
47. Durning, and Brough, "Taking Stock," p. 14. See also Ayres, Ed, "Will We Still Eat Meat? Maybe Not, If We Wake Up to What the Mass Production of Animal Flesh Is Doing to Our Health, and the Planet's," *Time,* November 8, 1999.
48. Halweil, "United States Leads World Meat Stampede."
49. "Cattle Feeding," in "Myths and Facts about Beef Production."
50. Lappé, Frances Moore, *Diet for a Small Planet,* 20th anniversary ed. (New York: Ballantine Books, 1991), pp. 69, 445–6.
51. National Cattlemen's Association, "Fact Sheet" Retort to the PBS Documentary, *Diet for a New America,*" 1991.
52. Brown, Lester, "Fish Farming May Soon Overtake Cattle Ranching as a Food Source," Worldwatch Institute Issue Alert 9, October 3, 2000.
53. Cheeke, Peter, *Contemporary Issues in Animal Agriculture,* 2nd ed. (Danville, IL: Interstate Publishers, 1999), p. 74.
54. Spedding, C. R. W., "The Effect of Dietary Changes on Agriculture," in Lewis, B. and Assmann, G., eds., *The Social and Economic Contexts Of Coronary Prevention* (London: Current Medical Literature, 1990), cited in World Cancer Research Fund and American Institute for Cancer Research, *Food, Nutrition and the Prevention of Cancer: A Global Perspective* (1997), p. 557. See also Pimentel and Hall, *Food and Natural Resources.*
55. Brown, "Facing Reality."
56. Pauly, Daniel, et al., "Fishing Down Marine Food Webs," *Science,* February 6, 1998, pp. 860–3.
57. Egan, Timothy, "U.S. Fishing Fleet Trawling Coastal Water Without Fish," *New York Times,* March 7, 1994, A-1.
58. Ayres, *God's Last Offer,* pp. 109–10.
59. Bogo, Jennifer, "Brain Food," *E,* July/August 2000, p. 42.
60. "Fishy Business," *New Internationalist,* July 2000, p. 11.
61. "Oceans Without Fish," *Rachel's Environment and Health Weekly,* February 26, 1998.
62. "Monoculture: The Biological and Social Impacts," *WorldWatch,* March/April 1998, p. 39.
63. Ibid.
64. Holt, S., "The Food Resources of the Ocean," *Scientific American* 221 (1969):178–94.

65. "Oceans Without Fish."
66. Cheeke, *Contemporary Issues in Animal Agriculture,* p. 205.
67. "Tyson Foods Target of Corruption Case," *Feedstuffs,* June 30, 1997.
68. *Feedstuffs,* Janury 5, 1998, p. 1.
69. St. Clair, Jeffrey, "Fishy Business," *In These Times,* May 26, 1997, pp. 14–6, 36.
70. Stevens, William, "Man Moves Down the Marine Food Chain, Creating Havoc," *New York Times,* February 10, 1998, C3. See also Pauly, et al., "Fishing Down Marine Food Webs," pp. 860–3.
71. Suzuki, David, and Dressel, Holly, *From Naked Ape to Superspecies* (Toronto: Stoddart Publishing, 1999), p. 19.
72. Suzuki and Dressel, *From Naked Ape to Superspecies,* pp. 20–1.
73. Brown, "Fish Farming May Overtake Cattle."
74. "The Facts of Fishing," *New Internationalist,* July 2000, p. 19.
75. McGinn, Anne Platt, "Blue Revolution—The Promises and Pitfalls of Fish Farming," *WorldWatch,* March/April 1998, pp. 10–9.
76. Naylor, R., et al., "Effect of Aquaculture on World Fish Supplies," *Nature,* June 29, 2000.
77. Ibid.
78. Atlantic Salmon in Short Supply, BBC News Online, May 31, 2000.
79. "Fishy Business," p. 11.
80. McGinn, "Blue Revolution," pp. 10–9.
81. Simopoulos, A. P., and N. Salem, Jr., "N-3 Fatty Acids in Eggs from Range-Fed Greek Chickens," *New England Journal of Medicine* (1989):1412; Crawford, M., "Fatty-Acid Ratios in Free-Living and Domestic Animals," *Lancet* 1 (1968): 1329–33; Simopoulos, Artemis, and Robinson, Jo, *The Omega Diet* (New York: Harper Collins, 1999), pp. 24–36; Robinson, Jo, *Why Grassfed Is Best* (Vashon, WA: Vashon Island Press, 2000).
82. "Farmed fish may be hazardous to your health," news release from the David Suzuki Foundation, Vancouver, BC, January 3, 2001.
83. "Fishy Business," p. 11.
84. "Facts of Fishing," p. 19.
85. "White Gold: The Social and Ecological Consequences of High-Intensity Shrimp Farming," *E,* May/June 2000, p. 11.
86. Cousteau, Jean-Michel, "Salmon Farming: The Great Fish Escape," Los Angeles Times Syndicate, October 16, 2000.
87. Naylor, et al., "Effect of Aquaculture."

chapter 16 Pandora's Pantry

1. Lappé, Marc, and Bailey, Britt, *Against the Grain: Biotechnology and the Corporate Takeover of Your Food* (Monroe, ME: Common Courage Press, 1998), p. 117.
2. Ibid.

3. Teitel, Martin, and Wilson, Kimberly, *Genetically Engineered Food* (Rochester VT: Park Street Press, 1999), pp. 20–2, 41.

4. Nash, J. M., "Grains of Hope," *Time*, July 31, 2000, pp. 39–46.

5. Shiva, Vandana, "Genetically Engineered Vitamin A Rice: A Blind Approach to Blindness Prevention," February 14, 2000; www.biotech-info.net/blind_rice.html.

6. Warwick, Hugh, *Splice*, March/April 2000; www.geneticsforum.org.uk.

7. Shapiro, Robert, Address to Greenpeace Business Conference, London, U.K., October 6, 1999.

8. "Seedless in Seattle," Rural Advancement Foundation International News Release, November 26, 1999.

9. Quoted in Suzuki, David, and Dressel, Holly, *From Naked Ape to Superspecies* (Toronto: Stoddart Publishing, 1999), p. 131.

10. Halweil, Brian, "Transgenic Crop Area Surges," *Vital Signs 2000*, Worldwatch Institute, p. 118.

11. Lappé and Bailey, *Against the Grain*, p. 23.

12. Halweil, "Transgenic Crop Area Surges," p. 118.

13. Pollan, Michael, "Playing God in the Garden," *New York Times Magazine*, October 25, 1998; see also Wrubel, R., et al., "Regulatory Oversight of Genetically Engineered Microorganisms . . .," *Journal of Environmental Management* 21:4 (1997):571–86.

14. Halweil, "Transgenic Crop Area Surges," p. 118.

15. Anderson, Luke, *Genetic Engineering, Food, and our Environment* (White River Junction, VT: Chelsea Green Publishing Company, 1999), p. 24; Lappé and Bailey, *Against the Grain,* p. 58.

16. "Monsanto Releases Seed Piracy Case Settlement Details," Monsanto Press Release 12, September 1998, cited in Anderson, *Genetic Engineering*, p. 23; Lappé and Bailey, *Against the Grain,* pp. 53, 57.

17. Anderson, *Genetic Engineering*, p. 24.

18. "Glyphosate: Environmental Health Criteria 159," World Health Organization, United Nations Environment Program, Geneva, Switzerland, 1994; cited in Anderson, *Genetic Engineering*, pp. 24–5; Abdel-Mallek, A., et al., "Effect of Glyphosate on Fungal Population, Respiration and the Decay of Some Organic Matters in Egyptian Soil," *Microbial Research* 149 (1994):69–73.

19. Pease, W., et al., "Preventing Pesticide-Related Illness in California Agriculture," Environmental Health Policy Program Report (Berkeley, CA: University of California School of Public Health; California Policy Summary).

20. Cox, C., "Glyphosate, Part 1: Toxicology, Herbicide Factsheet," *Journal of Pesticide Reform* 15:3 (Fall 1995), from the Northwest Coalition for Alternatives to Pesticides.

21. Lappé and Bailey, *Against the Grain,* p. 54; Presley, Amanda, "Reckoning for Roundup . . .," *E*, September/October 2000, p. 64.

22. Harden, Lent, and Eriksson, Michael, "A Case-Control Study of Non-Hodgkin Lymphoma and Exposure to Pesticides," *Cancer* 85:6 (March 15, 1999):1353–60.

23. Foreword to Lappé and Bailey, *Against the Grain*, p. viii.
24. Lappé and Bailey, *Against the Grain*, pp. 75, 125.
25. Suzuki and Dressel, *Naked Ape to Superspecies*, p. 114.
26. Quoted in Suzuki and Dressel, *Naked Ape to Superspecies*, p. 115.
27. Ibid.
28. Quoted in Anderson, *Genetic Engineering*, p. 27.
29. Anderson, *Genetic Engineering*, p. 24.
30. Cox, C., "Herbicide Factsheet: Glufosinate," *Journal of Pesticide Reform* 16:4 (1996):15–9; cited in Anderson, *Genetic Engineering*, p. 24.
31. Lappé and Bailey, *Against the Grain*, pp. 41–6.
32. Ibid.
33. Halweil, "Transgenic Crop Area Surges," p. 118.
34. Halweil, Brian, "Transgenic Crops Proliferate," *Vital Signs 1999*, Worldwatch Institute, p. 122.
35. Ibid.
36. Ibid.
37. Ibid.
38. Halweil, "Transgenic Crop Area Surges," p. 118.
39. Lappé and Bailey, *Against the Grain*, p. 147.
40. "Against the Grain," *Rachel's Environment and Health Weekly* 637, February 11, 1999; see also Lappé and Bailey, *Against the Grain*, pp. 88–9.
41. Holzman, David, "Agricultural Biotechnology: Report Leads to Debate on Benefits of Transgenic Corn and Soybean Crops," *Genetic Engineering News* 19:8 (April 15, 1999).
42. Lappé and Bailey, *Against the Grain*, pp. 82–4.
43. Lean, Geoffrey, "Research Backs Charles: GM Crops Don't Deliver," *Independent*, June 11, 2000.
44. Personal communication with author.
45. Quoted in Suzuki and Dressel, *Naked Ape to Superspecies*, p. 118.
46. Anderson, *Genetic Engineering*, pp. 55–57.
47. Quoted in Suzuki and Dressel, *Naked Ape to Superspecies*, p. 116.
48. Loving, Armory and Loving, Hunter, "A Tale of Two Obtains" (April 2000); www.wired.com/wired/archive/8.04/botanies.html.
49. Albright, Mark, "Biotech Battle Now a War of Words," *St. Petersburg Times*, May 10, 2000.
50. Anderson, *Genetic Engineering*, p. 66.
51. "Biotech: The Pendulum Swings Back," *Rachel's Environment and Health Weekly* 649, May 6, 1999.
52. "Terminator Terminated?" Rural Advancement Foundation International News Release, October 4, 1999; Brasher, Philip, "Terminator Seeds," Associated Press, October 31, 1999.
53. Anderson, *Genetic Engineering*, p. 68.
54. Ibid.
55. "Genetically Altering the World's Food," *Rachel's Environment and Health Weekly* 639, February 25, 1998.
56. Quoted in Anderson, *Genetic Engineering*, p. 88.

57. Ibid., p. 96.
58. Ibid., p. 32.
59. Hill, H., "OSU Study Finds Genetic Altering of Bacterium Upsets Natural Order," *Oregonian,* August 8, 1994.
60. Holmes, M., et al., "Effects of Klebsiella Planticola on Soil Biota . . .," *Applied Soil Ecology* 326 (1998):1–12.
61. Suzuki, and Dressel, *Naked Ape to Superspecies,* pp. 120–1.
62. Quoted in Anderson, *Genetic Engineering,* pp. 39–40.
63. Suzuki and Dressel, *Naked Ape to Superspecies,* p. 121.
64. Ibid., p. 122.
65. Quoted in Kemp, Christopher, "Hot Potato," *Cleveland Free Times,* June 14–20, 2000.
66. "Does the Biotechnology Industry Oppose Labeling of Biotech Foods?" Biotechnology Industry Organization Web site; www.bio.org/labeling_answer.html.
67. Suzuki and Dressel, *Naked Ape to Superspecies,* p. 144.
68. "Biotech In Trouble," *Rachel's Environment and Health Weekly* 696, May 11, 2000.
69. Quoted in Suzuki and Dressel, *Naked Ape to Superspecies,* p. 142.

chapter 17 Farmageddon

1. Suzuki, David, and Dressel, Holly, *From Naked Ape to Superspecies* (Toronto/New York: Stoddart Publishing, 1999), p. 102.
2. Ibid.
3. Ibid., p. 143.
4. Nash, M. J., "Jeepers! Creepy Peepers!" *Time,* April 3, 1995.
5. Ho, Mae-Wan, "The Unholy Alliance," *Ecologist,* July/August 1997, p. 153.
6. Quoted in Lappé, Marc, and Bailey, Britt, *Against the Grain: Biotechnology and the Corporate Takeover of Your Food* (Monroe, ME: Common Courage Press, 1998), p. 50.
7. Quoted in Anderson, Luke, *Genetic Engineering, Food, and our Environment* (White River Junction, VT: Chelsea Green Publishing Company, 1999), p. 35.
8. Quoted in Ticciati, Laura, and Ticciati, Robin, *Genetically Engineered Foods: Are They Safe? You Decide* (New Canaan, CT: Keats Publishing, 1998), pp. 4–5.
9. Suzuki and Dressel, *Naked Ape to Superspecies,* p. 106.
10. Shapiro, Robert, "The Welcome Tension of Technology: The Need for Dialogue about Agricultural Biotechnology," Center for the Study of American Business, CEO Series 37, February 2000.
11. Nordlee, J. D., et al., "Identification of a Brazil Nut Allergen in Transgenic Soybeans," *New England Journal of Medicine* 334:11 (March 14, 1996): 688–92.
12. Ibid.
13. Ticciati, *Genetically Engineered Foods,* p. 44.

14. Mayeno, A., et al., "Eosinophilia-Myalgia Syndrome and Tryptophan Production . . .," *Tibtech* 12 (1994):346–52; cited in Anderson, *Genetic Engineering*, p. 17.

15. Raphals, P., "Does Medical Mystery Threaten Biotech?" *Science* 249 (1990):619; see also Love, L., et al., "Pathological and Immunological Effects of Ingesting L-tryptophan . . .," *Journal of Clinical Investigation* 91 (March 1993):804–11.

16. Anderson, *Genetic Engineering*, p. 18.

17. Quoted in "Genetically Engineered Foods—Are They Safe?" *Safe Food News;* 500,000 copies of this newsmagazine were distributed in late 2000 to health food stores and other venues in the United States.

18. Teitel, Martin, and Wilson, Kimberly, *Genetically Engineered Food: Changing the Nature of Nature* (Rochester, VT: Park Street Press, 1999), p. 56.

19. Mepham, T., Challacombe, D., et al., "Safety of Milk from Cows Treated with Bovine Somatotrophin," *Lancet* 344 (1994):197–8; Epstein, S., "Unlabeled Milk from Cows Treated with Biosynthetic Growth Hormones: A Case of Regulatory Abdication," *International Journal of Health Services* 26:1 (1996):173–85; Epstein, S., "Potential Health Hazards of Biosynthetic Milk Hormones," *International Journal of Health Services* 20:1 (1990):73–84.

20. Chan, J. M., et al., "Plasma Insulin-Like Growth Factor-I and Prostate Cancer Risk: A Prospective Study," *Science* 279 (1998):563–6; see also Cohen, P., "Serum Insulin-Like Growth Factor-I Levels and Prostate Cancer Risk: Interpreting the Evidence," *Journal of the National Cancer Institute* 90 (1998):876–9.

21. Hankinson, S. E., et al., "Circulating Concentrations of Insulin-Like Growth Factor-I and Risk of Breast Cancer," *Lancet* 351 (1998):1393–6.

22. Juskevich, J., et al., "Bovine Growth Hormone: Human Food Safety Evaluation," *Science* 249 (1990):875–84.

23. Daughaday, William, et al., "Bovine Somatotropin Supplementation of Dairy Cows: Is the Milk Safe?" *Journal of the American Medical Association* 264 (1990):1003–5.

24. Epstein, "Unlabeled Milk"; Epstein, "Potential Health Hazards"; Mepham, Challacombe, et al., "Safety of Milk"; Coghlan, Andy, "Arguing Till the Cows Come Home," *New Scientist,* October 29, 1994, pp. 14–5; Juskevich, et al., "Bovine Growth Hormone."

25. Keeler, Barbara, and Lappé, Marc "Some Food for FDA Regulation," *Los Angeles Times,* January 7, 2001.

26. Keeler, Barbara, and Lappé, Marc "Some Food for FDA Regulation," *Los Angeles Times,* January 7, 2001.

27. "Biotech: The Pendulum Swings Back," *Rachel's Environment and Health Weekly,* #649, May 6, 1999; Rampton, Sheldon, and Stauber, John, *Trust Us, We're Experts!*, Jeremy Tarcher/Putnam, New York, 2001, p. 153.

28. Rampton, Sheldon, and Stauber, John, *Trust Us, We're Experts!*, Jeremy Tarcher/Putnam, New York, 2001, p. 154.

29. Stanley, W., Ewen, S, and Pusztai, A., "Effects of diets containing genetically modified potatoes . . . on rat intestines," *Lancet*, Vol. 354, No. 9187, October 16, 1999.

30. Rampton, Sheldon, and Stauber, John, *Trust Us, We're Experts!*, Jeremy Tarcher/Putnam, New York, 2001, p. 154.

31. Quoted in "FDA Genetic Food Policy Denies Americans the Right to Know What They Are Eating," Greenpeace, January 17, 2001.

32. "Against the Grain," *Rachel's Environment and Health Weekly*, 637, February 11, 1999.

33. Lappé, M., et al., "Alterations in Clinically Important Phytoestrogens in Genetically Modified, Herbicide Resistant Soybeans," *Journal of Medicinal Food* 1: 4 (1998/1999): pp. 241-5

34. Quoted in Ticciati, *Genetically Engineered Foods*, 14.

35. Pollan, Michael, "Playing God in the Garden," *New York Times Magazine*, October 25, 1998; see also Wrubel, R., et al., "Regulatory Oversight of Genetically Engineered Microorganisms . . . ," *Journal of Environmental Management* 21:4 (1997): pp. 571–86.

36. November 12, 1999; see Biotechnology Industry Organization Web site, www.bio.org/food&ag/1112letter.html.

37. Kemp, Jack, "Resistance Dropping Toward Biotech Foods," *Chicago Tribune*, August 25, 2000.

38. This list, and others, found in Anderson, *Genetic Engineering*, pp. 93–6.

39. These industry ties were widely discussed in the European media. See *The Guardian*, February 1, 2001.

40. Ibid.

41. Lambrecht, Bill, "Outgoing secretary says agency's top issue is genetically modified food," *St. Louis Post-Dispatch*, January 25, 2001.

42. Eichenwald, Kurt, et al., "Biotechnology Food: From the lab to a debacle," *New York Times*, January 25, 2001.

43. Halweil, Brian, "Transgenic Crop Area Surges," *Vital Signs 2000*, Worldwatch Institute, p. 118.

44. "Compilation and Analysis of Public Opinion Polls on Genetically Engineered Foods," Center for Food Safety, 2000.

45. "Monsanto Picks Up Its BGH and Goes Home," *Good Medicine* (Spring 1999), p. 22.

46. Nader, Ralph, and Smith, Wesley, *No Contest: Corporate Lawyers and the Perversion of Justice in America* (New York: Random House, 1996), pp. 186–92.

47. Quoted in Suzuki and Dressel, *Naked Ape to Superspecies*, p. 150.

48. Quoted in *Splice* 4:6 (August/September 1998).

49. Statement signed by Mike Batchelor, Quality Systems Director of Granada Food Services Limited, Fall 1999; see also Kirby, Alex, "Monsanto's Caterers Ban GM Foods," BBC Online, December 22, 1999.

chapter 18 The Emperor's New Foods

1. Anderson, Luke, *Genetic Engineering, Food, and Our Environment* (White River Junction, VT: Chelsea Green Publishing Company, 1999), p. 50.
2. "Farmer's Plight Shows GM Trouble," Environment News Service, June 20, 2000.
3. Ibid.
4. Ibid.
5. Ibid.
6. Woolf, Marie, *Independent,* April 18, 1999, quoted in Suzuki, David, and Dressel, Holly, *From Naked Ape to Superspecies* (Toronto/New York: Stoddart Publishing, 1999), pp. 112–3.
7. "Sustainability and Ag Biotech," *Rachel's Environment and Health Weekly* 686, February 10, 2000.
8. Anderson, *Genetic Engineering,* p. 40.
9. Muir, Ward and Howard, R., "Possible ecological risks of transgenic organism release when transgenes affect mating success," *Proceedings of the National Acdemy of Sciences,* 96; 13853–56, 1999.
10. Quoted in "Genetically Engineered Foods—Are They Safe?" *Safe Food News;* 500,000 copies of this newsmagazine were distributed in late 2000 to health food stores and other venues in the United States.
11. Carol Kaesuk Yoon, "Altered Salmon Lead the Way to the Dinner Plate, but Rules Lag," *New York Times,* May 1, 2000.
12. MacKenzie, D., "Can We Make Supersalmon Safe?" *New Scientist,* January 27, 1996, pp. 14–5; "New Prospects for Gene Altered Fish," *New York Times,* November 27, 1990.
13. "New Zealand Salmon Research Halted," Associated Press, February 26, 2000.
14. Metzger, H. Peter, *The Atomic Establishment* (New York: Simon and Schuster, 1972), p. 227.
15. "Against the Grain," *Rachel's Environment and Health Weekly* 638, February 18, 1999.
16. "In the last 40 years, the percentage of the annual crops lost to insects and disease in the U.S. has doubled"—Lappé, Marc, and Bailey, Britt, *Against the Grain: Biotechnology and the Corporate Takeover of Your Food* (Monroe, ME: Common Courage Press, 1998), p. 102.
17. Suzuki and Dressel, *Naked Ape to Superspecies,* p. 140.
18. Quoted in Pollan, Michael, "Playing God in the Garden," *New York Times Magazine,* October 25, 1998.
19. Halweil, Brian, "Transgenic Crop Area Surges," *Vital Signs 2000,* Worldwatch Institute, p. 118.
20. Lappé and Bailey, *Against the Grain,* p. 70.
21. Ibid., pp. 63–72.
22. Anderson, *Genetic Engineering,* p. 28.
23. Shapiro, Robert, Address to Greenpeace Business Conference, London, U.K., October 6, 1999.

24. Hilbeck, A., et al., "Effects of Transgenic Bt Corn Fed Prey on the Mortality . . .," *Environmental Entomology* 27:2 (1998):480–87; Hilbeck, A., et al., "Toxicity of Bt . . .," *Environmental Entomology* 27:4 (August 1998).

25. Gledhill, Matthew, and McGrath, Peter, "Call for a Spin Doctor," *New Scientist,* November 1, 1997, pp. 4–5; see also Tirch, A., et al., "Tri-Trophic Interactions Involving Pest Aphids, Predatory 2-Spot Ladybirds, and Transgenic Potatoes . . ." *Molecular Breeding* 5:1 (1999):75–83; and Birch, A., "Interaction between Plant Resistance Genes, Pest Aphid Populations and Beneficial Aphid Predators," *Scottish Crops Research Institute Annual Report* (1996–1997), pp. 70–2.

26. Anderson, *Genetic Engineering,* p. 29.

27. Losey, J., et al., "Transgenic Pollen Harms Monarch Larvae," *Nature,* May 20, 1999; see also, Ho, David, "Genetically Engineered Corn Proves Toxic to Monarch Butterflies," Associated Press, August 23, 2000.

28. Saxena, D., et al., "Insecticidal Toxin in Root Exudates from Bt Corn," *Nature,* December 2, 1999.

29. Massey, Rachel, "Biotech: The Basics," *Rachel's Environment and Health Weekly,* January 18, 2001.

30. Ayres, Ed, *God's Last Offer: Negotiating for a Sustainable Future* (New York/London: Four Walls Eight Windows Publishers, 1999), p. 259.

31. Goldberg, Carey, "1,500 March in Boston to Protest Biotech Food," *New York Times,* March 27, 2000, A-14.

32. Halweil, "Transgenic Crop Area Surges," p. 118.

33. Lappé and Bailey, *Against the Grain,* p. 52.

34. Halweil, "Transgenic Crop Area Surges," p. 118.

35. Ibid.

36. Ibid.

37. Ibid.

38. Ibid.

39. Lappé and Bailey, *Against the Grain,* p. 147.

40. Ibid., p. 55.

41. Ibid., p. 147.

42. "McDonald's Dumps GM-Fed Meat," BBC News, U.K., November19, 2000.

43. Murphy, Dan, "Bogus Battle Against Biotechnology Lesson in 21st Century Conflict," www.meatingplace.com, November 10, 2000.

44. Nottingham, Stephen, *Eat Your Genes* (London: Zed Books, 1998), p. 99.

45. Quoted in Suzuki and Dressel, *Naked Ape to Superspecies,* p. 147.

46. Ibid., pp. 152–3.

chapter 19 The Turning of the Tide

1. Halweil, Brian, "Organic Farming Thrives Worldwide," *Vital Signs 2000,* Worldwatch Institute, p. 120.

2. Ibid.

3. European totals and growth from Halweil, "Organic Farming Thrives," p. 120.

4. Halweil, "Organic Farming Thrives," p. 121.

5. Ibid.

6. Canadian and U.S. organic acreage from Halweil, "Organic Farming Thrives," p. 120.

7. Halweil, "Organic Farming Thrives," p. 120.

8. Ibid.

9. Burros, Marian, "U.S. Imposes Standards for Organic-Food Labeling," *New York Times,* December 21, 2000.

10. Quoted in Charman, Karen, "Saving the Planet with Pestilent Statistics," *PR Watch* 6:4 (4th Quarter 1999).

11. Ibid.

12. Quoted in "Organics: The Blurred Vision of ABC's 20/20," EarthSave newsletter 11 (Spring 2000), pp. 2, 10.

13. *New York Times* article published July 31, 2000, reported in FAIR (Fairness and Accuracy in Reporting) Action Alert, August 1, 2000.

14. "Distorted News," *USA Today,* August 13, 2000.

15. Quoted in the *Oregonian,* October 26, 1994.

16. "Stossel's Distortions Finally Catching Up with Him?" FAIR (Fairness and Accuracy in Reporting) Media Advisory, August 7, 2000.

17. Halweil, Brian, "Cultivating the Truth about Organics," *San Francisco Chronicle,* August 21, 2000.

18. "Food Safety and Quality as Affected by Organic Farming," UN Food and Agriculture Organization (FAO) report, July 2000; www.fao.org/organicag/frame2–e.htm; see also Halweil, "Cultivating the Truth."

19. Study published in *New Scientist,* October 7, 2000; www.newscientist.com/.

20. "Organic Foods vs. Supermarket Foods: Element Levels," *Journal of Applied Nutrition* 45 (1993):35–39.

21. "Farming Systems Trial," Rodale Institute, Kutztown, Pennsylvania, 1981–1995; www.enviroWeb.org/publications/rodale/usrarc/fst.html. See also: Proceedings from USDA, ERS, Farm Foundation Workshop, "The Economics of Organic Farming Systems: What Can Long-Term Cropping System Studies Tell Us?", Washington, DC, April 21, 1999; see also Welsh, Rick, *The Economics of Organic Grain and Soybean Production in the Midwestern United States,* Policy Studies Report 13, Henry A. Wallace Institute for Alternative Agriculture, May 1999.

22. Fillip, J., "American Farmers and USDA Start to Take Organic Seriously," *Not Man Apart,* September 1980.

23. Greenpeace Press Release, "Leaked Document from Monsanto Reveals Collapse of Public Support for Genetically Engineered Food," November 18, 1998, quoted in Anderson, Luke, *Genetic Engineering, Food, and our Environment* (White River Junction, VT: Chelsea Green Publishing Company, 1999), p. 115.

24. Genetix Update, March, 1999, quoted in Anderson, *Genetic Engineering,* p. 115.

25. "Genetically Altering the World's Food," *Rachel's Environment and Health Weekly* 639, February 25, 1998.
26. "Monsanto's Cremation Starts in Karnataka," Karnataka State Farmers Association Press Release, Sindhanoor, India, November 28, 1998.
27. "Biotech: The Pendulum Swings Back," *Rachel's Environment and Health Weekly* 649, May 6, 1999.
28. Ibid.
29. Halweil, Brian, "Portrait of an Industry in Trouble," Worldwatch News Brief 2000–2001.
30. Petersen, Melody, "New Trade Threat for U.S. Farmers," *New York Times,* August 29, 1999, A1, A18.
31. Luoma, Jon, "Pandora's Pantry," *Mother Jones,* January/February 2000.
32. Burros, Marian, "Eating Well: Different Genes, Same Old Label," *New York Times,* September 8, 1999, F5; Burros, Marian, "Eating Well: Chefs Join Effort to Label Engineered Food," *New York Times,* December 9, 1998, F14; Burros, Marian, "U.S. Plans Long-Term Studies on Safety of Genetically Altered Foods, *New York Times,* July 14, 1999, A18.
33. Charman, Karen, "The Professor Who Can Read Your Mind," *PR Watch,* 6:4 (4th Quarter 1999).
34. In 2000, USDA scientists in Raleigh, N.C., announced that using conventional breeding methods—not genetic engineering—they had developed a new soybean that's healthier for the heart because the oil need not go through a process that produces artery-clogging trans fatty acids, and it has less than half the saturated fat of conventional soybeans. See Brasher, Philip, "Healthier Soy Oil Coming," *Santa Cruz Sentinel,* March 29, 2000, B-5.
35. Personal communication with author.
36. "Biotech."
37. Ibid.
38. Burros, "U.S. Plans Long-Term Studies," A18.
39. Lambrecht, Bill, "Outgoing secretary says agency's top issue is genetically modified food," *St. Louis Post-Dispatch*, January 25, 2001.
40. Cheddar, Christina, "Tales of the Tape: Seed Co. May Yet Reap/What They Sow," *Wall Street Journal,* January 7, 2000.
41. Barboza, "In the Heartland, Genetic Promises," *New York Times,* March 17, 2000, C1.
42. "State's Ag Exports Could Be In Danger," *Santa Cruz Sentinel,* D-5, October 27, 2000; see also Halweil, "Portrait of an Industry."
43. Eichenwald, Kurt, et al., "Biotechnology Food: From the lab to the debacle," *New York Times*, January 25, 2001.
44. Halweil, "Portrait of an Industry."
45. Dorfman, Brad, "Many Americans Say Stop Planting Gene-Altered Crops," Reuters, Chicago, November 3, 2000.
46. "Biotech in Hot Oil," *Wall Street Journal,* May 2, 2000.
47. Kilman, Scott, "McDonald's, Other Fast-Food Chains Pull Monsanto's Bio-Engineered Potato," *Wall Street Journal,* April 28, 2000, B4.

48. "Frito-Lay Won't Use Genetically Altered Corn," Associated Press, February 1, 2000; "Eating Well: What Labels Don't Tell You (Yet)," *New York Times,* February 9, 2000, F5.

49. Lyman, Eric, "Pope Expresses Opposition to GMOs, Cites Need For 'Respect for Nature,'" Vatican City, November 15, 2000; Center for Food Safety.

50. Greenpeace Press Release, "Leaked Document from Monsanto Reveals Collapse of Public Support for Genetically Engineered Food," November 18, 1998, quoted in Anderson, *Genetic Engineering,* p. 121.

51. Quoted in Barboza, David, "Monsanto Faces Growing Skepticism on Two Fronts," *New York Times,* August 5, 1999, C1.

52. Goldberg, Carey, "1,500 March in Boston to Protest Biotech Food," *New York Times,* March 27, 2000, A14.

53. Re: Financial Support from Monsanto: "Biotech: The Pendulum Swings"; Blair's turnaround and quotes cited in Halweil, Brian, "Politically Modified Foods," *WorldWatch,* May/June 2000, p. 2.

54. Halweil, "Politically Modified Foods."

55. "Taking It to Main Street," *Time,* July 31, 2000, p. 42.

Index

About John Robbins

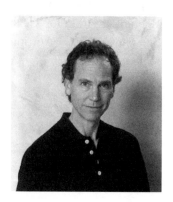

John Robbins is widely considered to be one of the world's leading experts on the link between diet, environment, and health. He is the author of several books, including the international bestseller *Diet for a New America*, and his work has been the subject of cover stories and feature articles in the *San Francisco Chronicle*, the *Los Angeles Times*, *Chicago Life*, the *Washington Post*, the *New York Times*, the *Philadelphia Inquirer*, and many of the nation's other major newspapers and magazines. His life and work were also featured in an hourlong PBS documentary entitled, "Diet for a New America."

The only son of the founder of the Baskin-Robbins ice cream empire, John Robbins was groomed to follow in his father's footsteps, but chose to walk away from Baskin-Robbins and the immense wealth it represented to ". . . pursue the deeper American Dream . . . the dream of a society at peace with its conscience because it respects and lives in harmony with all life forms. A dream of a society that is truly healthy, practicing a wise and compassionate stewardship of a balanced ecosystem."

John serves on the boards of many non-profit groups working toward a thriving and sustainable way of life. He is the founder and board chair emeritus of EarthSave International, an organization dedicated to healthy food choices, preservation of the environment, and a more compassionate world. John is also the active board chair of Youth for Environmental Sanity (YES!), which educates, inspires and empowers youth to take positive action for all life on Earth.

John Robbins can be reached through the mail, c/o The John Robbins Institute for Health and Compassion, 420 Bronco Road, Soquel, CA 95073. For information about his work, see *www.john-robbins.info*.

To Our Readers

Conari Press, an imprint of Red Wheel/Weiser, publishes books on topics ranging from spirituality, personal growth, and relationships to women's issues, parenting, and social issues. Our mission is to publish quality books that will make a difference in people's lives—how we feel about ourselves and how we relate to one another. We value integrity, compassion, and receptivity, both in the books we publish and in the way we do business.

Our readers are our most important resource, and we value your input, suggestions, and ideas about what you would like to see published. Please feel free to contact us, to request our latest book catalog, or to be added to our mailing list.

Conari Press
an imprint of Red Wheel/Weiser, LLC
with offices at
665 Third Street, Suite 400
San Francisco, CA 94107
www.redwheelweiser.com